Teaching and Learning in Medical and Surgical Education
Lessons Learned for the 21st Century

Edited by

Linda H. Distlehorst
Gary L. Dunnington
J. Roland Folse
Southern Illinois University School of Medicine

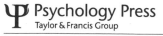 Psychology Press
Taylor & Francis Group

New York London

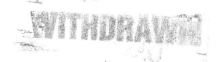

First Published by
Lawrence Erlbaum Associates, Inc., Publishers
10 Industrial Avenue
Mahwah, NJ 07430

Taylor & Francis
711 Third Avenue, New York, NY 10017
2 Park Square, Milton Park, Abingdon, Oxfordshire OX14 4RN

The final camera copy for this work was prepared by the author, and therefore
the publisher takes no responsibility for consistency or correctness of typo-
graphical style. However, this arrangement helps to make publication of this
kind of scholarship possible.

Cover design by Kathryn Houghtaling Lacey

First issued in paperback 2011

Library of Congress Cataloging-in-Publication Data

Teaching and learning in medical and surgical education : lessons learned
for the 21st century / edited by Linda H. Distlehorst, Gary L. Dunnington,
J. Roland Folse.
          p.   cm.
Includes bibliographical references and index.
ISBN 0-8058-3542-3
1. Surgery—Study and teaching. 2. Medical education.   I. Distlehorst,
Linda H.   II. Dunnington, Gary L.   III. Folse, J. Roland.
[DNLM: 1. Education, Medical. 2. Surgery—education.
    W 18 T25093 2000]
RD28.A1 T43   2000
610'.71'1—dc21   99-052564
                                                            CIP

Publisher's Note
The publisher has gone to great lengths to ensure the quality of this
reprint but points out that some imperfections in the original may
be apparent.

ISBN 978-0-805-83542-7 (hbk)
ISBN 978-0-415-51565-8 (pbk)

Dedication

This book is dedicated to Terrill A. Mast, PhD
1945-1998

Contents

Foreword

This book was initially the idea of Terrill Mast, developed in conversations with Roland Folse. Mast was dedicated to the belief that all teachers in medicine should be generalists with skills and knowledge in all aspects of the field. Before his untimely death, he had recruited many of the contributors to this book. Linda Distlehorst, Gary Dunnington, and Roland Folse have handsomely carried out this orientation by providing us with the insights of experienced educators working in the wide areas of medical education.

Medical education emerged as a recognized field in the early 1960's, heralded by the ground breaking, seminal book, *Teaching and Learning in Medical School* (Miller, 1996). To those of us heavily involved in teaching medical students, residents, and physicians in continuing medical education as part of full-time academic responsibilities, along with patient care and research, it came as an exciting and welcome revelation. Two of the authors of that book, Steve Abrahamson and the late George Miller, were the founding fathers of the medical educational movement in this country. Much of the expanding developments in medical education are from those who have worked with or were influenced by those giants, either primarily or secondarily. It seems appropriate that the opening chapter of this book is by Steve Abrahamson.

In the first medical educational workshop I ever attended, two years into my first academic appointment, Steve made the point that just because most of us in the workshop were experts or "-ologists" of some type or other, we could not conclude that we knew how to teach our "-ology." Now 40 years later, with the even more complex demands of practicing medicine, this truism is even more valid. There is no place in medical education for faculty to teach by the seat of the pants, the way they were taught, not questioning what or how they should teach, any more than there would be a place for such an approach in research or patient care. Anyone with responsibility for educating students, residents, and physicians should be skilled and well informed about medical education--as preparing these learners to provide safe, humane, and effective care for the members of our society is a heavy responsibility. This book provides both new and established medical teachers with rich information on the present state of medical education.

Howard S. Barrows, MD
Southern Illinois University School of Medicine

REFERENCE

Miller, G. E. (Ed.), (1961). *Teaching and learning in medical school*. Cambridge, MA: Harvard University Press.

ACKNOWLEDGMENTS

We wish to acknowledge the many persons who have contributed ideas to this book, particularly Melinda Mast who did much of the early correspondence with the authors and ensured that progress was made. We also wish to acknowledge the excellent technological assistance of Linda M. Sigrist who prepared the camera ready copy of each chapter.

Linda H. Distlehorst
Gary L. Dunnington
J. Roland Folse

Contributors

Stephen Abrahamson, PhD, ScD
Division of Medical Education
University of Southern California
   School of Medicine
1975 Zonal Avenue, KAM 200
Los Angeles, CA 90033
stephen@hsc.usc.edu

M. Brownell Anderson, MEd
Association of American
   Medical Colleges
2450 N. Street, NW
Washington, DC 20037
mbanderson@aamc.org

William A. Anderson, PhD
Michigan State University
   College of Human Medicine
East Lansing, MI 48824
ander113@pilot.msuedu

Louise M. Arnold, PhD
University of Missouri at Kansas City
2411 Holmes
Kansas City, MO 64108
larnold@med.umkc.edu

Howard S. Barrows, MD
Department of Medical Education
Southern Illinois University
   School of Medicine
PO Box 19622
Springfield, IL 62794-9622
hbarrows@siumed.edu

Nancy Bennett, PhD
Department of Continuing Education
Harvard Medical School
641 Huntington Avenue
Boston, MA 02115
Nancy_bennett@hms.harvard.edu

Robert G. Bing-You, MD, MEd
Department of Internal Medicine
Maine Medical Center
22 Bramhall Street
Portland, ME 04102
bingyb.mail@mmc.org

Jerry A. Colliver, PhD
Division of Statistics and Research
Southern Illinois University
   School of Medicine
PO Box 19622
Springfield, IL 62794-9622
colliver@siumed.edu

Erik J. Constance, MD
Office of Student Affairs
Southern Illinois University
  School of Medicine
PO Box 19624
Springfield, IL 62794-9624
econstance@siumed.edu

Debra A. DaRosa, PhD
Northwestern University Medical
  School
250 East Superior, Suite 201
Chicago, IL 60611-2950
ddarosa@nmh.org

Anna M. Derossis, MD
Northwestern University Medical
  School
250 East Superior, Suite 201
Chicago, IL 60611-2950
a-derossis@nwu.edu

Gary L. Dunnington, MD
Southern Illinois University
  School of Medicine
Department of Surgery
PO Box 19638
Springfield, IL 62794-9638
gdunningto@surg800.siumed.edu

Jack Ende, MD
University of Pennsylvania
  Health System
Presbyterian Medical Center
39th & Market Streets, Suite W-285
Philadelphia, PA 19104-2699
ende@mail.med.upenn.edu

Janine C. Edwards
Associate Professor and Vice Chair
  for Academic Affairs
Texas A & M University
  College of Medicine
College Station, TX 778-43-1114
jcedward@medicine.tamu.edu

Charles E. Engel
Centre for Higher Education Studies
University of London
55-59 Gordon Square
London WC1H ONT
United Kingdom

J. Roland Folse, MD
Department of Surgery
Southern Illinois University
  School of Medicine
Springfield, IL 62794-9638
jfolse@siumed.edu

Earl Loschen, MD
Department of Psychiatry
Southern Illinois University
  School of Medicine
Springfield, IL 62794-9642
eloschen@siumed.edu

Linda J. Morrison, MSW
Department of Medical Education
Southern Illinois University
  School of Medicine
PO Box 19622
Springfield, IL 62794-9622
lmorrison@siumed.edu

Richard H. Moy, MD
Southern Illinois University
  School of Medicine
PO Box 19620
Springfield, IL 62794-9620

Eileen Reynolds, MD
University of Pennsylvania Health System
Presbyterian Medical Center
39th and Market Streets
Philadelphia, PA 19104-2699
reynolds@mail.med.upenn.edu

Quinn Mast-Cheney
NE Lake Street, # 619
Hopkins, Minn. 55343
quinn.mast@dfait-maeci.gc.ca

Richard K. Reznick, MD, MEd
The Toronto Hospital
Eaton North 9-237
200 Elizabeth Street
Toronto, Ontario M5G 2C4 CANADA
reznick@inforamp.net

Linda Perkowski, PhD
Office of Educational Programs
University of Texas - Houston Medical
School
6431 Fannin, Suite G 024
Houston, TX 77030
lperkows@dean.med.uth.tmc.edu

Kenneth Roberts, PhD
University of Missouri at
  Kansas City School of Medicine
2411 Holmes Street
Kansas City, MO 64108
kroberts@streck.com

Krishan Rajaratnam, MD, MEd
Resident, University of Toronto
Centre for Research in Education
BW6666, 585 University Avenue
Toronto, Ontario, Canada
M5G 2C4
k.rajaratnam@utoronto.ca

Ajit Sachdeva, MD
Medical College of Pennsylvania
3300 Henry
Philadelphia, PA 19129
sachdeva@AUHS.edu

Glenn Regehr, PhD
Centre for Research in Education
BW6666, 585 University Avenue
Toronto, Ontario, Canada
M5G 2C4
g.regehr@utoronto.ca

John H. Shatzer, PhD
The Johns Hopkins University
  School of Medicine
600 N. Wolfe Street, Blalock 402
Baltimore, MD. 21287-4461
jshatzer@jhmi.edu

Deborah E. Simpson, PhD
Medical College of Wisconsin
8701 Watertown Plank Road
Milwaukee, WI 53226
dsimpson@post.its.mcw.edu

Michael Whitcomb, MD
Division of Medical Education
Association of American Medical
    Colleges
2450 N Street NW
Washington DC 20037
mwhitcomb@aamc.org

Mark H. Swartz, MD
Mount Sinai School of Medicine
One Gustave Levy Place
New York, NY 10029
mswartz@smtplink.mssm.edu

LuAnn Wilkerson, EdD
Center for Educational Development
    and Research
UCLA School of Medicine
Box 951722
Los Angeles, CA 90024
lwilker@deans.medsch.ucla.edu

Ara Tekian, PhD
University of Illinois at Chicago
Department of Medical Education
808 South Wood Street
Chicago, IL 60612-7309
Ara.Tekian@uic.edu

Ken Williamson, PhD
Director of Educational Programs
Radiology Department
Indiana University Medical School
Indianapolis, IN 46202-5120
KenWilli@iupui.edu

Richard G. Tiberius
Department of Psychiatry
University of Toronto, Clarke Institute
    of Psychiatry
250 College Street
Toronto, Ontario M5T 1R8 CANADA
r.tiberius@utoronto.ca

PART I

THE EVOLUTION OF MEDICAL AND SURGICAL EDUCATION

CHAPTER ONE

Medical Education: The Testing of A Hypothesis

Stephen Abrahamson
University of Southern California

There are many ways to consider medical education. In this chapter, medical education is conceptualized as the complex of processes by which a medical student is changed from a medical school applicant to a medical school graduate--with all that is implied: from unknowing to knowing, from unskilled to skilled, from layman to professional--in summary, from medical student to physician. The complex of processes includes the following: learning by the medical students, teaching by the faculty members of a medical school, and governance by the administrators of the medical school. How these three processes are interwoven to form medical education as we know it today warrants critical review.

THE SCIENCE OF LEARNING

Education can be thought of as a profession, and as such it includes a set of practices and a body of sciences underlying those practices. Those who have studied education maintain that the sciences provide the basis for the practices. Thus, a brief review of some principles of learning should precede any discussion of practices of teaching.

Time and space do not permit the presentation of learning theory in detail. Indeed, there are different theories of learning, each with a body of research supporting it. But extant learning theories all agree on some basic principles which the good teacher knows and attempts to apply.

1

Learning is an Individual Matter. No two students learn in exactly the same way. What may help one student to learn may not help another. What may help one student may even hinder another's learning. Some students report that when they are intimidated by the teacher, they cannot learn well. Others report that such a stimulus "forces" them to learn. Some students cannot listen to a lecture and take notes at the same time. Others find note-taking to be a necessary aid to their concentration.

The application of this basic principle of learning suggests that the teaching program should include a variety of teaching techniques. It suggests further that the good teacher tries to get to know his or her students as individual learners. Of course, if the teacher is merely a lecturer to a large group of students, the opportunities to treat students as individual learners is quite limited. But even in this case, the skilled teacher prepares lectures and delivers them in such a way as to maximize the opportunity for students to be active participants rather than passive listeners: through rhetorical questions, through question-and-answer periods, through "programmed" lectures, through "six-by-six" discussions--in other words by abandoning the "55-minute lecture" in favor of varying the learning activities in an attempt to meet different learning styles of different students.

In fact, there are "learning styles" conceptualized by educational psychologists concerned with learning. Different students have different "styles" of learning, and helping students discover their respective learning styles may itself be a significant aid to their education. When students are aware of how they learn, their learning is facilitated.

Learning is More Efficient and More Effective When the Learners are Motivated. Motivation is difficult to define but generally is "regarded as a process internally seated which, once aroused by an appropriate stimulus, leads to more intensive (learning) activity than otherwise would have been present (Miller, Abrahamson, Cohen, Graser, Harnack, et al., 1961). Motivation, in other words, is something within the learner: his or her drive to learn, desire to learn, need to learn. The teacher cannot "motivate the student." Instead, the teacher can offer incentives--positive (rewards, praise, recognition) or negative (failing grades, reprimands, ridicule). In other words, the teacher can take advantage of the student's motivation. Of course, the teacher needs to know what that motivation is and how to use that information in planning and conducting the teaching-learning exercise. Once again, there is this connection between the art of teaching and the science of learning--in this case, planning learning activities which capitalize on the student's motivation.

It has been postulated that it is not possible to prevent a person from learning what he or she is motivated to learn--up to, of course, physiologic limits to that learning. The challenge for the teacher--the good teacher, that is--is to discover the motivation of individual students and work from there, rather than to demand that the student learn what the teacher thinks he or she ought to learn. The key for the teacher is to find ways to help the student develop that motivation by recognizing the need for learning. In other words, the teacher should start with students' perceived needs and help the student recognize other needs--which then, in turn, become perceived needs of the students.

Learning is More Efficient When the Learning Experience Has Meaning to the Learner. In some ways, this principle of learning is so obvious as to obviate the need for elaboration. Students become "lost" when what is to be learned is so foreign to them that it has little or no meaning to them. Sometimes, teachers assume that students are at a certain level of understanding of a given topic, only to discover that they, in fact, are not nearly up to that level. When that situation occurs, the good teacher backs up and ensures that students become familiar enough with the subject to move ahead. The poor teacher forges ahead with the apparent assumption that "it's not my fault that they're not ready."

In a related manner, plunging students into a learning milieu which is totally foreign to them will slow the learning process, if not inhibit it totally. For students who have never seen the inside of an operating room, a learning experience scheduled there may pose serious learning blocks. Their first experience in that setting should be an orientation, not a "training run."

Learning is More Efficient When There is "Feedback" for the Student. Research is very clear on this matter: students learn far better when they receive feedback from the teacher: information about how well they--the students--are doing, how much they are learning, whether they are achieving the desired goals of the learning exercise.

Application of this principle of learning demands that the teacher know what those goals and objectives are and, in addition, how well individual students are achieving. The teacher then has the obligation to let the student know those same facts: what the goals are and how the student is doing. All too often in medical education this obligation is met by giving each student his or her test score, rather than by meeting with the student and reviewing how he or she did and in what ways he or she met or did not meet the goals.

The challenge for the teacher goes beyond merely understanding these principles. The real challenge is to apply these principles in planning and carrying out teaching-learning activities.

THE ART OF TEACHING

As just mentioned, education can be thought of as a profession. Thus, the practices constitute the "part of teaching," and they are amenable to examination by students of education processes. These practices include, or should include, both familiar and less well-known techniques of teaching. In medical education, the familiar practices, of course, are lecture, seminar, laboratory supervision, ward rounds, conferences, and case presentations, among others. The less well-known or less frequently used (or even considered for use) practices include problem-based tutorials, student-led discussions, and self-instructional programs designed by faculty for purposes of student learning.

For each of the techniques of teaching, there are skills which teachers develop throughout their careers. These skills are learned by teachers, although there is very seldom a systematic effort to teach them to new faculty members. It is generally assumed that the acquisition of an advanced degree automatically qualifies a person for the role of teacher in higher education. If nothing else, it is expected that the new graduate--MD or PhD--will emulate his or her own teachers and thus become a "practitioner" of education. This avoidance of systematic preparation of a teacher for his or her teaching role in a medical school ensures that good teaching will appear by chance and that bad teaching often will serve as a model for new teachers.

To defend the lack of teacher preparation, false premises often are advanced and assumed by the medical education establishment to be true. One such false premise is that "good teachers are born that way." The fallacy here is patent! Teaching involves a set of skills which can be learned and therefore are not innate. The false premise simply obscures the need for teacher preparation and, further, provides a defense for bad teaching. It also obviates the need for medical school teachers to devote more of their academic time to preparation for teaching--time which can then be used on higher priority institutional goals which, in their turn, mandate that medical school teachers concentrate on clinical practice and/or research, and not on teaching. After all, it is clear that the careers of medical school teachers depend on their productivity in practice and/or research, not on their excellence in teaching.

Another false premise is related to Abrahamson's Myth #1: It doesn't matter what curriculum a medical school uses (Abrahamson, 1996). This time, however, the false premise would be: "These students are so damned smart that it doesn't matter what kind of teaching they get!" In fact, medical students are so intelligent and so highly motivated that the premise is almost true! (It would be true if it were stated: "These students are so intelligent and so motivated that they might learn despite the bad teaching.") In this case, however, there is an important corollary: Medical students would learn more effectively and more efficiently with good teaching.

In addition to these false premises, there are several misconceptions about teaching which should be explored. The first of these is "Teaching = Learning." That is, if the teacher has "taught" something, the student must have (or should have) "learned" it. The misconception is heard in the expression: "We have already covered that ground." (There are only two occupations which use the expression, "cover the ground": farming and teaching!) The expression is clearly a misconception. Just because something has been "covered" in class (i.e., included in a lecture) does not necessarily mean that it has been learned.

The second of these misconceptions is "Lecturing = Teaching." All too often, the lecture is the only method of teaching considered. Although lecturing is one technique of instruction, it is but one of many and not nearly so effective as apparently assumed by medical school teachers. The severest critics of the lecture describe it as a process by which information is transmitted from the notes of the teacher to the notes of the student without going through the minds of either! But most critics, not so severe, are not condemning the lecture or advocating that it not be used. They are simply raising questions about the excessive number of lectures used in medical education and their assumed effectiveness in producing learning. But because the lecture is used so much, they are also concerned with the substantial number of lecturers who are not skillful in using the technique.

But what is "teaching," anyway? Teaching is providing activities, materials, and guidance which facilitate learning. The teacher is the person who provides the "activities, materials and guidance which facilitate learning." Thus, although lecturing is one of the "activities," there are many others. Whereas slides or transparencies are one form of "materials," there are others, and "guidance" is often a neglected area of the teacher's art. Using this definition of teaching, we must shift our thinking from the teacher to the learner because the outcome, learning, is the raison d'etre for the input, teaching.

With this definition of teaching, it would be expected that teachers plan for their teaching with the student in mind. How do they learn? What will help them learn? What can I do to facilitate that process for them? Sometimes the activities will be teacher centered. At other times, the activities may be student centered. On occasion, the materials may be teacher controlled. Often, the materials might be managed by the students themselves. But the guidance of student learning is the critical role of the teacher. The art of teaching is helping students learn--by whatever means prove to be most effective and most efficient. The good teacher is one who performs a number of tasks which are expected to produce learning.

The Teacher Must Have Thorough Knowledge of the Subject. The teacher must know his or her subject well enough to feel free to explore teaching processes, to react in a flexible manner to what takes place in the teaching-learning situation, and to understand what is taking place among his or her group of learners. There is no substitute for the teacher's mastery of his or her subject. "Educationists" (those concerned with the study of educational processes) often are accused by their detractors of being so preoccupied with techniques of instruction that they denigrate or otherwise minimize the need for the teacher to be knowledgeable of his or her subject. This accusation is another means of evading the need for improving skills of teaching. Educationists start with the assumption that the teacher must be a master of his or her subject. Otherwise, the teacher would not be in a position to concentrate on skills of teaching.

The Teacher Must Have a Thorough Knowledge of the Students. The teacher must know his or her students well in order to know how to work with them, to help meet their needs, and to offer challenges to them--all to facilitate their learning. As difficult as this may seem when there is a large class, there are techniques which can be used to enable the teacher to "get to know" his or her students. Unfortunately, these techniques demand the dedication of some time and, thus, are usually ignored in favor of applying that time to other institutional goals: research and clinical practice.

The Teacher Must Match His or Her Teaching Techniques to the Learning Objectives. Obviously, those learning objectives must be defined first! Only by knowing the learning objectives is the teacher in a position to select appropriate activities and/or materials. That is, if the objectives are to help students learn specific information, then certain techniques of instruction are best suited for that purpose, quite possibly the lecture or self-instructional materials. If the objectives are to help students gain a deeper understanding of basic principles or relationships, then the teacher may want to use some different techniques: small-group discussion, problem-based tutorials. If the objectives are to help the student develop clinical skills, the techniques should undoubtedly involve demonstration by the teacher and supervision of the student practicing those skills.

Thus, we have the picture that teaching includes a set of skills to be used by the teacher, skills that must be learned and practiced by the teacher. But if the practice of teaching is to bring about learning, the teacher--as a professional--should become conversant with the sciences underlying learning, or at least with some basic principles of learning that have clear implications for the teacher.

GOVERNANCE OF THE MEDICAL SCHOOL: THE SETTING

Thus far, the model is simple: students who learn and faculty who teach (i.e., help students learn). But all these activities take place in an institution: the medical school. Any institution requires some system to make it operate.

Today's medical school is a far cry from what it was originally. The medical school of yesteryear was a simple model: a faculty who planned curriculum, admitted students, taught the classes, tested the students; a dean who presided over the faculty, ensured that faculty received needed resources, and implemented educational decisions made by faculty. Even as faculty began to spend more time on their respective research interests, the school remained just that: an institution dedicated to helping young people prepare for a career in medicine.

But during the second half of the 20th century, dramatic changes have taken place. The fact that these changes have been so gradual has made them truly insidious.

There Has Been a Significant Shift in the Role of the Teacher. Fifty years ago (forgive me, Gertrude Stein!), a teacher was a teacher was a teacher! Fifty years ago, faculty members were almost exclusively educators. Today, faculty members are entrepreneurs in research, clinical practice, or both.

A Shift Has Occurred in the Mission of the Medical School. Fifty years ago (forgive me again, Gertrude Stein!), a medical school was a medical school was a medical school. Fifty years ago, the medical school was an institution in which the goal was to prepare young people for the practice of medicine. Today, the medical school is a research institute, a tertiary-care hospital, and a health maintenance organization (HMO)--and only incidentally, a school.

The Number of Medical Students Has Increased Dramatically. Fifty years ago, there were 88 medical schools; in 1999, there are 126. Fifty years ago, the number of medical students in those 88 medical schools was half the number in those same schools in 1999.

There Has Been a Shift in Sources of Funding for Medical Schools. Fifty years ago, medical schools were supported essentially by tuition fees and endowment (or in public schools, the state). Today, medical schools derive most of their support from research grants and contracts, and clinical practice.

The Number of Faculty in Each Medical School Has Dramatically Increased. Fifty years ago, in existing medical schools the faculty-to-student ratio was less than half that ratio in those same medical schools today. For example, in one medical school, there were 154 full-time faculty and 72 students, a faculty-to-student ratio of two. Today, that same medical school has 960 full-time faculty and 160 students, a faculty-to-student ratio of six!

The Nature of Medical Practice Has Changed. Hospital stays are significantly shorter. Solo practice has all but disappeared in urban areas. Managed care is replacing fee-for-service medical reimbursement, and more and more patients are "covered" by insurance plans or the government.

Each of these changes has had--and continues to have--a significant impact on undergraduate medical education. These respective impacts, however, have not been sudden. Rather, they have been cumulative over time and contributory to one another. The result is that on the surface, today's medical education may resemble what it once was, but the system is dramatically different in ways which are beginning to have a substantial effect on students and their learning.

A Shift Has Occurred in the Role of the Teacher. Today, many faculty members do not even see medical students, let alone teach them. As recently as the 1960s, most faculty members knew all the medical students by name. Today, almost no faculty member, particularly in the clinical departments, knows the medical students.

Because today's medical school teacher does not teach, he or she has little interest in all the educational activities normally associated with being a faculty member: planning courses; preparing learning materials; constructing, administering, and grading examinations; advising students; and observing students, to mention a few. How much should those faculty members be involved in decisions which affect the educational program? An accepted truism among educationists is that "the curriculum 'belongs' to the faculty." The system thus continues to operate with the underlying philosophy that all faculty should have an equal voice in determining curriculum and instruction. But in the case of faculty members who literally never are in contact with medical students, departmental vested interests and narrow emotional responses to innovation in education can come to govern the program. If faculty members do not teach, what is their proper role in the governance of the curriculum?

Moreover, there is an interesting corollary to be considered. In the basic sciences, more and more of the remaining supervision in teaching laboratories has been turned over to graduate students in those basic sciences. In the clinical disciplines, house officers and fellows in specialty areas have replaced faculty in supervising and, therefore, teaching students.

The Mission of the Medical School Has Shifted. Although it is true that the medical school has always been home to scientific research and to patient care, these activities were secondary to the basic mission of the institution: preparation of young people for the practice of medicine in one of its many forms. Indeed, teachers were expected to do some research as part of their maintaining "scholarship," particularly the basic science faculty members. But with the growth of "outside funding," this activity has burgeoned to its present importance and has become part of the financial structure of the medical school. Basic science teachers are expected to "bring in" a significant portion of their own salaries--in some cases as much as 100%. How can such a faculty member be expected to give any significant portion of his or her time to educational matters? The result is that the curriculum runs the risk of becoming a form of perpetual motion machine. Benign neglect is almost the best that might be expected.

Furthermore, it is not very much better in the clinical areas. Here, faculty members are expected to "bring in" revenues through patient care, either in a medical-school HMO practice or in high-tech procedures conducted in the medical school hospital. Again, these clinical teachers are better advised to devote their time, effort, and energy to the practices that will earn them respect, renown, and other rewards from the system than to engage in activities which the system does not prize or reward.

The Number of Medical Students Has Increased. During the decade of expansion (1968-1978) in response to what was perceived as a "doctor shortage," existing medical schools doubled their respective class sizes. (Interestingly enough, at that same time, these schools tripled or quadrupled the number of faculty members. Since that time, of course, when class sizes were "frozen," the number of faculty has continued to grow at an even faster rate!) The increase in the number of medical students makes the lecture all the more attractive as a method of teaching--all too often to the exclusion of other methods. With a class size of 160 instead of 80, for example, recommendations for more small-group learning activities or more one-to-one teaching experiences are rejected by a faculty subject to all of those other institutional pressures with the cry of "we-don't-have-enough-faculty" or "we-don't-have-enough-time"! In the very school in which that claim is made, however, the number of full-time faculty alone might very well be more than 1,000--more than enough to provide for that small-group or one-to-one teaching.

Thus, the very existence of larger numbers of medical students has a marked influence on teaching-learning activities: always in the direction of the status quo, thus contributing to the notion of the undergraduate medical education as a perpetual-motion machine.

The Sources of Funding Have Shifted. There is a famous and possibly overused wheeze which goes: "He who pays the piper calls the tune." When the medical school was supported by tuition and "hard money" sources, it was possible to commit funds to educational activities. Now, in an era in which department chairs (and even many faculty members) have more institutional money at their personal disposal than does the dean, faculty recruitment is dramatically affected in the direction of those who might enhance the revenue-producing capabilities of the department rather than those who might enhance the educational efforts. Furthermore, even the medical school's "hard money" is seen as being better invested in the entrepreneur type of faculty member rather than one concerned with education.

Moreover, these pressures on faculty members to "bring in" more money dictate a justifiable self-preservation response from faculty members. They cannot be faulted for protecting their careers by declining any expanded participation in educational endeavors. Thus, once again, the gradual change in the ethos of the medical school as an institution has had and continues to have a profound impact on medical education.

The Number of Faculty Has Increased. With the increase in number of faculty members, the question of governance of the curriculum becomes a crucial one. How is it possible for more than 1,000 full-time, part-time, and volunteer faculty to be involved in decision making with regard to curriculum and instruction? Fifty years ago all faculty members--at least all full-time faculty--were consulted when decisions were to be made, usually through departmental representation on committees whose members truly functioned as representatives, taking issues back to departmental meetings. Now with the number of faculty so large, that system seldom functions well. Departmental meetings are attended by large numbers of faculty whose major interests seldom include undergraduate medical education. The departmental representatives on the curriculum committees, therefore, tend not to bring matters to the department members until some decision is needed. Thus, those faculty members are ill prepared to render a thoughtful response.

Departmental self-interests frequently act to prevent the establishment in each department of a "special" faculty whose major responsibility would be the education of medical students--with appropriate recognition (e.g., promotions, salary increases) for their efforts. For similar reasons, department chairs also reject another possible solution which has been proposed: an administration and budget dedicated to undergraduate medical education.

Change Has Occurred in Medical Practice. Once medical students learned from patients whose hospital stays were long enough for students to study their problems over some time, even to the extent of "getting to know" those patients. Today, with hospital stays severely curtailed by improved medical and surgical techniques and by the economic pressures of managed care, insurance companies, and even the government, those opportunities for learning are sharply reduced. Newer teaching techniques are called for--but in an atmosphere in which faculty members are under pressure not to spend time on development of newer educational approaches!

The general response has been an effort to shift much of the clinical learning activities to the outpatient setting. This effort is thwarted by the absence of a "teaching model" because the inpatient clerkship is not applicable.

Furthermore, even the charity patients, who once formed the population which served as learning sources, are now often "covered" by some form of government or other insurance. Thus, even short-term inpatients may choose not to be available for students' learning activities.

One interesting facet to the changes in medical practice, of course, is the disappearance of solo practice, which once formed the practice model for which students were being prepared. All too often, however, that model still exists in the minds of many faculty members, thus providing still one more problem for medical education. How to prepare students to assume a role in managed-care settings is a major curriculum-planning problem that must be addressed by the very faculty members whose clinical load virtually prevents them from doing so.

MEDICAL EDUCATION: THE TESTING OF AN HYPOTHESIS

This chapter provides a sketch of the three components in the complex process called undergraduate medical education: the science of learning and the art of teaching in the setting of a medical school governed by an administration also responsible for many activities other than teaching and learning.

What a simple paradigm! Students learn; faculty teach; administrators govern. But the preceding pages suggest that there is much to be desired in the relationships among the three components. Students try to learn what they think is expected of them, only to discover that memorizing information for examinations is only a very small part of what they ultimately need to learn. Moreover, they find themselves mired in a system which appears not to place high priority on their education. The faculty, in turn, find themselves judged for advancement in the system by a set of criteria not related to medical education at all, thus providing no real incentive for them to excel in their educational efforts. The administrators, strangely enough, are no better off in this system. They are under great pressure to have their respective schools excel in research and grantsmanship, provide extensive clinical services, and sponsor cutting-edge clinical procedures as a means of generating revenues. Can this strange--almost surrealistic--set of conditions be managed so as to provide high-quality education for medical students? There is one approach that might give medical education at least a better chance of getting the attention and support it needs and deserves.

It has been said that all education should be treated as the testing of an hypothesis.[1] The hypothesis, of course, is quite straightforward: Students learn what the faculty want them to learn as a result of the curriculum and instruction provided for them by the faculty in the medical school under the governance of the administration. The medical school, then, might very well treat the entire program of medical education as an experiment, thus involving the testing of an hypothesis.

The idea is intriguing. Medical school faculty members hold science in the highest esteem. Can we not expect them to apply scientific principles to their role as educators? As the medical educators go about the tasks involved in providing medical students with their learning experiences, thus applying the sciences of learning through the art of teaching, the setting (the medical school itself) becomes the laboratory for the study of student learning.

Thus, defining the desired outcomes is the first step in stating the hypothesis of the educational experiment. For example, one desired outcome might be: "The student should be able to meet a new patient and obtain a relevant and focused history, no matter what the chief complaint." (Here we have the dependent variable.) The hypothesis then becomes: "The program of teaching and learning provided by the faculty will produce the desired outcome in the students." The task for the faculty is to design a set of learning experiences best calculated to produce the "desired outcome." (And here we have the independent variable.) Appropriate measures must be made, preferably both before and after the teaching-learning experiences.

Such an approach demands attention, time, and effort from faculty members. The investment of that effort, however, will undoubtedly result in better education for the students because the testing of the hypothesis will provide information concerning the effectiveness of the learning experiences and over time permit objective comparisons of different curricula and different methods of teaching.

In this way (i.e., treating education as the testing of an hypothesis) the medical school will be acknowledging that there are scientific principles of learning, that applying these principles constitutes the art of teaching, and that the school recognizes research in medical education as an appropriate activity for its faculty members. By recognizing medical education in this way, the school would be providing legitimacy to its mandate: the education and training of medical students. Many believe that undergraduate medical education is the primary purpose of the medical school. Of course, others challenge this belief. But whether it is the primary purpose or not should not be the subject of argument or discussion. Brandt (1989) said it best when he urged medical educators not to engage in "fruitless and divisive debates" on this issue, but instead to remember that no other institution in our society

---

[1] This statement is attributed to Edwin F. Rosinski, EdD recently retired after more than 40-years of a career in medical education, which included service as Deputy Assistant Secretary of Health, Education, and Welfare (HEW), Executive Vice Chancellor of the University of California, San Francisco (UCSF) Medical School, and founding director of offices of research in medical education at the Medical College of Virginia, the University of Connecticut School of Medicine, and the UCSF Medical School.

is permitted to educate and train young people to practice medicine. It is incumbent on medical educators to provide the best curriculum and instruction so that tomorrow's practice of medicine will, in turn, be the best possible. Applying the sciences of learning through the arts of teaching and treating the entire system as the testing of an hypothesis could be the way to achieve these goals.

POSTSCRIPT: THE FUTURE

What of the future? What will medical education be like in the 21st century? When one considers the remarkable changes in health care, in the role of the physician, in the sciences underlying the practice of medicine, in the technological advances available to educators, one must also wonder whether there will be changes in medical education. Although there is no presumption here of clairvoyance, I propose the possibility of three different scenarios.

Scenario 1

Matters will continue to worsen in an insidious manner. In this scenario, the total control of the education of medical students will remain in the hands of those whose major concerns do not include the education of those medical students, and thus the insidious drift will continue. For instance, there are many medical faculty members, particularly department chairs, who believe that modern technology available to educators will solve all problems. Some of them refer to the new technology almost as a shibboleth: "All of medical education will be under computer management." "The Internet will provide basic medical education." The allegiance to such shibboleths demonstrates an utter lack of recognition that the computer will do what it is instructed to do (by faculty members), and that the Internet will carry what is placed there (again, by faculty members). Therefore, faculty members will have to engage in the time-consuming activities of sound educational planning and preparation of materials for "the computer" and "the Internet."

If medical school faculty members are lulled by those shibboleths into even less involvement and less participation, medical education will continue its steady deterioration in quality, losing even more of the one-to-one and small-group instruction that once was its hallmark. Students will have less contact with faculty in a system that will place increased emphasis on acquisition of information rather than development of cognitive processes. As long as medical education remains the lowest priority in a medical school, it will continue to suffer.

Scenario 2

Today's medical education will change. That is, thanks to continued pressures deriving from current Liaison Committee on Medical Education (LCME) accreditation procedures and from critiques of undergraduate medical education, (Association of American Medical Colleges, 1984; 1992), no more "damage" will accrue from the system that places responsibility for medical education in the hands of those who are then judged and rewarded for accomplishments not in medical education.

Under this scenario, the steady decrease in small-group and one-to-one instruction will stop taking place, and the shibboleths about the new technology available to education will be recognized for what they are: slogans attractive to medical school faculty members under severe pressure to "produce" in areas other than education. At least, things will not get worse!

Scenario 3

Medical education will respond thoughtfully to all of the recent criticism. It is possible that reform in medical education will begin with reform of the system which provides the governance of medical education. Teachers will be recognized and rewarded for dedicating time to preparing for a career in teaching, for participating in sound educational planning, and for filling the role of educator: teaching, counseling, role-modeling, assessing student performance.

The realization of this scenario depends in large part on establishing control of undergraduate medical education in the hands of faculty who are not subject to the current pressures of "publish-or-perish," "grantsmanship," and/or "show-me-the-money" derived from institutional clinical practice plans. Unfortunately, this scenario, therefore, depends on a change in the ethos of medical education. Medical education can realize such a dramatic change (remember Abraham Flexner?), but strong leadership is required along with some form of subsidy (remember Flexner's support from Carnegie?). American medical education experienced a modest--but significant--reform in the 1960s, thanks to forward-looking medical educators in key deanships and support from a variety of sources, most notably the Commonwealth Fund. It can happen again. Maybe it will.

REFERENCES

Abrahamson, S. (1996). *Essays on medical education*. Lanham, MD: University Press of America.

Association of American Medical Colleges: (1984). *Physicians for the Twenty-First Century, the GPEP Report*. Washington, DC: The Association of American Medical Colleges.

Association of American Medical Colleges. (1992). *ACME-TRI Report. Educating medical students: Assessing change in medical education--the road to implementation*. Washington, DC

Brandt, Jr., E. N. (1989). "Medical school survival versus social responsibility: Finances as a driving force." *The Pharos*. (Based on an address delivered at the Annual Meeting of the Association of American Medical Colleges, 1997.)

Miller G. E., Abrahamson S., Cohen, I. S., Graser, H. P., Harnack, R. S., & Land, A. (1961). *Teaching and learning in medical school*, (pp. 51-52). Cambridge, MA: Harvard University Press

CHAPTER TWO

Medical Education in the 20th Century

Richard H. Moy
Southern Illinois University

Having sat through many presentations on the progress of medical education during the 20th century, it seems to the author that the inevitable cliché is to start with a genuflection to the Flexner Report of 1910. The impression given is that Abraham Flexner, by his own efforts, brought about the demise of the terribly defective proprietary schools and launched the era of modern medical schools and medical education that led directly over time to whatever innovation the presenter was describing or promulgating. In his superb and scholarly book, *Learning to Heal*, Ken Ludmerer (1985) describes the origins and evolution of the modern medical school over the last third of the 19th century, the decade before Flexner, in excellent and cogent detail.

The great German universities with their strong research departments were being copied in this country, thus bringing about the modern university. This raised the question inevitably that medicine here as in Germany should be part of a university with clear expectations for research and scholarship. The model was being evolved at Harvard, Pennsylvania, and Michigan, finally reaching its culmination with the establishment of the Johns Hopkins Medical School in 1893, where college graduates were taught by full-time research faculty. In addition, the advent of progressive education by John Dewey enforced the Hopkins model that students should learn by doing. Osler's[1] ideal curriculum was what he called self-education under guidance, with the guide (professor) just further along in the process of

---

[1] Quoted in Reid, E. G. (1931). *The Great Physician: A short life of Sir William Osler*, 230-231. London: Oxford University Press.

learning. This, of course, sounds very much like problem-based learning, with which we are now finishing this century.

The story of medical education in the 20th century is a rich one involving dedicated and innovative teachers, some famous, some now forgotten, and above all the perseverance of bright, dedicated students who at times have displayed a profound capacity to learn medicine despite the teachers and the curriculum, for there were times when the former were not very attentive and the latter was uncoordinated drudgery. Just as the development of medical education in the 19th century was shaped and molded by other forces in society, so also in the 20th century, progress, lack of progress, and reform often were strongly influenced by what was going on around us.

While the modern medical school was taking shape at the beginning of the 20th century, proprietary schools still existed in large numbers. These were schools with very short terms of instruction in which almost anyone could enroll, and in which the faculty of practicing physicians anticipated making a profit from tuition. The early decades of the 20th century were times of reform, and the reformers were working also in medicine. The American Medical Association (AMA) from its origins in the 19th century had been very much concerned about the quality of education for doctors, and in 1906 established the Council on Medical Education (COME), which for many years was dominated by six professors from "modern" medical schools. The Association of American Medical Colleges (AAMC), was established when sixty-six schools banded together in 1890, began inspection of medical schools in 1903. Both the AAMC and the COME pushed the primacy of research in medical schools as well as the dogma that full-time faculty were the best teachers. This, of course, is not necessarily true, but you have to remember that they were out fighting the Philistines of the proprietary schools.

As Ludmerer pointed out, the AMA Council on Medical Education had already carried out a survey of medical schools in the United States, but realized that publication of their findings under AMA aegis could be troublesome. Therefore, along with other leaders in medical education, they convinced the Carnegie Foundation to take on the study and thus the Flexner Report. One cannot help but assume that Flexner was assisted greatly by the previous work done by the AMA and the AAMC and by their staff work. Otherwise, it would have seemed physically impossible to visit and meaningfully comment upon 166 medical schools over one year. The report, however, was pure Flexner and, as Ludmerer points out, was a classic of the muckraking reform style of the period.

Many states had been trying to improve the quality of medical licensure in the late 19th century. Flexner's report was a great prod to this important social function. To assist in this process, in 1914 the AMA Council on Medical Education began the process of accrediting medical schools, ranking them A, B, or C. An A school was acceptable because it approached the Hopkins model, with the characteristics that it had an endowment to underwrite the costs of medical education, owned or had an affiliation with a teaching hospital, rated as a C and had teaching that included full-time research faculty. A school in the B category was one that could be improved. A school rated as C was one that needed a complete overhaul and reorganization or one that should get out of the business.

With licensure now a significant barrier to getting into practice, students were very reluctant to attend class C schools and sought those with more substance. Because one could not finance an A school from tuition alone, this spelled the inevitable end of the proprietary schools, so by 1930, there was essentially a single model, and the number of medical schools had dropped from more than 160 to 76.

During the late 19th century and the first third of the 20th century, many graduates of American medical schools would spend a year in Europe, frequently in Germany, to further their education and enhance their ability to establish a practice or join a medical faculty. Progressively, as the number of modern medical schools increased in size and sophistication post-MD training opportunities became available in this country, starting what we now call graduate medical education. Some states began to require a year of internship before licensure. Even by 1920 the Council on Medical Education called for universities to control these expanding training programs. However, a difficulty arose from the fact that hospitals had become proprietors of these programs, the employers of the interns, and most universities did not own their teaching hospitals. Thus, graduate medical education evolved along separate paths slowly and without coordination.

Ophthalmology was the first to set national standards. Medicine was the first, in 1939, to organize formal accreditation under the aegis of the Council on Medical Education, the teaching hospitals, the American College of Physicians, and the American Board of Internal Medicine. Surgery followed this model in 1950, and by 1953 the other major medical specialties had established their residency review committees (RRCs). The Millis Report in 1966 called for better coordination of graduate medical education, and in 1973 the Liaison Committee on Graduate Medical Education was formed. It still met with resistance from the RRCs, however, which did not wish to give up their autonomy. Finally, under the reorganized Accreditation Council for Graduate Medical Education, progress began to be made, and in 1988 general requirements for all residencies were published. The fact that the relationship between medical schools and their teaching hospitals was immature in 1920 resulted in a delay of approximately 70 years in bringing these important programs under the formal general oversight of medical school faculty and administration.)

Meanwhile, the strengthening of licensing standards by the various states resulted at times in microprescription of curriculum, which became exceedingly trying for medical schools, particularly those that drew students from all across the country. Gradually, the states began to coordinate better together with the advent of the Federation of State Medical Boards in 1912, and to rely on the accreditation process of the Association of American Medical Colleges and the AMA Council on Medical Education. These latter two finally came together in 1942 to establish the Liaison Committee on Medical Education, which continues to accredit schools in the United States and Canada. Many states, however, continued to have their own state licensure examinations however until 1968 when working with the National Board of Medical

Examiners (NBME) they evolved the Federation Licensure Examination (FLEX). The NBME (National Boards) had begun in 1915 to provide an examination for licensure of such high quality that it would be accepted by all of the states, thus facilitating the ability of graduates who passed this examination to be eligible for licensure anywhere in the country. This began the saga of the National Boards.

As any reasonably bright student recognizes very quickly, the examination drives the educational system. For convenience, in 1922 the National Board was broken into three parts. Part I, covering the basic sciences, usually was given at the end of two years, part II, covering the clinical sciences, at the end of medical school, and part III after a of internship. For many years, parts I and II were essay and part III oral. The state examinations, and later the FLEX examination, were one examination given after graduation. Increasingly, most students, assuming that it would be best to take the basic science part of the examination right after they had finished their basic science courses, signed up to take the National Boards, and medical schools were willing to facilitate this process by providing space and proctors for the examinations.

In 1951, the National Boards shifted to a multiple-choice exam, which greatly increased their reliability, but at the expense of validity. Difficulties began to arise as some schools began to require that their students take the National Board and indeed pass part I before proceeding to the clinical years. National Board scores began to be included as part of the grading system in medical schools as the National Boards provided shelf examinations in each of the major subjects. Residency program directors started asking students to provide their part I National Board scores, often as a filter to reduce the number of applicants interviewing for a residency program. The LCME began looking at the school's overall performance on the National Boards as an indicator of the quality of its educational program.

The examinations, in many respects, were high quality and well conceived. The questions were derived by a hard-working committee of acknowledged experts in each subject area who, working with psychomericians at the National Boards, would evolve high-quality and reliable questions covering their respective fields. The problem was that the examination was norm referenced, which with the ebb and flow of quality of applicants to medical schools caused problems from time to time. In addition, to get a spread, many of the questions were highly esoteric. Also, there was little integration among the parts or within the parts. Finally, to achieve superb reliability, the validity of the examination had been limited primarily to recall of facts and some limited problem solving or about one fourth of what you really would like to know about a progressing or graduating medical student. The discussion shall return to this problem later.

World War II had a profound effect on medical education in several ways. First, it demonstrated that the process of medical education could be shortened considerably under the exigencies of wartime, and that the participants in these programs turned out to be good doctors. Another major factor was the Manhattan Project, in which the mobilization of great scientific and research effort resulted in the atomic bomb. Many of the returning veterans wanted to go to medical school, which stressed the capacity of existing institutions and further enhanced the importance of good undergraduate grades for acceptance into medical school. In addition, the booming economy after World War II and the spread of health benefits to employees changed the economic expectations of those practicing medicine.)

The drama of the Manhattan Project had created the mentality in Congress that with enough effort in research, almost any problem could be solved. This contributed to the expansion of the National Institutes of Health during the Truman administration, with a high influx of new dollars made available to medical schools and institutes for biomedical research.

For the next 20 years, research appeared to be the number one preoccupation of medical schools. Institutional reputation was based on research productivity, which led to more grants as well as gifts. Tenure and promotion at many medical schools was based almost completely on research productivity (the publish or perish syndrome). Inevitably, teaching took on a lower priority, because committing any great time to it could be perilous to one's career. The author knows of a person recruited as a full professor in a midwestern medical school who had written into his contract that he would not have any obligation to teach anybody unless he felt like doing so.

As the priority of teaching began to fall, the faculty, pressed for time, looking for the most efficient way to fulfill this distraction, began to lean heavily on lectures and to spread them out among all faculty available. In some institutions in the 1960's and 1970's, medical students were spending almost 40-hours a week in this passive form of learning. Obviously, to further enhance efficiency, to meet the students' needs, and to give the impression of doing a good job, the lectures became increasingly focused on the National Boards. During this period, big-name institutions with large research budgets consistently were given a maximum 10-year span of accreditation by the LCME because it was unthinkable to question the quality of education in such prestigious institutions. Besides, their students "did so well on the National Boards."

Pressures to get into medical school were having a negative influence on the undergraduate experience as well. Students and their premedical advisors, and focusing on the Medical College Admissions Test (MCAT) provided by the Association of American Medical Colleges looking toward surviving the first-year of medical school, took primarily premed subjects and advanced science subjects beyond those required so they would appear more competitive. The end result was that some of our brightest young people attended some of our finest universities without getting a college education. They then entered a medical school, where for the next two years they attended lectures and demonstrations. Often, it was not until they arrived in the clerkships that they began to feel they really were in medical school, experiencing at least something of what Osler had in mind. But even here, the real bedside teaching, by default, often was given by interns and residents. In many institutions, after the introduction to clinical medicine course in the sophomore year, the senior faculty never did watch the students do a history and physical examination.

In the middle 1960s Congress passed Medicare and Medicaid, greatly increasing entitlement for health care and the demand for physician services. During this same time, the United States entered the Vietnam War. The demand for places in medical school increased dramatically. From 1960-1980, forty new schools developed. But even with expansion, many students during the 1970s were unsuccessful in gaining admissions to American medical schools, and hundreds took advantage of new off-shore schools being established to help them meet their desires. When the dust settled and the demographics were analyzed, it became quite clear that much of the apparent interest in medical school during the late 1960s and early 1970s to which the educational establishment magnificently responded, was really a desire of young men to avoid service in Vietnam. In fact, if it had not been for the significant increase in the number of women matriculants in the late 1970s, there would have been an embarrassing excess of medical school places much earlier and much more dramatic than that which occurred in the late in 1980s. With excess capacity in the system, it certainly would have seemed reasonable not to start any new schools, and to put to rest any that could not consistently provide a quality educational experience for their students.

The Vietnam experience did have one very positive influence on medical education, however. This was a period of great social unrest, especially for our young people as they challenged authority and the status quo, demanding "accountability" from university presidents and deans. Part of the reaction in educational institutions was a heightened sensitivity to the students' needs and increased flexibility in trying different ways of meeting them.

That this change of attitude in educational institutions occurred over the time span that many of the 40 new medical schools were started was fortuitous and very positive. It meant that these new schools not only had the opportunity for a new beginning (which can be refreshing in its own right), but that they were evolving in an era that permitted more innovation and experimentation than had occurred since the first decades of the century. The community-based schools found that it was now safe to use high-quality practitioners in private practice as teachers and models for medical students and residents. The new schools, particularly during the 1970s, produced some distraction and annoyance among the establishment, and were at times a challenge to the LCME such that there was pressure,. at times not too subtle, to conform.

In the late 1960s the Coggeshal Report had called for the reorganization of the Association of American Medical Colleges which indeed took place in the early 1970s with the establishment of the Council of Deans, the Council of Teaching Hospitals, the Council of Academic Societies, and medical student representatives. (Resident representatives were added in the 1990s--late as usual.) In addition, a variety of interest groups were established, including those representing faculty who were medical education professionals, many of whom were working in the newer medical schools helping to evolve and measure the effectiveness of their new curricula. These, through their demonstrations and presentations, began to enhance the respectability of what the new schools were doing. In addition, a subsection of the Council of Deans, called the Deans of New and Developing Medical Schools, was established not only for mutual support, but also to remind the AAMC that it was a representative of all of the medical schools in the United States and to push for a stronger educational agenda.

At the 1979 Council of Deans meeting in Scottsdale, Arizona, a debate was scheduled between the dean of a traditional medical school and the dean of a new community-based medical school regarding important issues in medical education. The result was not so much as debate as it was a mutual call for a refocusing and reform of the medical school curriculum. The response from the deans was a vigorous and positive discussion that ran well over the time allotted and resulted in a call that next years meeting of the Council of Deans should be devoted to educational topics (something long neglected). The subsequent meeting in 1980 again was very successful and challenging, resulting in the leadership of the AAMC calling for an in-depth study of undergraduate medical education which resulted several years later in the General Professional Education of the Physician (GPEP) Report in 1984 financed by the Kaiser Family Foundation. Educational reform now became respectable. The GPEP harvested much of the best from the ferment of the 1970s and laid out clear directions for medical schools to follow. Some of these have now evolved into standards of the LCME such as the need for a strong central control of the curriculum and a decrease in the passive learning of the lecture system.

Some of the experiments of the 1970s were unsuccessful. The three-year curriculum, which had spread to many schools, was rapidly abandoned because of fatigue and disappearance of incentives. The six-year program from high school to MD status was not copied. A major problem was jurisdictional disputes between college and medical school administrators.

In the 1980s and into the 1990s a new external force began to exert itself on medical schools. A decrease in direct federal funding for medical education, as well as a dropoff in the largess of research grant support caused schools to look elsewhere for revenue. The answer was found in expanding the practice of medicine, and in some schools by raising tuition to levels previously unthinkable. As the pressure for practice income increased and research dollars decreased, it was clear that some faculty, particularly clinical faculty, could not proceed academically by the usual career path of research and publication. Accordingly, most schools during the past decade have evolved a program of two tracks: the traditional research track and a clinical track with different criteria for academic promotion.

In recent years, with competition among medical centers and decreased revenues resulting from managed care, the overall financing of medical education is again in difficulty. Some clinical faculty members now wonder where they will find time to teach. The pressures of big-time practice could have the same onerous effect on medical education that big-time research did. This is the challenge for the current faculties. Hopefully, with such advances as problem-based learning and standardized patients, medical students can be brought along at a much higher level of clinical sophistication so that during their clinical years they can be an asset to patient activities rather than a burden slowing them down.

Finally, returning to the National Boards, after years of trying to explain that they were just providing a service and that others were using their examinations inappropriately, the Board finally underwent a thorough review resulting in dramatic changes. The three parts of the old NBME, which were essentially an academic achievement examination, gave way to the Steps of the United States Medical Licensing Examination (USMLE), which asks important questions and is criterion referenced, thus becoming a real licensure examination. The steps are integrated within the Steps and across the Steps, and with the approval of the Federation of State Medical Boards in 1990, there finally is only one path to licensure in the United States. With the hoped-for advent of direct clinical skills assessment for Step 2 and Step 3, the National Board Examination, which has always had high reliability, will now have significantly greater validity. If the examination is going to drive the system, we will finally have a good examination that drives it in the right directions. We might even get back to where we started a 100 years ago--self education under guidance.

What have we learned in a 100 years? First, a medical school is primarily an educational institution, and the education of our medical students deserves the same scholarship and discipline that we bring to the laboratory bench and the bedside. Second, we are part of a larger system that is capable of profoundly influencing our activities, positively or negatively. Scholarship in medical education cannot be passive or merely reactive to these changes. Our faculties must be very alert to avoid or ameliorate the negative influences and not become so enamored of our habits that we miss the benefits of the positive influences.

The saga continues.

REFERENCES

Lundmerer, K.. M. (1985). *Learning to Heal*. New York: Basic Book, Inc.

CHAPTER THREE

Medical Education in Australia, Great Britain, and New Zealand in the 21st Century

Charles E. Engel
Centre for Higher Education Studies
University of London

The development of medical education during the 20th century in Australia, Great Britain, and New Zealand needs to be seen in the context of the century as a whole. In the early 1900s, these three countries were key partners in the British Empire, together with Canada, India, and South Africa. The Victorian era and the reign of Edward VII had been periods of essential economic and social stability. There thus seemed to be no pressing reasons for major change, not even in response to the American scholar Abraham Flexner and his suggestion that medical education would benefit from a fusion of the German emphasis on theory with the British more pragmatic focus on practical experience (Flexner, 1910).

Yet even before World War I, the blossoming of scientific research and growing advances in technology caused voices to be raised in support of change in medical education. For example, Sir William Osler, the Regius Professor of Medicine at Oxford, with wide experience in both the United States and Canada, warned medical students at St. George's Hospital Medical School in London (Osler, 1913):

> The chief difficulty is the extraordinary development in every subject of the curriculum--a new anatomy, a new physiology, a new pathology, new methods of practice, to say nothing of phenomenal changes in physics, chemistry, and biology. The truth is, we have outrun an educational system framed in simpler days and for simpler conditions. The pressure comes hard enough upon the teacher, but far harder upon the taught, who suffer in a hundred different ways.

23

Nevertheless, only minor changes occurred in the education of doctors. Communication still was at a leisurely pace, and travel between the dominions of the empire could occupy many weeks at sea. Even so, the first tentative, political decisions were made in Britain, and therefore in the dominions, toward the creation of a national safety net for those citizens who could not afford the attention of a doctor or subsistence in old age.

World War I saw the first major infusion of North American influence, as well as the decline of the Pax Britannica, together with the abandonment of the gold standard. Hyperinflation in Germany and worldwide mass unemployment bred political extremism, fueled by the revolution in Russia.

Yet, it was not until the cataclysmic events of World War II, a mere 20 years later, when the British Empire changed into the Commonwealth of independent nations, that the research, practice and education in medicine of these nations gradually began to develop in separate ways. The age of rapid and mass travel was born, together with the age of electronics and satellites, which spawned computers, television, and instantaneous, worldwide communication. Vast funds were expended on the space race and a renewed armaments race, which included nuclear war heads.

All these developments have had a major influence, not only on the continuing social and economic changes in societies across the world, but also on the exponential development of medical science and technology. This, then, is the context in which the development of medical education in Australia, Great Britain, and New Zealand during the second half of the 20th century needs to be viewed.

MEDICAL EDUCATION IN GREAT BRITAIN

While World War II was still at its height, with a total involvement of the entire population in the war effort and the horrendous destruction of habitation and civilian lives, the British coalition government developed postwar plans for a national health service that would be free of charge at the point of delivery. This was quickly followed by a government enquiry (Goodenough, 1945) that concerned itself with the education of the doctors who would staff this comprehensive health service. Among other consequences, the report accelerated the incorporation of the historically freestanding, hospital-based medical schools of London within the University of London.

By the 1960s these schools also had been persuaded to appoint professors in clinical disciplines. These moves reinforced the academic emphasis in medical education leading to university qualifications rather than the diplomas granted by examination of the Royal Colleges and the Society of Apothecaries, that ancient guild of the City of London. The Royal Commission on Medical Education (1968) ensured that medical education would focus henceforth on a general education, to be followed by postgraduate education in specialties, including family medicine.

By the late 1970s it had become clear that the veritable explosion of knowledge and the related brief shelf life of knowledge in medical science had imposed an intolerable and irrational information overload on students (Dornhorst, 1981). Stirred by the examples of radical change in Canada (Hamilton, 1976) and Australia (Clarke, 1977), the King's Fund Centre organized a Delphi Conference to identify the views of senior medical academics, as well as officers of the main medical institutions and associations. The report identified 11 aspects that had received widespread agreement among the respondents (Towle, 1991):

- reduction in factual information
- active learning (to produce inquiring doctors)
- principles of medicine (core knowledge, skills, attitudes)
- development of generalizable competencies (e.g., critical thinking, problem solving, communication, management)
- integration (vertical and horizontal)
- early clinical contact
- balance between hospital/community and curative/preventive experience
- wider aspects of health care (e.g., medicolegal/ethical issues, health economics, political aspects, medical audit)
- interprofessional collaboration.
- methods of learning/teaching to support the aims of the curriculum
- methods of assessment to support the aims of the curriculum.

These recommendations were incorporated in the Recommendations of the General Medical Council (GMC, 1993). The GMC is legally responsible for the quality of medical practice and hence for the quality of medical education. Its recommendations should therefore be considered seriously. However, traditional conservatism, and a number of constraints tend to handicap major change. Government funding for British universities has been reduced, despite political pressure to admit more students. At the same time, basic scientists are under pressure to increase their "research productivity," and clinical teachers practicing in the National Health Service are called on not only to increase their clinical activities, but also to intensify their teaching of the postgraduate staff (National Health Service Executive, 1996). The various medical schools of the University of London also have been faced with the additional organizational upheaval of amalgamation and incorporation in multifaculty colleges of the University.

Nevertheless, all British schools are undertaking some curricular reform, mainly with a degree of integration, early patient contact, rearrangement of "core" content, and the addition of "special study modules" (GMC, 1993). With a few notable exceptions, most schools have established active units of medical education, initially with financial support from the government for the salaries of "facilitators for curriculum change."

The medical schools of the Universities of Glasgow, Liverpool, and Manchester stand out as models of radical reform in well-established institutions. Glasgow is about to celebrate its 500th anniversary. All three schools have adopted entirely new, problem-based learning curricula (Barrows & Tamblyn, 1980).

Medical education is university based and as such subject to the wider traditions and regulations of its respective parent institution. In Great Britain, as in Australia and New Zealand the universities derive the bulk of their income from the government. In the United Kingdom, government funds are distributed through the Higher Education Funding Councils of England, Wales, Scotland, and Northern Ireland, respectively. The Dearing Report (National Committee of Inquiry Into Higher Education [NCIHE], 1997), a government-initiated inquiry into higher education, will thus exert a major influence on the future of medical education. All university students must now, for the first time, contribute an annual tuition fee of £1,000 (U.S. $1,650), a significant addition to the cumulative debt of the newly graduated doctor. Another result of the Report is the introduction of training in education for all new academics. However, there still is no formal policy that would ensure due recognition and reward for creativity and effort in education as opposed to research and/or clinical practice (Chaput de Saintonge, Elzubeir, & Towle, 1997).

MEDICAL EDUCATION IN AUSTRALIA AND NEW ZEALAND

Both Australia and New Zealand based their university education on that of the "mother country" until the end of World War II. Since then, Australia, even more than New Zealand, has tended to explore its own paths to reform and innovation. As the General Medical Council of Great Britain withdrew from overseas visits as part of its accreditation of medical schools, the Australian Medical Council (AMC) was established with close links to the New Zealand Medical Council. The accreditation procedures of the AMC have adopted the best aspects of the North American and United Kingdom systems (Australian Medical Council, 1992; Hamilton, 1993).

Even before the cutting of the apron strings, the new medical school at the University of Newcastle, New South Wales, Australia, had created the first problem-based learning curriculum in the Southern Hemisphere (Engel & Clark, 1979). This stimulated the older of the two New Zealand medical schools and also one of its clinical schools (Lewis, Buckley, Kong, & Mellsop, 1992) to experiment with problem-based learning (Schwartz, Heath & Egan, 1994). Most recently, the medical schools at the Australian Universities of Flinders, Sydney, and Queensland have taken the major radical step to accept only university graduates into their new, problem-based learning and shortened curricula (Sefton, 1997). Much of their approach to the selection of students and their educational thinking are based on the Newcastle experience. The admission of graduates alone, although similar to North American practice, is unique within Commonwealth countries and unknown in

Europe. These developments in Australia and New Zealand should be seen in the context of the urge in these countries for change in the last quarter of the old century.

The foundation dean at Newcastle, New South Wales, sounded the first trumpet call for urgent action (Maddison, 1978). The state of Queensland produced an erudite report on the need for change and a thoughtful set of recommendations (Medical Board of Queensland, 1981). An imaginative initiative by the New Zealand Department of Health (Committee of Inquiry, 1985) involved the public in defining the future roles of doctors and thus their education. A national conference was convened in the same year to discuss the Report with members of the New Zealand public. The resulting Summary Report "issued by the conference participants" was published in both Maori and English.

This Summary Report was followed by a discussion paper from the Advisory Committee on the Medical Workforce (1987) in New Zealand. In the following year, a report on the education of medical students was published by the Medical Council of New Zealand (1988). Since then, changes of governments and increasing curtailment of government funding have led to substantial changes in the organization and administration of New Zealand's pioneering national health service. This, in turn, has imposed constraints on the reform of medical education (Hornblow, 1997).

Also in 1988, the Australasian and New Zealand Association for Medical Education published the results of its Delphi Conference (Marshall & Engel, 1988) on changes to be implemented in medical education. The responses from around Australia were included in the evidence used by the Committee of Inquiry into Medical Education and Medical Workforce (1988) by the Australian Federal Government. This report legitimized the innovations in student selection and curriculum design at Newcastle, New South Wales, and thus reinforced their influence on the three medical schools that changed to a graduate entry with problem-based learning curricula in the late 1990s.

TOWARD THE NEXT 40 YEARS

A number of trends can be identified even now. Perhaps some of the more important trends may be the following:

- continuing growth in the world's population--eight-billion by 2050 (World Health Organization [WHO], 1998)
- overuse of irreplaceable resources and pollution leading to conflicts over water and adverse affects on the environment because of increased population combined with continuing growth in technology
- rapid spread of disease across continents, because of mass air travel
- new diseases (WHO, 1996) and growing resistance to antibiotics

- increasing ability of medicine to preserve life, balanced by increasing cost of health care
- a plethora of ethical challenges resulting from scientific developments, such as genetic engineering, and cloning
- progressively aging populations with increasing needs for health care, to be provided by a shrinking pool of young people, with those under 20 years of age constituting 32% of the population by 2050 as compared with 40% in 1997 (WHO, 1998)
- growing inability to support large numbers of doctors financially (Abel-Smith, 1986a, 1986b), while the other health professions receive advanced education and are permitted to undertake tasks that used to be reserved for licensed medical practitioners (Spitzer, Sacket, Sibley, Roberts, Gent, Kergin, Hackett, & Olynich 1974).

In addition to the educational requirements listed in the King's Fund Delphi Conference Report (Towle, 1991), the next century will need to see rigorous developments in an overt development of social responsibility (Ewan, 1985) as well as community-oriented and community-based education (Hamilton, 1993), with the creation of professorial chairs for community-based education, as at the University of Manchester, UK (Whitehouse, 1996), and an emphasis on rural and remote-location practice (Hays, Strasser, & Wallace, 1997).

Much has been written about the desirability of interprofessional "shared" learning for interprofessional collaboration (Barr, 1996). A great deal of careful research will be needed before appropriate educational interventions can be identified and applied.

Governments as primary funding agencies in the three countries discussed exert a significant influence on institutions of higher education, yet with short-term political imperatives. For example, in Great Britain the government wishes medical schools to add another 10% to their annual intake of students, with some financial incentive. This leads to ever larger classes of students.

What ethical responsibility will medical schools accept for their individual students and for the population that these students will come to serve? Will such students continue to be treated as an anonymous crowd to be herded through a sequence of examination obstacles? What will the medical schools do to plan and implement a carefully graded maturation process--from late adolescent lay people into caring, empathic young adult professionals?

Will these medical schools accept a continuing responsibility for their graduates, who will still be in active practice almost up to the middle of the new century? Will all the doctors now being trained be affordable by the 2020s and 2030s?

Perhaps the greatest challenge for the universities and their medical schools is to ensure that their graduates are able to adapt to change and that they are able to participate in the management of change.

The intricate and interrelated problems that affect our planet will require interprofessional and, indeed, intersectoral, long-term planning and intervention that politicians alone cannot be expected to accomplish. The special competencies required for this overarching task will need to be developed in the context of developing profession-specific competencies (Engel, 1995). Faculties of medicine and health sciences also will need to shoulder the special responsibility of fostering and preserving human values in a time that is likely to be even less caring than the 20th century has turned out to be.

REFERENCES

Abel-Smith, B. (1986a). The world economic crisis: Part I. Repercussions on health. *Health Policy and Planning, 1*, 202-213.

Abel Smith, B. (1986b). The world economic crisis: Part II. Health manpower out of balance. *Health Policy and Planning, 1*, 309-316.

Advisory Committee on the Medical Workforce. (1987). *The development of medical practitioners: A discussion document.* Wellington, New Zealand: Ministry of Health.

Australian Medical Council (AMC). (1992). *The assessment and accreditation of medical schools by the Australian Medical Council.* Melbourne, Australia: AMC.

Barr, H. (1996). Ends and means in interprofessional education: Towards a typology. *Education for Health, 9*, 341-352.

Barrows, H. S., & Tamblyn, R. M. (1980). *Problem-based learning.* New York: Springer.

Chaput de Saintonge, D. M., Elzubeir, M., & Towle, A. (1997). Promoting policies and recognition of teaching excellence in UK universities and medical schools. *Education for Health, 10*, 153-164.

Clarke, R. M. (1977). The new medical school at Newcastle, New South Wales. *The Lancet, 1*, 434-435.

Committee of Inquiry. (1985). *The role of the doctor in New Zealand and implications for medical education.* Wellington, New Zealand: Department of Health.

Committee of Inquiry into Medical Education and Medical Workforce. (1988). *Australian medical education and workforce into the 21st century.* Canberra, Australia: Federal Ministry of Health.

Domhorst, A. C. (1981). Information overload: Why medical education needs a shakeup. *The Lancet, ii*, 513-514.

Engel, C. E. (1995). Medical education in the 21st century. *Capability, 1*(4), 23-29.

Engel, C. E. & Clarke, R. M. (1979). Medical education with a difference. *Programmed Learning and Educational Technology, 16*, 70-87.

Ewan, C. (1985) Objectives for medical education: Expectations of society. *Medical Education, 19*, 101-112.

Flexner, A. (1910). Medical education in the United States and Canada. *Carnegie Bulletin, 4.* Reproduced (1960) Washington, DC: Science and Health Publications.

General Medical Counsel (GMC). (1993). *Tomorrow's doctors.* London, UK: General Medical Council.

Goodenough, W. (1945). *Goodenough Report.* Interdepartmental Committee on Medical Schools. London, UK: His Majesty's Stationery Office.

Hamilton, J. D. (1976). The McMaster curriculum: A critique. *British Medical Journal, 1*, 1191-1196.

Hamilton, J. D. (1993). Community orientation: Ups and downs at Newcastle. *Annals of Community-Oriented Education, 6*, 35-42.

Hamilton, J. D. (1993). Medical accreditation: The Australian experience. *Annals of Community-Oriented Education, 6*, 231-242.

Hays, R. B., Strasser, R. P., & Wallace, A. (1997). Development of a national training programme for rural medicine in Australia. *Education for Health, 10*, 275-286.

Hornblow, A. (1997). New Zealand's health reforms: A clash of cultures. *British Medical Journal, 7098*, 1892-1894.

Lewis, M. E., Buckley, A., Kong, M., & Mellsop, G. W. (1992). The role of evaluation in the development of a problem-based learning programme within a traditional school of medicine. *Annals of Community-Oriented Education, 5*, 223-234.

Maddison, D. C. (1978). What's wrong with medical education? *Medical Education, 12*, 97-102.

Marshall, J. R., & Engel, C. E. (1988). *Enquiring into medical education for capability and change*. Occasional Paper No 1. Monash University, Clayton, Australia: Australasian and New Zealand Association for Medical Education.

Medical Board of Queensland. (1981). *Committee of Inquiry into Future Needs and Training for Medical Practice in Queensland*. Brisbane, Australia: Medical Board of Queensland.

Medical Council of New Zealand (MCNZ). (1988). *The education of medical undergraduates in New Zealand*. Wellington, New Zealand: Medical Council of New Zealand.

National Health Service Executive. (1996). *A guide to specialist registrar training*. London, UK: Department of Health.

National Committee of Inquiry Into Higher Education (NCIHE). (1997). *Higher education in the learning society*. Report of the NCIHE. London, UK: Her Majesty's Stationery Office.

Osler, Sir W. (1913). Examinations, examiners, and examinees. *The Lancet*, 1047-1050.

Royal Commission on Medical Education. (1968). *Todd Report*. London, UK: Her Majesty's Stationery Office.

Schwartz, P. L., Heath, C. J., & Egan, A. G. (1994). *The art of the possible: Ideas from a traditional medical school engaged in curricular revision*. Dunedin, New Zealand: University of Otago Press.

Sefton, A. J. (1997). From a traditional to a problem-based curriculum: Estimating staff time and resources. *Education for Health, 10*, 165-178.

Spitzer, W. O., Sacket, D.L., Sibley, J. C., Roberts, R .S., Gent, M., Kergin, D. J., Hackett, B. C., & Olynich, C. A. (1974). The Burlington randomized trial of the nurse practitioner. *New England Journal of Medicine, 291*, 251-256.

Towle, A. (1991). *Critical thinking: The future of undergraduate medical education*. London, UK: King Edward's Hospital Fund for London.

Whitehouse, C. R. (1996). Planning for community-oriented medical education at Manchester. *Education for Health, 9*, 45-59.

World Health Organization (WHO). (1996). *World Health Report 1996*. Geneva, Switzerland: WHO.

World Health Organization (WHO). (1998). *World Health Report 1998*. Geneva, Switzerland: WHO.

CHAPTER FOUR

Teaching and Learning in Medicine and Surgery in the 21st Century: Challenges to the Developing World

Ara Tekian
University of Illinois at Chicago

The developing world faces enormous challenges. Such an opening statement, however, is not intended to mislead anyone into believing that it is prudent to conceive of a developing world as if it were a single static entity with unity and well-defined boundaries. In fact, it is neither judicious nor practical to refer to a sizable portion of the earth's human population in this way. The nations that comprise the developing world are in no way homogeneous. Vast diversity exists in their cultures, religions, resources, and social systems. The idea of grouping countries implies a comparison akin to that of the proverbial apples and oranges.

Whereas many of the challenges facing the developing world are quite specific to individual countries, others are common to all. The World Health Organization (WHO) has declared that the protection and promotion of its citizens' health is one of the most important functions of government. After all, without a healthy population, any country's hopes for economic prosperity and productivity, social justice, and education are quickly diminished.

Classifying problems in such a dichotomous fashion, of course, may be overstating the case. Even a problem common throughout the entire developing world is bound to have a strong local component. The very differences in culture, religion, resources, and social fabric mentioned previously mandate it. Directing attention to the variety of medical establishments already in place in different regions of the developing world gives a sense of the complexity of forces that can be expected to influence their further development. The determinative social textures existing in such geographically diverse locations as Asia, South America, and Africa are in a constant state of flux, and changes are likely to be driven by a complex interaction of factors including economics, cultural particularities, issues of the environment, changes in governmental structure, national priority shifts, availability and distribution of resources, and critical regional issues. Clearly, an in-depth understanding of these local factors is required before any assessment or change to an institution of health care can be properly made.

However, several themes central to the issue of effecting change in the health of developing countries may provide at least a cursory understanding and appreciation of the current state of affairs. First and foremost, medical education should be thought of as the base of health care, and any assessment will be incomplete without considering the role played by institutions that train future health care personnel. It also goes without saying that looking at systems of health care delivery is of utmost importance to the goal of understanding the situations of developing countries. Both of these issues, however, must be examined in light of the diversity that so much of this introduction has emphasized. In searching for universal recommendations, it must be kept in mind that a course of action that provides the perfect solution to the problems in one region of the world may be entirely unfeasible in another. As such, any global recommendations must transcend the cultural, social, religious, and economic boundaries presented throughout the developing world.

The goal of this chapter is to work within a simplified model of the fluid interactions between medical education and health care delivery, and to discuss the importance of the anticipated changes to health care over the next few decades, including changing distribution of resources, humanization of care, integration of care, issues of finance and cost control, and issues of technology. Similarly, the changes necessary in medical education to meet the needs of the world's population are discussed. These changes are likely to correspond to changes in health care delivery, and include normative, curricular, methodologic, and evaluative changes. A series of recommendations are proposed, the goal of which is to establish applicability across cultural, economic, and political boundaries.

THE WORLD HEALTH ORGANIZATION: GLOBAL ASSESSMENT AND IMPETUS FOR CHANGE

In September 1978, WHO's International Conference on Primary Care was held at Alma-Ata in the former Soviet Union (Alma-Ata, 1978). Among the most important accomplishments of that landmark conference was the compilation of the Declaration of Alma-Ata, which would come to be seen as a seminal event toward effecting change in worldwide medical education and health care delivery. The Declaration called on all governments, health and development workers, and the world community to protect and promote the health of all the people of the world. Health was deemed a fundamental human right.

Alma-Ata did more than plead for the health of the world's citizens. As if possessing the ability to foresee future ambiguity resulting from misinterpretation, the International Conference on Primary Health Care, in the first article of the declaration, clearly defined health as a state of complete physical, mental, and social well-being, and not merely the absence of disease or infirmity.

The conference determined the health status of the world's nations to be grossly unequal, with a particularly wide gap between the health of developed nations and the health of developing nations. In 1960, the richest 20% of the world had more than 30 times the wealth of the poorest 20%. Currently, the richest have 60 times more than the poorest (United Nations Development Program, 1991). Furthermore, in the 1990s, the world's 50 poorest countries contained roughly 75% of the world's population and occupied half of the world's land mass, yet had only 25% of the world's wealth (United Nations Development Program, 1994).

Finding this gap politically, socially, and economically unacceptable, the Alma-Alta delegates agreed that the resolution of the world health problem was not to be the sole responsibility of the individual nation. Rather, a collective international effort was assigned the task of helping the people of the world attain the highest possible level of health. Economic and social development, both on a local level and in the context of the emerging international economy, was declared to be a strong contributor to health. In turn, the promotion and protection of health was declared to be essential to sustained economic prosperity and social well-being. In this cyclical relationship between health and socioeconomic status, health is a fastening pin that, when pulled, uncouples the process and uniformly causes a decline in quality of life.

The course of action recommended by the conference at Alma-Ata was simply increased reliance on primary health care. The Declaration of Alma-Ata says of primary care:

> Primary health care is essential health care based on practical, scientifically sound and socially acceptable methods and technology made universally accessible to individuals and families in the community through their full participation and at the cost that the community and country can afford to maintain at every stage of their development.

Medicine's first level of contact with the individual, then, was to be the focus of improving the world's health. The advantages of the primary care approach were many. These were enumerated in the seventh article of the declaration.

The greatest advantage afforded by primary care to the developing world is its universality because it reflects and evolves from the economic conditions and sociocultural and political characteristics of the country and is based on the relevant results of social, biomedical, and health services research and public health experience. In other words, the primary care approach will do away with many of the difficulties imposed by diversity across developing nations because, by definition, primary care is heavily rooted in local customs. Similarly, the statement implies the use of relevant technologies as a means of raising the health status without incurring huge costs.

After endorsing the recommendations of the International Conference at Alma-Ata, four months later, WHO (1979) initiated Health for All by the Year 2000 (HFA-2000). The proceedings at Alma-Ata formed the basis of the program. The goals of Health for All were not well defined, and the program was initially viewed as a continuing process toward improving the health of the world at large. Among the process objectives listed in the introduction to Formulating Strategies for Health for All by the Year 2000 were the 1990 worldwide immunizations of children against the main infectious diseases and the provision of safe drinking water to the entire world population. Providing worldwide access to primary care was another goal, although the document professed that it was a longer range goal that would require unprecedented efforts on the part of all of the world's nations, both individually and collectively.

Changes in Health Care Delivery in the 21st Century

The interaction between medical education, medical practice, and health care is strong (Boelen, 1994). Change one just slightly, and there likely will be a waterfall effect, with proportional reverberations in the other two. Therefore, in recommending changes toward increased reliance on primary health care, WHO was not proposing only changes to the existing systems of health care delivery, but also corresponding changes to institutions of medical education (Garcia-Barbero, 1995). To be effective, changes to health care must be coordinated across these two areas, or any successful changes might have to be attributed to chance.

In essence, recommending changes to medical education is conditioned on the model projecting that changes to the educational institutions will result in commensurate changes to health care delivery. After all, if, in effect, nothing has been altered in the actual practice of medicine, then changes to medical education will have accomplished nothing. However, care should be taken not to make the mistake of modeling the interaction between delivery and education as a relatively simple chain of causality. Rather, just as changes in health care will result not only from changes in medical education, so changes to education will result similarly from new developments in health care delivery. Ignoring the health care delivery component of the model seems to be a quick way to diminish the value of any situational assessments and subsequent implementations. In this section, anticipated as well as already emerging concerns and challenges to health care delivery in developing nations are addressed.

Resource Allocation

The factor that will exert its effect on the state of health care delivery, regardless of other details, is resource allocation. Because the world contains a finite amount of capital and labor, delivery systems must be streamlined, interventions must be cost effective, and the results of research must have valuable applications. Wisely rationing existing resources, and searching for new and more efficient ways of using labor and capital are among the chief concerns concerning the future of health care. Unfortunately, at this point, resource allocation is more art than science, and to complicate matters, resource allocation is subject to change in accordance with the political wind.

The issues of resource distribution can be approached on two levels. The first level is among countries, and this perspective offers description of the differences in resource availability internationally. Second, resource distribution can be viewed from within a specific country. Of course, addressing resource distribution on a nation-to-nation basis is an assignment too great for this discussion. Several salient points remain to be made concerning resource allocation in individual nations.

The pattern of global resource distribution was originally cited by WHO as one of the major obstacles to achieving Health For All. The difference between the "haves" and "have nots," particularly across developed and developing countries, currently is staggering, and any efforts in the area of resource allocation should be directed toward bridging this gap. Originally, WHO called for international social support. After an enormous period of economic growth from 1945 to 1974, however, the organization may have made the mistake of viewing the industrialized world's support for programs promoting social equity as not yet fully developed. It now appears that in the future, international support in the forms of capital and labor will severely fall short of what is needed. As a result, WHO has reformed its own process of allocation to give resource priority to the most seriously deprived nations, or the least-developed countries (LDCs) (Changes and Reform at WHO, 1997). Mechanisms other than state-sponsored donations will need to be called on to bridge the gap.

Fortunately, the void that politics has failed to fill may soon be occupied by economics. Globalization (Kickbusch, 1997), the term used to denote the current trend toward economic and social interdependence, may aid in resolving global resource inequity. In the future, corporations will be the nations' diplomats, and hopefully will serve as ambassadors of goodwill. Globalization, however, is expected to demonstrate both positive and negative effects on population health. For example, increased trade and communications are bound to bring new economic opportunities to areas of the world abandoned a century ago by the burgeoning industrialized nations. Used appropriately, these new resources could serve to improve the social, political, and economic condition, and by extension, the health status, of the country's people. However, economic globalization left unchecked may afflict rather than aid people in developing countries, for example, by making wage-slaves of people who have nowhere else to turn for sustenance. It is of primary concern that the governments of both developed and developing countries monitor the international activities of corporations.

Integration

The effects of resource distribution on health care delivery can be seen more easily if it is examined on a national level. Following the analogous reforms at WHO, nations can give resources to the places where they are most needed, although this probably will not raise the mean population health status, and most likely will only reduce the standard deviation. A second approach is to distribute resources by population density, although this will involve increased reliance on a nationwide primary health program, which will require political support. This second method of distributing resources to the regional health care establishments appears to be promising, with recent success in its implementation by Iran (Marandi, 1995). Only part of the health reforms in Iran, however, can be attributed to resource distribution. Another contributing factor in the Iranian experience was the merging of the medical education institution with the health care delivery systems.

This integration of health care delivery and medical education appears to contribute favorably toward improving the general health of the citizens in developing nations. This approach emphasizes service to the community along with a new manifestation of hierarchical regionalism. In the case of Iran, two centralized ministries were merged into a single Ministry of Health and Medical Education. The results appear promising to other developing countries.

Bringing together medical education and health care delivery is critical to further development of health care in any society. As remarked in the journal *Medical Education*, the two systems should be as indivisible, as the two sides of the same coin (Integration of Medical Education and the Health Care System, 1996). Medicine, the same editorial says, is too theoretical and unapplied in medical schools, and opportunities for learning in the clinical setting are far too often overlooked. Within integration lies an inexpensive way to improve the institutions that are largely responsible for determining the health status of a nation.

Information Management

In the same vein, however, it is essential to recognize that the acceleration and expansion of the medical knowledge base has had an enormous impact on the educational procedures currently in place at most of the medical schools in the developed world. In addition, this knowledge explosion poses many problems for the future of the medical profession and its educational requirements. Knowledge, now doubling every five to eight years, is reliably predicted to begin doubling every year. Perhaps for this reason medical educators bemoan the fact that medicine has become too theoretical and unapplied in medical schools, and that opportunities for learning in the clinical setting are far too often overlooked. This is the reason why the practice of simply adding to an already overcrowded curriculum will no longer suffice. Medical schools, institutions, practitioners, and students all need to be helped in developing strategies for dealing with the sheer volume of information, concepts, and skills that health providers must have at their disposal. Some of these new strategies slowly making headway in medical schools are discussed later.

The expanding knowledge base may, however, hold very different implications for nations of the developing world. The worst-case scenario is that because developing countries lack both the technology to access the new wealth of information and the resources to import the technology, they may remain in the dark with regard to medical advances. A better scenario would involve a delayed reaction, in which nations of the developing world initially would lag behind (as is the case today), but would approach information levels approximating those of developed countries over several decades. Of course, the amount of time spent catching up will depend on several factors. For instance, the mind-set of individuals in the developing world may undermine the acquisition of new technologies. Persons who have lived their lives without a dominant technological presence may not be sufficiently prepared for an introduction to personal computers. It seems quite likely that before the game of informational catch-up can begin, extensive technological upgrading will have to take place.

Prevention

Another trend that health care delivery likely will be undergoing in the coming century is the shift from tertiary care to preventive medicine. A common saying is that an ounce of prevention is worth a pound of cure, although, as Jeremiah Stamler (1987) pointed out, this may be underrating the value of prevention, because many diseases are incurable once a patient is afflicted. The axiom, however, should be credited for establishing a fairly accurate portrayal of the relative costs of the two commodities: It is estimated that for every dollar spent on prevention, three dollars are saved in acute and rehabilitative costs (Turnock, 1997). This economic incentive seems already to have been recognized, especially in Western industrialized countries, by private health organizations, although their effectiveness in promoting health, and their over inflated interest in cutting costs have been criticized by the public. Prevention, a prerequisite for health, must be applied continuously in different stages. The direction for prevention in developing countries depends on their current demographic state. Following are the steps to prevention that developing countries must undertake over the course of the next century.

In least-developed countries, a good starting point, as it was for the United States in the 19th century, might be a sanitation movement. The value of clean water and proper refuse disposal can hardly be overstated, yet water-borne infectious diseases such as cholera and dysentery take appalling tolls in terms of morbidity and mortality in the developing world.

The next step in prevention may involve immunization campaigns. Science is producing an ever-expanding arsenal of vaccines, and although the newest vaccines may prove to be outside the financial reach of most developing countries, many of the older, less-expensive vaccines are available and needed. Significant proportions of the population in developing countries are unvaccinated against rubella, (a significant cause of morbidity in newborns), measles and mumps, (both incur economic costs from the inactivity of those who are sick), polio, and hepatitis B (the second leading carcinogen after tobacco, known to cause a vast majority of the world's liver cancer cases).

After the successful routing of infectious diseases, prevention efforts need to be directed toward combating chronic, noninfectious diseases. Much of the developed world is now struggling at this point, and the developing world is expected to arrive here shortly in the next century. Chronic diseases present a different challenge, in that the etiology of most chronic diseases is not well understood, and many of the diseases involve a behavioral component not as simple to address as sanitizing of water supplies or vaccination. Diet is a major risk, for instance, in type II diabetes, cardiovascular diseases, and several cancers. Similarly, smoking has been found to be associated with lung cancer and coronary heart disease. (An unfortunate health outcome of globalization, as mentioned before, is that much of the developing world may fall prey to tobacco companies whose sales may have reached a dead end in industrialized nations.) Therefore, decreasing mortality and morbidity from chronic diseases appears, in part, to require a societal change in behavior, the magnitude of which is unprecedented. Nevertheless, steps, however infinitesimally small, to this end are being made.

A second component of chronic disease prevention focuses on reducing environmental or occupational risks. Pollution, including lead and other metallotoxins, organochlorines, and inappropriate waste disposal, poses a serious problem in all countries, although the most severe effects in the future may be seen in developing nations that lack adequate industrial controls. Given the rate at which the environment is being poisoned, students and physicians alike must be trained in managing the effects of pollution and its health consequences. This is a prime example of the changing role of the physician, from personal care to social responsibility.

The future of prevention also will depend largely on the diseases that society produces. Infectious diseases are reemerging as a major problem worldwide because of medication misuse (which has generated new strains of antibiotic resistant bacteria) as well as social movements. For instance, the sexual revolution, while credited with bringing increased liberty to men and women alike, also has aided in the spread of sexually transmitted diseases. However, to make medicine affordable and to extend medicine throughout a population, prevention must become the dominant form of medicine early in the next century.

Economics

Another way that health care delivery can be expected to evolve both in the developed and developing world is in the mechanism of paying for services. A first look at developed countries, shows the magnitude of change that has occurred in finances over the past 60 years, and there is no reason to believe that this evolution will not continue into the next century.

Greenlick (1995) examined the changing nature of financing health care, providing a summary through three cross-sectional assessments of health care and projections for the future. In 1935, services were provided primarily on a fee-for-service basis, with the payment coming directly from the pocket of the patient. Government had no role in health care financing, and in the United States, 30 years would elapse before the instatement of Medicare. By 1985, 50 years later, the situation had changed substantially. The role of private insurance as the payer had been increasing steadily, but reached the peak at around this time. Still, some medical expenses were paid out-of-pocket. Similarly, the method by which physicians were paid was undergoing a metamorphosis from fee-for-service to capitation and salary, as the practice of medicine became assembled into small-to moderate-size organizations. The role of the government became slightly ambiguous, with government appearing to pick up the tab when no other source of payment was possible.

Greenlick (1995) predicts that these trends will extend into the early 21st century. The tendency away from out-of-pocket payment and the increasing numbers of uninsured people will result ultimately in socially organized mechanisms of payment, in which government will have to act as the principal organizer of financing. The vast majority of physicians will be paid on a capitation or salary basis. Hand in hand with these new developments in health care financing, evaluation based on cost effectiveness can be expected.

The developing world is, for the most part, mired in the fee-for-service, out-of-pocket stage that many of the developed nations experienced earlier in the 20th century. It would be foolish, though, to think that they will remain there in times to come. Although the health care delivery systems of developing countries are not likely to change overnight, it should be expected that their health care systems over time will face the same financial challenges that have plagued health care finance in Western countries for the past century.

The progression of finances in developing nations might be viewed as analogous to the previous discussion regarding the shifting emphasis of prevention (i.e., that each stage is a necessary precursor to the next). In this case, a developing nation would need only to follow the paths trod by developed countries toward satisfactory health care finance. This type of plan, however, falls short in that a developing nation would be committing itself to both the triumphs and failures of the Western experience. It seems to be far more efficient for the developing world to analyze the Western systems and identify the decisions that brought about the most desired results, as well as the pitfalls. With this information in hand, developing nations could, with reasonable confidence, construct health care finance policy demonstrated in the past to produce successful results, thus avoiding undesired effects.

Technology

The application of high technology to medical care also should be closely coordinated with the proper health care financing policies, especially in the developing world where it is increasingly difficult to justify or obtain funds for superspecialties based on high technology when resources usually are insufficient for even the most basic primary health care. Even the more affluent countries of the developed world are faced with the dilemma of rapidly changing technological advances and the relative inability of their health care delivery systems adequately to keep pace. Advances in technology have been coming so fast that medical practitioners can hardly catch their breath.

Along with progress and technological advancement, however, comes the inevitable rise in the cost of medical care. Unfortunately, governments of the developing world are faced with the burden of adapting their respective medical practices to meet the needs of their populations and health-care systems better while dealing with the critical problem of limited resources. The problems of high-priced technology in developing countries, as outlined by Elmeligy (1996), include difficulties in: (a) obtaining money for the initial equipment purchase, (b) determining the best choice of equipment available within the allocated budget, (c) obtaining money to cover maintenance costs for the equipment, and (d) obtaining money to cover the additional costs of peripheral and other related equipment that may be required. In addition, the discrepancy between what a medical practitioner learns in a developed country and what can be done on return to one's own country is almost always a problem.

The concept of appropriate technology provides some answers to the problems posed by the technology gap between developed and developing nations. Nations need to use technology that fits their economic and demographic profile. Consider, for instance, a project completed by the University of Gezira in Sudan (Mohi, Eldin, & Magzoub, 1995). Determining that the major health threat to a village was malaria, the medical students and the community constructed a drainage bridge. After this well-planned intervention, incidence of malaria rapidly declined. One of the lessons to be learned from this project is that the level of technology required to raise the health of the villagers substantially was rather low: All of the knowledge required could be obtained from a rudimentary civil engineering text, and the materials for the bridge were readily available.

How then does a community or nation determine what level of technology is most appropriate for their situation? One line of thought is that technology should follow a linear progression (e.g., Do not purchase the computed tomography [CT] scan unless you have done all you can with the x-ray, and do not purchase magnetic resonance imaging [MRI] until the effectiveness of the CT scan has reached its upper limit). The argument has its limitations, however, and perhaps a better method of determining exactly what technology is appropriate is determination by cost effectiveness.

FROM HEALTH CARE DELIVERY TO MEDICAL EDUCATION

To be effective, changes to health care must be coordinated across health care delivery and medical education, or any successful changes to health care would have to be attributed to chance. Defining the highest priorities must be a national issue, because no two countries are likely to be experiencing the exact same conditions within and surrounding their medical establishments. For example, in the United States, prevention may be the highest priority, when all factors are considered. In the United States, the major causes of mortality are heart disease, stroke, and cancer. The major threats to health care in the United States are runaway costs and a population that is living longer and in need of increasing amounts of health care. Under such circumstances, prevention may be the most effective measure, as it has been proven to cut costs and decrease incidence of disease.

In another country, however, prevention may not be the major concern. For example, various nations dealing with high rates of infant mortality may concentrate efforts on maternal and child health, nutrition, or immunization. Countries faced with the increased threat from malaria may concentrate their efforts on drug and antibiotic development to limit the spread of malaria parasites throughout the population. Nations dealing with acquired immune deficiency syndrome (AIDS) and other sexually transmitted diseases (STDs) may wish to stress education as a means of controlling the spread of infection. Ultimately, the highest health care priority is a function of local factors, and bound to vary from area to area. Regarding decisions about prioritizing, though, one statement is universal: Highest priorities must be established.

With the preceding illustrations in mind, it is easy to make the mistake of recommending health care priorities that would apply only to certain areas. Rather than address matters that are of relevance to a specific national priority, recommendations must be made that are universal and can be applied across national boundaries, however difficult that might be.

Policy

To help ensure universality, the policies of the medical education establishments should parallel the policies of health care delivery, with both factions moving toward achieving the national priority. Similarly, medical education and health care delivery should establish a close, coordinated relationship. In this way, a cogent transition from student to practitioner can be made by health care providers, which in the long run may conserve resources that might otherwise have been diverted into changing basic classroom knowledge into applied clinical knowledge. In an analogous manner, transitions between differing levels of medical education, for example undergraduate to graduate or graduate onward, might be examined and smoothed in order similarly to conserve resources. In compliance with WHO's recommendation that many diverse sectors be included in the primary health care approach, new departments specializing in areas such as social and community medicine should become common in institutions of medical education.

Curriculum

In addition, the curriculum content of medical schools also should focus on national priorities. Failing to acknowledge this principle almost certainly will result in disaster. If a country were to educate physicians without regard for the pressing national health problems, it is likely that entire graduating classes of doctors would be inadequately prepared to confront the nation's ailments. Consider, for example, the generic case of a developing, undernourished society ravaged by infectious diseases and unsanitary conditions. Now, suppose this nation chose to import its medical education from the United States or some other developed world country. Rather than addressing the largest endemic problems (malnutrition and sanitation), the medical establishments would be training physicians most adept at dealing with high-cost acute-care cases. Furthermore, lack of health promotion and disease prevention in the medical school curricula of industrialized nations casts doubt on whether current medical education in the developed world actually is addressing its own needs. Clearly, importing medical education at this point is a lost cause: A nation's system of medical education must be built from the ground up.

Another important point is made in the preceding discussion. Many would make the mistake of equating improvement of medical establishments in developing countries with the Westernization of medicine. Those who would support extending the Western model into the developing world fail to account for the many differences existing from country to country and region to region. National priority must be the major consideration with regard to the establishment of medical education and health care delivery. The availability of resources such as appropriate technology and finance programs is another such consideration.

It was the suggestion of the World Summit on Medical Education in Edinburgh, Scotland (1993) that curricular changes involving increased attention to ethics, social diseases, AIDS, and chronic diseases might contribute to the accomplishment of the goals of Health for All. The goal of such changes in developing countries is almost certainly to strike preemptively at problems that have evolved as a result of medical establishments in the developed world. For instance, the problem of stigmatizing sexually transmitted diseases such as syphilis, gonorrhea, and AIDS is not likely to be as pressing in underdeveloped countries as it is in Western societies. However, if the medical establishments, including medical schools, are given the chance to grow in the same direction as Western establishments have, these issues are likely some day to be the problems posed. In this context, teaching ethics, social diseases, and diseases of the elderly will put emerging medical establishments in a better position to deal with these problems than their Western predecessors. In a matter of speaking, they will have learned from the experienced.

Community Responsibility

In a larger sense, physicians must be taught responsibility to the community. This may be more difficult in some regions than in others. For instance, for centuries in the now industrialized countries (particularly the United States), physicians were taught that their primary responsibility was to the patient. In addition, physicians now have to place the health of the communities they serve at the same level they would place their individual patients. The global phenomenon in the developing world, however, seems to be the privatization of health care previously financed by the government. The reliance on market exchange to dictate the organization, financing, and delivery of health care and services has led to the increased reliance on private clinical practices as the sole means of health care delivery. This flies in the face of any notion that physicians should place the health of the community on a par with their individual paying patients.

If medical education does not provide the basis for community responsibility, physicians are not likely to develop it at all. Consider China's experience, which holds several lessons for other developing nations (Hsiao, 1995). Chinese macro-health policy shifted its health care financing and delivery toward a free market system. It encouraged all levels of health facilities to rely on user fees to support their operations. The Chinese government continued to operate hospitals and administer prices, however, and the implemented financing, pricing, and organizational policies were left uncoordinated. Irrational prices distorted medical practices, which resulted in the overuse of drugs and high-technology tests. Market-based financing created more unequal access to health care between the rich and poor. Public control of hospitals and poor management caused inefficiency, waste, and poor quality of care. Physicians no longer considered the communities they served. Their only obligation became their individual patients.

This example helps to illustrate the importance of instituting specific national priorities for health care delivery in the developing world, not relying on factors such as the free market to establish such priorities. Furthermore, China's experience shows how laissez-faire policy reinforces the division between physician and community, something that could effect disastrous results in the developing world.

Prevention

In considering reformation of medical school curricula, it is universally important to teach aspects of health promotion and disease prevention. As developed countries are discovering, the most effective and efficient way to treat disease is to prevent it from occurring in the first place. Developing countries should not make the same mistake of undergoing the acute care route, only to find decades later that their health establishments not only are failing to address the dominant problems, but are doing so at exorbitant costs. Making cognitive curricular changes to include health promotion and disease prevention (e.g., emphasizing classes in epidemiology, statistics, decision analysis, and clinical evaluative sciences), however, is just the beginning.

Continuing Medical Education

The length of medical education in many developing countries might be considered inadequate. The typical path to becoming a physician has been characterized as follows: four to five years of undergraduate medical education followed by one year of clinical experience resulting in receipt of the medical degree. The decision to continue into postgraduate residency is, at this point, completely voluntary, and the alternative is to go into the practice of general medicine (Alma-Ata, 1978). Continuing medical education is critical to the widespread application of new discoveries as an effective method of keeping the physician informed about the latest developments in medicine. At this point, continuing medical education may hold special significance. In an age wherein medical discoveries are out pacing the ability to implement proper interventions, keeping physicians informed and up to date is an arduous task. This applies across the boundary between developed and developing nations, although the former may use considerably more advanced and prolonged programs in continuing education. Developing nations must, however, institute more advanced programs in medicine, establish tighter regulation of practice and licensure (to encourage higher levels of professional competency in practice), and develop continuing education programs. Of course, it is recommended that such developments take place at the local level to account for diverse situations, and that national priority be used as a guide in establishing such programs.

Education Methodology

In addition to changing what is taught, consideration must also be given to changing how it is taught. New innovations in learning have been made recently, including new ways of integrating the basic sciences and clinical sciences with practice. Currently, one of the most dramatic developments is the effort to shift the paradigm from passive to active learning. Problem-based learning (PBL) is perhaps the best example of the new active learning. A shift from lectures to students working independently or in small groups is tied to the institution of PBL, and the goals such programs provide include an overall contextual framework for learning, enhancement of student recall ability, and the continued development of the thinking process.

Why then should developing countries herald PBL as an answer to the problems overwhelming their medical systems? For one reason, in a developing nation where medical education resources are precious and must be conserved, any means of conserving energy in the process of training a physician is greatly needed. One of the advantages of PBL, undoubtedly, is its ability to ease the transition from student to practitioner, a task that requires an inordinate amount of training, and one that needs to be addressed in both the developing and developed nations. Second, active learning provides a solution to one of the newer problems in medical education: The exponential increases in medical knowledge. To make optimal use of the latest medical information, let alone avoid being buried in the vast sea of new observations and discoveries, students are prepared by problem-based learning to extract the information relevant to a case. The learning habits called on repeatedly throughout a physician's career are acquired long before graduation from medical school. At the current rate, physicians with these organizational tools will inevitably become valued public servants throughout both the developed and developing world.

In considering changes to the learning process, medical education must become more horizontal. Health care is an interdisciplinary field, more so now than ever. In preparing physicians for the complicated environment surrounding medical practice, joint learning and collaborations with nonhealth personnel might be considered a wise decision. Improving communications across the many fields also is necessary because nearly any foray into research will prove that no discipline is an island.

Standards

Similarly, accreditation, licensure, and cross-licensing needs to become more horizontal as well. Every country has some mechanism for identifying approved medical schools. However, uniform international standards are nonexistent. In addition, medical practitioners licensed in one country rarely have extended practice privileges in another. Persons trained or licensed in one country are usually required to undergo additional training and examination to obtain licensure in another. Some countries, such as Egypt, do not allow foreign medical graduates to practice within their borders (Garg & Seefeldt, 1998).

Admissions

Admissions policies are yet another area of medical education requiring reexamination, according to the primary health care approach of Health for All. Two questions need to be answered: What are the qualities in a candidate that will best accomplish the goals of Health For All, and which qualities will make for the best physician?

Working toward the goal of raising the health status of all people to a level at which they may be socially and economically productive requires a local approach. As such, it seems logical that a good candidate might have a predisposition for practicing in a certain area. Such predispositions are likely to arise from growing up or living in such an area. Thus, it has been recommended that native candidates be given special consideration for admission. However, the idea that physicians will practice medicine in their home region is offset by a trend in continuing medical education. Unable to obtain adequate continuing education in a developing nation, international medical graduates may seek training abroad in a developed nation, and then either fail to return or return with training that does not optimally serve local needs.

Two conferences in medical education, one in Edinburgh in 1988 and one in Crete in 1990, have agreed that selection of candidates should transcend simply evaluating their intellectual abilities. Although rooted firmly in the scientific tradition, medicine has become as much a social science endeavor as a purely scientific endeavor. As a result, candidates who are intellectually superior yet lack creativity or compassion may not best serve the health needs of their nation as a physician. Almost certainly, the qualities in a candidate best suited for medicine are bound to vary by local needs and culture. Therefore, making generalizations about which qualities are predictors of successful physicians would be nothing more than a waste of time. However, both developed and developing countries should be encouraged to forgo strict adherence to the admissions models presented by other nations, and to be creative in developing new criteria for evaluating candidates in a way that best suits their unique situation.

CONCLUSION

Clearly, this chapter just begins to scratch the surface of the issues that currently confront medical education and health care delivery in the developing world. Hopefully, though, the reader will glean some ideas about the complexity of the situation and the intertwining of the social, economic, political, and religious forces that influence the health care of an individual in any part of the world. Diversity cannot be examined on a single level: The differences across individual nations are far too large for this approach to be feasible. Therefore, nations must examine their own unique situations and prioritize accordingly, all the while bearing in mind the experiences of other countries, both developed and developing. Only in this way can a bright future for the health of a developing nation be ensured. This chapter also presents some alternatives that should be pondered by those in the business of educating those who deliver health care. If these notions or other rational alternatives are not implemented during the next century, then the goals of the Alma-Ata Conference will never be realized.

REFERENCES

Alma-Ata 1978: Primary health care. (1978). Geneva: World Health Organization.

Boelen, C. (1994, June). First Global Conference: International Collaboration on Medical Education and Practice, Rockford, Illinois. *WHO Daily News.*

Changes and Reform at WHO. (1997). Geneva: World Health Organization.

Elmeligy, M. R. (1996). Cost effectiveness of radiology: Economic and diagnostic considerations in developing countries. *Academic Radiology, 3,* S125.

Formulating strategies for Health For All by the year 2000. (1979). Geneva: World Health Organization.

Garcia-Barbero, M. (1995). Medical education in the light of the world health organization health for all strategy and the European Union. *Medical Education, 29*, 3-12.

Garg, M. L., & Seefeldt, M. (1998). A new focus for medical education in the 21st century: Chaotic pathways after graduation in developing countries. *University of Illinois at Chicago Department of Medical Education Bulletin, 4*, 1-3.

Greenlick, M. R. (1995). Educating physicians for the twenty-first century. *Academic Medicine, 70*, 179-185.

Hsiao, W. (1995). The Chinese health care system: Lessons for other nations. *Social Science Medicine, 41*, 1047-1055.

Integration of medical education and the health care system. (1996). Editorial. *Medical Education, 30*, 1-2.

Kickbusch, I. (1997). *Creating a global web for health: Challenges for WHO and its collaborating centres.* Presented at 1st Meeting of U.S. Collaborating Centres, Washington, DC., June 12-14.

Marandi, A. (1995). Integrating medical education and health services: The Iranian experience. *Medical Education, 30*, 4-8.

Magzoub, M. E. (1995). The challenges of innovation in medical education and practice: The experience in Gezira, Sudan. *Changing Medical Education and Practice, 8*, 1,3-4.

Stamler, J. (1987). Epidemiology, established risk factors, and the primary prevention of coronary heart disease. In W. W. Parmley, & K. Chatterjee (Eds.), *Cardiology*, (p. 1). Lippincott, Philadelphia: J. B.

Turnock, B. J. (1997). What is public health? In *Public Health* (Ch. 1). Gaithersburg, MD: Aspen.

United Nations Development Program. (1991). *Human Development Report.* New York: Author.

United Nations Development Program. (1994). *Human Development Report.* New York: Author.

PART II

THE ART AND SCIENCE OF MEDICAL EDUCATION

CHAPTER FIVE

Models of Learning: Implications for Teaching Students and Residents

Glenn Regehr
Krishan Rajaratanam
University of Toronto Faculty of Medicine

The training of medical students and residents is arguably one of the most important and rewarding roles of the academic physician. Many faculty members fill this teaching role very effectively. Yet, as with any skill, reflection on the process of teaching is important if teachers are to be as effective as possible. For example, whether explicitly or implicitly, each teacher develops his or her own theory of the learning process. Understanding and reflecting on this theory can be helpful to one's success as a teacher. One's model of learning substantially influences both one's views regarding the role of a teacher and one's definition of successful teaching. It is only when the model is explicit that one can examine it for its strengths and weaknesses and use it strategically for the purposes of teaching.

To this end, three theories of learning are briefly presented in this discussion. For each model is described the theory of learning, its implications for how one might view the role of the teacher, and its implications for the definition of teaching success. None of these models is necessarily correct or incorrect. The point is *not* to indicate the correct way to view the process of learning, but to provide a series of explicit examples against which each individual can compare his or her own theory of learning, and to provide some alternative ways of viewing the learning process that might not have been considered previously.

BEHAVIORISM

Behaviorist theory (or operant learning theory) describes the learner as a relatively passive recorder of events in the world. This model suggests that the human learning hardware does not have much built into it, merely the capacity to notice events and record connections between these events. Beyond such basic capacities, the learner is a clean slate on which experience writes. As a result, the behaviorists would argue that the rules of learning that determine all human behavior are very simple. In short, learning is a process whereby actions or behaviors are performed and the consequences noted. If the consequences are desirable to the individual, the behavior is more likely to be repeated. If the consequences are undesirable, then the behavior is less likely to be repeated. Thus, all behavior is dictated by the anticipated rewards or punishments that result from the behavior, and learning of appropriate behaviors is increased by rewarding correct responses and/or punishing incorrect responses.

Behaviorism is so named because of its focus on behavior. The behaviorists chose to ignore notions of consciousness or understanding, claiming that these concepts had no direct evidence or explanatory power in describing human learning. Thus, for the behaviorist, true learning is being able to provide the appropriate response to a given stimulus. Behavior is not the evidence of what is learned. Rather, behavior is what is learned. In short, the point of teaching is to ensure that the student can flawlessly repeat the information or actions being taught under the appropriate circumstances.

Several laws of learning were generated out of this paradigm, and even if one does not subscribe to the basic tenets of the theory, these "laws" of learning are worth keeping in mind. For example, research in the tradition of behaviorism demonstrated that rewarding appropriate behavior is a more effective training strategy than punishing inappropriate behavior. Furthermore, evidence suggests that feedback regarding behavior is more effective if it is delivered close to the time of the behavior itself, and if the reason for the reinforcement is explicit and unambiguous.

At the same time, however, behaviorists noted that learning is somewhat slower but substantially more enduring if the reward for a particular behavior is intermittent. In other words, immediate, powerful reward after every appropriate behavior will lead to rapid learning, but behavior learned in this way will require continued immediate, powerful reward if it is to be maintained. Therefore, the effective teacher will use reinforcement strategically, determining the particular level and frequency of reward that maximizes and maintains performance for each individual learner.

COGNITIVE LEARNING THEORY

In contrast to the behaviorist model of learning, cognitive learning theory views learners as active constructors of knowledge. That is, the learner is constantly trying to understand the world and incorporate new information into his or her current worldview. Motivation for learning comes not so much from the desire to obtain rewards or avoid punishment as from desire to expand one's understanding and to become more competent. Such a model of learning places a very high importance on the meaning and relevance of the knowledge and skills the learner is to be taught. New knowledge or skills will be properly learned only if they are fitted sensibly into the learner's existing framework of knowledge, and new knowledge will be sought and properly integrated only if the relevance of this new knowledge is obvious to the learner. If the information provided is not effectively tied into the learner's existing knowledge structures, then it is far less likely to be remembered, and even if it is remembered it, will be isolated and therefore inert and unusable.

For the cognitive learning theorist, true learning is not merely the capacity for rote responding when cued. Rather, true learning involves gaining an understanding of the information and its implications. Although evidence of learning clearly must be obtained by observing appropriate behaviors, the behavior itself is not sufficient. Behavior without understanding is not a success, as the behaviorists might claim, but a clear failure of learning and potentially dangerous. Thus, for example, the capacity to recite a set of facts is not helpful if those facts cannot be put to use, and they cannot be put to use unless the knowledge of those facts is situated in a larger framework of understanding.

Cognitive learning theory leads to learner-centered models of teaching, in which the teacher is a facilitator of learning, not the source of all knowledge. Learning is a highly individualistic process. New knowledge must be incorporated into existing knowledge, yet each individual's existing knowledge base is bound to be different. In addition, new knowledge must be seen as relevant by the learner, yet each individual's motivation for learning is bound to be slightly different. The teacher therefore cannot structure the information beforehand and present it formulaically with the expectation that it will be understood and learned in a meaningful, and therefore useful, way. If the teacher is to present information, it must be adapted to the individual to ensure that the information is timely, relevant, and meaningful.

Yet it may not even be appropriate for the teacher to provide information in the classic sense. In fact, learning is likely to be better if the learner seeks the knowledge and discovers information for him- or herself. Therefore, the effective teacher does not merely transmit information. Rather, the effective teacher creates situations in which the learner sees a need for the information and is motivated to seek it. The job of the teacher is to ensure that the information is elaborated and understood in the relevant context. In short, the point of teaching is to ensure that the student develops his or her own useful understanding of the information. A critical aspect in this development is enabling and encouraging the learner to take the time to reflect on current knowledge and to elaborate this knowledge in the context of practice, drawing connections between the current situation and previous situations, noting similarities and differences between experiences, and in doing so, developing a rich understanding of the domain while recognizing where further knowledge and understanding are still required.

SOCIAL LEARNING THEORY

Like cognitive theories of learning, social learning theory describes humans as dynamic, information-processing, problem-solving organisms who actively seek to understand their world. In addition, however, social learning theory sees the human learner as a social creature, emphasizing the fact that almost all learning takes place in a social setting. With this emphasis comes the recognition that learning need not always be the result of direct personal experience. Instead, the individual can, and often will, learn vicariously through observing the performance of others. The learner will observe another's behavior, draw inferences regarding the motivation for the other's actions, and note the consequences of those actions for the individual. Furthermore, what is learned from such observation is not merely the relation between behavior and consequences. The learner also will draw inferences about the actor's attitudes, beliefs, motivations, and standards of behavior. These inferences, too, are important aspects of what is learned.

Several factors determine what the learner will do with this information. On the basis of the learner's beliefs about the similarity between him- or herself and the individual being observed, the learner will draw inferences about how the behavior and its consequences might apply to him or her. Furthermore, to the extent that the learner likes, respects, and views the other individual as competent, the learner will attempt to model him- or herself after the individual and incorporate the behaviors, attitudes, beliefs, motivations, and standards of behavior that were observed and inferred.

Viewed from the social learning theory model, the learner is no longer just a repository of information and skills that will be evoked when the proper stimulus occurs. Nor is the learner merely an information-processing module seeking to develop and integrate knowledge and skills through interaction with the world. Similarly, the teacher is not merely a dispenser of information or a manipulator of circumstance to maximize learning. Here the student and teacher are viewed from an interactive, humanist perspective. The student is a protégé of the teacher, and the teacher is a mentor for the student. In successful learning and teaching, the student adopts the appropriate values, attitudes, knowledge, skills, and standards from the teacher. The definition of success for the teacher must include the development of an individual with whom the teacher is proud to be associated in all aspects.

As a consequence, the responsibility of the teacher becomes far more comprehensive. It is not just a matter of reinforcing the repetition of an appropriate response. Nor is it merely a matter of orchestrating circumstances to ensure that the student seeks out and obtains the appropriate knowledge in a meaningful manner. Instead, effective teaching involves providing an appropriate role model for the student to follow. To use an old saying, a teacher must recognize that actions speak louder than words. The manner in which the teacher treats colleagues, support staff, patients and the students themselves, the manner in which the teacher approaches difficulties in his or her own practice and tries to learn from experiences, the manner in which the teacher accepts challenge and promotes open discussion of issues, all these behaviors and their implied attitudes will have a profound impact on the learner as an individual and as a professional. As Tosteson (1979) eloquently stated: "We must acknowledge that the most important, indeed, the only thing we have to offer our students is ourselves. Everything else they can read in a book." (p. 693)

SUMMARY

In the preceding sections, three models of learning and their implications for teaching were provided. It is important to note that although these models are contrasted here, they are not necessarily contradictory or mutually exclusive. It is the authors' belief that each has something to contribute to an understanding of learning and teaching processes. The good teacher is not necessarily one who selects the "right" model and uses it consistently. Rather, the good teacher is one who views any model of learning as a useful metaphor that is appropriate for some circumstances and inappropriate for others. Similarly, one need not accept or reject a model of learning as a whole and thus accept or reject the implications for teaching represented in the model as correct or incorrect. Again, the lessons for teaching generated from each model all are likely to be useful in certain circumstances and inappropriate in others. Each of the implications discussed should be considered as one more tool in the teacher's repertoire of educational strategies. The point of this chapter is to highlight the theory behind these various tools and some of the implications for using them. It is hoped that the teacher will use these tools strategically, purposefully, and effectively to the maximum benefit for the individual learner.

As we approach the 21st century, the authors have every reason to believe that the strategic use of teaching tools such as those described in this discussion will become more rather than less important. A variety of forces are pressuring for more efficient and economical use of learning time for trainees. At the same time, a variety of technologies such as computer-based learning and virtual reality-based simulators are promising delivery of this efficiency and economy. With increasing demands on the clinician's time and increasing competition for the trainee's attention, the interactions between teachers and learners will become more and more precious. Hopefully, through the careful development and use of teaching strategies, the clinician educator can ensure that these interactions also will be valuable.

REFERENCES

Tosteson, D. C., (1979). Learning in medicine. *New England Journal of Medicine. 301*: 690-694.

CHAPTER SIX

Applying Instructional Principles to the Design of Curriculum

Debra A. DaRosa
Anna Derossis
Northwestern University Medical School

The Curriculum Committee at Whatsamatta University Medical School has been charged by the dean to plan and integrate a new primary care longitudinal experience into the curriculum. Your role and mission, should you choose to accept it, is to chair the committee and produce a draft proposal for the dean's approval before its implementation in next year's curriculum.

The purpose of this chapter is to outline basic phases of curriculum development, applying both change theory and instructional principles requisite to a sound and balanced clinical and basic science curriculum. The preceding scenario is used to demonstrate how these principles might be applied to an actual situation. Although the developmental procedures outlined in different curriculum planning models can vary, the steps outlined in the following discussion are typical of those in most curriculum development efforts. The process for developing curriculum may appear to be fairly logical and sequential. In reality, however, curriculum designers do not progress through the process in a linear mode, but rather work on several steps simultaneously with intermingling decisions, details, and deadlines.

SIX PRELIMINARY CONSIDERATIONS TO CURRICULUM DEVELOPMENT PLANNING

At the start of any new curriculum initiative it is critical to take the following six steps:

1. Establish a carefully thought out organizational plan that ensures an efficient use of faculty time and a collaborative working environment. Because faculty time is expensive, each curriculum meeting should include a formal agenda with highlighted action items so responsibilities are clear. Minutes should be distributed beforehand and a notebook containing all meeting minutes should be available for reference at the meeting. A supportive organizational culture is crucial so those involved feel a sense of confidence in the leader's process and progress. Members need to view themselves as a team and function accordingly. This is imperative to quash boundaries and traditional "turf wars" that often create circular and nonproductive arguments. The common aim must be emphasized to reinforce collaboration among disciplines, to encourage positivism and enthusiasm, and to maintain a forward momentum.

2. Anticipate criticisms and resistance to any changes in the curriculum. Faculty members who argue from a philosophical or logical standpoint will pose the type of challenges that can enhance the possibilities of successful development and implementation. Those who argue with reactionary "shooting from the hip" arguments will frustrate and stagnate the process, if allowed.

3. Negotiate with the dean for support of professional (educator-type) and clerical personnel. Expect that any curriculum development effort will not be done well without sufficient time and support. If no support is made available, expect the process to take longer, require even more time of the committee and chair, and pose risks of momentum loss and inattention to significant details.

4. Explore the availability of resources needed for new curriculum initiatives from the individuals empowered to delegate dollars, curriculum time, educational space, and the like. It is of paramount importance to be aware of one's resources when developing a curriculum. It may be necessary to plan curriculum changes to occur in stages should resources not be available at the time designated for the new curriculum to start. For example, if planning for a new primary care longitudinal experience to occur throughout a four-year curriculum, learning in advance that insufficient general medicine ambulatory facilities exist may prompt recruitment of pediatricians or other generalists. The curriculum would likely look quite different for a multidisciplinary primary care program than for a pure general medicine ambulatory experience. Building a curriculum without knowing what

resources exist would be like planning to build a house without knowing how much money or land is available.

5. Follow a "change management plan" to navigate through the pitfalls surrounding the human elements of change. The literature abounds with descriptions of new courses or curriculum initiatives that were the innovative brainstorms of an individual or groups, but lacked sufficient endorsement and involvement of others to continue once the initiators moved on to other places or projects. Change theory provides a basis for planning curriculum additions or modifications that more likely will result in permanent, yet dynamic changes. For example, Galpin (1996) offers a model of the change management process that defines nine stages for creating and implementing "grassroots" change. The stages are the following: (a) establish the need/rationale to change, (b) develop and disseminate a vision of change, (c) diagnose/analyze the current situation, (d) generate general recommendations, (e) detail the recommendations, (f) pilot test recommendations, (g) prepare recommendations for rollout, and (h) measure, reinforce, and refine changes. The last is a critical and often neglected stage in curriculum change. One change management process model is not advocated over another, but it is strongly recommended that one be selected for use.

6. Use learning theory and adult learning principles. Another important first step is to decide the set of learning theories on which the curriculum will be based. Although there exists numerous theories on how humans best learn, most can be categorized into three classifications: behaviorism, cognitivism, and humanism. Each set of theories is premised on underlying assumptions of what best facilitates learning. In general, behaviorism assumes that learning is optimally accomplished with specific learning objectives developed by the faculty, opportunities to learn at one's own pace, intermittent feedback to learners before progressing on to the next sequential block of instruction, no competition among learners, and criterion-referenced evaluation systems. In contrast, cognitivism, encourages competition, because it tends to rank learners according to scores or other performance measurements. It makes use of learning objectives that articulate "roads to travel" rather than terminal behaviors, and prefers a norm-referenced evaluation system. Humanistically oriented curricula arrange for faculty and learners to negotiate individually tailored learning objectives, often makes use of self-directed learning strategies and small-group instruction, and prefers a self-referenced type of evaluation system.

Although few curriculum foundations are completely purist in application, their instructional design tends to favor one educational orientation over another. The key is that the features of the curriculum and their theoretical underpinnings should be known by the faculty and learners and consistent with the institution's educational and management philosophy. As cautioned by Knowles (1990), if you are not clear about the theoretical basis for your curriculum, the chances are the curriculum will end up a hodgepodge. He cautions:

> You will use different theories in different times or situations, or conflicting theories for different decisions in the same situation. You won't know why you are doing what you are doing. There is a cliché in the applied social sciences--often attributed to Kurt Lewin--that nothing is as practical as a good theory to enable you to make choices confidently and consistently, and to explain or defend why you are making the choices you make. (p. 110)

In other words, establishing a clear theoretical foundation that articulates the main features of your curriculum will provide a blueprint for planning, future decision making about the curriculum, and evaluation of the curriculum under design. Deviations from the chosen foundation are certainly acceptable, but should be purposeful rather than based on convenience or instructor bias.

STEPS IN THE CURRICULUM DEVELOPMENT PROCESS

Assess Needs

One of the first steps of the Whatsamatta University Medical School's Curriculum Committee is to identify what medical students need to know about primary care that is not addressed or fully addressed already in the existing curriculum. This step verifies the existence of learning needs and prioritizes them. A needs assessment can be accomplished a number of ways. Examples include examining the literature, consulting with medical schools with similar missions who already have implemented comparable programs/curriculum, reviewing the Association of American Medical College's (AAMC's) Medical School Objectives Project (MSOP), or reading results of published surveys that examine learning needs relevant to primary care.

Other options include expert consensus achieved through surveys, guided interviews, or faculty retreats. The results of the needs assessment provide a blueprint or "map" for planning the content of the curriculum. As stated by Dunnington, (1998, p. 26) "Foregoing needs assessment in curriculum planning is like writing a prescription before completing the history and physical examination." In another context, a curriculum designer is somewhat like a new house contractor. Before building the house, the contractor needs to learn from the future tenants how many will be living in the home, their hobbies, whether or not there are special needs, and so forth. The house then can be planned according to the needs of the owners. Likewise, a curriculum needs to be premised on learners' needs.

Although there are times when a needs assessment is unnecessary, (e.g., when curriculum content is required for accreditation), most new curriculum initiatives benefit from this step being completed. A needs assessment does not guarantee a successful educational program, but the curriculum will more likely be on target, less biased by individual instructors' biases about what should be learned, and justified in terms of time needed in the curriculum. Results of the needs assessment should be documented and presented to the curriculum committee to ensure that the findings are actually used. The proposed scenario, would involve consulting with medical schools that already have longitudinal primary care experiences, inquiring as to why they developed one, how it works, and what its strengths and weaknesses are in its current format. It also would involve exploring through a retreat or survey with the faculty in primary care specialties what clinical skills and patient problems already are adequately addressed and which they advocate including in the new curriculum.

A second consideration in completing a needs assessment is determining the incoming skills and knowledge of the learners so the curriculum can be targeted to the appropriate learning level. Written assumptions of what the students should know and be able to do before starting the curriculum should be clarified.

Develop and Document Curriculum Goals and Objectives

On the basis of the needs assessment results, objectives should be developed. The level of specificity (i.e., terminal performance objectives or general learning expectations) will depend on the theoretical premise of the curriculum, but all learners and faculty members should have in writing what participants will be able to do by the end of the curriculum experience. Some faculty feel terminal performance objectives, such as those advocated by Mager (1997), work fine for simple skills. However, more complex skills and knowledge are articulated better in whatever format is most meaningful to the faculty and students: content acquisition, terminal behaviors, or directions of growth. Flexibility is the key, so participants, whenever possible, can incorporate their own learning agendas given that students' past knowledge and experiences, motivation levels, and readiness to learn may differ.

Develop Performance and Program Evaluation Plans

Systems should be designed that will provide information for judging the quality of the curriculum, the faculty involved in teaching, and student performance. The evaluation approaches should be specified, as should how the data will be collected, who will collect it, when and how it will be summarized, who will receive the summarized reports, and how judgments will be made about the success and shortcomings of the curriculum/learner. All curriculum stakeholders should approve the evaluation system. Accountability for the quality of the curriculum will be realized only with sound performance and program evaluation systems.

Identify Learning Activities and Teaching Methods

This step involves outlining how the objectives will be accomplished. For the longitudinal primary care program referenced earlier, most of the learning activities may occur in light of patient care experiences. According to the literature, however, independent learning modules, electronically posted case problems, practice chart review exercises, and other types of methods or materials could be developed to supplement the experience depending on the learning objectives (DaRosa, Dunnington, Stearns, Ferenchick, Bowen, et al. 1997; Ferenchick, Simpson, Blackman, DaRosa, & Dunnington, 1997).

Relevant literature should be provided to the curriculum committee members involved in determining teaching and learning methods for the curriculum being planned. The key is to choose feasible instructional techniques that match the focus of the proposed learning outcomes and that your institution is capable of supporting.

Coordinate Schedules, Faculty, Staff Needs, and Facilities

For example, the longitudinal primary care curriculum would require staff for attending to details associated with orienting students, patients, office/clinic staff and faculty; sending necessary correspondence; responding to inevitable clinic/office schedule changes; and managing documents for curriculum, faculty, and student performance evaluation systems. Who has the locus of control over these functions must be clarified in advance. Traditionally, these responsibilities fell to individual departments, but new centralized curriculum efforts require negotiation and clarification concerning who will take responsibility for interdepartmental communications and coordination.

Identify Enhancers and Barriers to the Transfer of Learning

Transfer of learning is the effective application of what is learned from participating in a curriculum. Learning is an additive process. Before implementation, the curriculum committee needs to examine the variables that will support or impede the planned curriculum. Examples of variables in the proposed scenario that could impede or enhance the curriculum's ability to result in a positive learning transfer might include the following:

- *Faculty*: Do the faculty at the various teaching sites possess the necessary knowledge and teaching/mentoring skills? Do they have the time and motivation to integrate learners properly in their ambulatory care settings? Do they view the program as important? Have they been oriented to the curriculum so they know what should be taught/learned, how to evaluate learners, and so forth?

- *Students*: Will students be given time to attend their assigned longitudinal primary care offices? Once they reach their third-year, will they be discouraged by faculty and residents from attending because of conflicting service demands? Will they have the opportunity to practice the skills they are learning? Do they view the curriculum positively or negatively? Do operational problems exist such as transportation, geographic proximity to the medical school, language barriers, and the like?

- *Curriculum design and execution*: Do the actual instructional methods and learning activities reflect those intended? Does the curriculum include application exercises as a major part of the instructional activities? Is transfer of learning strategies well executed or unrealistic? Is there a balance between teacher and learner-centered learning activities?

- *Curriculum content*: Are the knowledge and skills expected to be learned realistic in terms of level, volume, and scope? Are they relevant and practical? Do they build on previous knowledge and experience?

- *Opportunities required to apply learning*: Is enough time allotted to accomplish curriculum expectations? Does the curriculum take place in an environment conducive to learning? Is the curriculum too disruptive to competing responsibilities such that it will not be given adequate attention and focus? Are information type resources available at the various sites? Are learners, regardless of site, receiving adequate feedback? Is there sufficient opportunity for learners to process (i.e., engage in organized reflection), conceptualize, and apply what they are learning?

- *Organizational context*: Is a reward system needed to recognize those site preceptors doing an exceptional job, and does a system exist to assist or drop ineffective site mentors? Is there support from key leaders in the school, faculty, students, and where appropriate, the community? Is there an ongoing communication channel to ensure that participants have input and are informed of accomplishments, program changes, and/or problems? Are sufficient financial and other types of resources available?

- *Environmental forces*: Are there people openly hostile to the new curriculum? Does a receptive "political" climate exist? Are space and time conditions reasonable for those involved? Is there support and appropriate involvement from the various primary care faculty members?

This list is not exhaustive but reflects types of barriers that can detract the best laid curricular plans. Some barriers can be anticipated and addressed before curriculum implementation, whereas others can be identified only after implementation. Although the barriers are not all resolvable, being able to address those that can be addressed is important. According to Cafferella (1994), these seven key factors, depending on how they play out in the transfer of learning process, can be barriers or enhancers to the success of the curriculum.

Communicating the Value of the Curriculum

A report should be generated at least annually that communicates to stakeholders how the curriculum fared and any future modifications being planned. This can be done via a poster or media presentation, written report, or simply a letter from either the dean or individuals directing the curriculum. Follow-up should be planned to clarify any questions or concerns about the curriculum. This step is part of the reinforcement stage described by Galpin (1996) and reflects the dynamic, nonstatic nature of a formal curriculum. It also reaffirms the curriculum principles and serves to refine changes to ensure the curriculum's effectiveness.

SUMMARY AND PREDICTIONS

It has been said that chairing any committee is akin to taking a dozen dogs for a walk together. Leading a curriculum committee charged with developing or modifying a curriculum is an adventure, but with fewer pools of troubled waters when a methodic approach is taken and sufficient numbers of faculty and students are involved. The resulting curriculum "product" is never finished, because curriculum should be an ongoing development, freshened regularly. Ensuring a high-quality curriculum is a critical responsibility of the faculty, who should possess a keen sense of pride and ownership of what is taught, how, and when.

Changes in how physicians practice medicine and its growing complexity will have an impact on how the curriculum of tomorrow is progressively developed and managed. It is important that the changes do not take the approach of some curriculum reform efforts of the past in other areas of higher education, which have been conceived on the Tinkertoy model. The Tinkertoy curriculum model occurs when the key elements of the curriculum remain the same, the only change being the arrangement of these elements. It is akin simply to taking different routes to the same end.

Looking ahead, changes in curriculum will likely involve modifications of what is included in the curriculum, the forces that influence curriculum content, the way it is taught/learned, the way it is managed and evaluated, and the environment in which the curriculum is implemented.

The content or the knowledge and skills prioritized in the curriculum likely will move from a departmentally developed and controlled curriculum to more centralized development efforts. The territoriality or "turf" battles over blocks of time, number of lectures, and content priority fought by departments unfortunately are still prevalent at curriculum committees around the world, which explains why curriculum continues to be fractionated. Departmentally based curriculum will yield to interdisciplinary teaching, creating an integrated program. The authors have long thought that medical schools should contain caution statements that read: "Caution: Department organizational structure could prove harmful to your education." For example, some departments of surgery include general surgery and three or four additional surgical disciplines, with the remaining disciplines having separate department status. Typically, clerkships then are designed to include only those disciplines in the main surgery department, although it is shown that other surgical specialties are critical to the general professional education of medical students.

A centralized curriculum approach, however, will require that thought be given to ensure that lost ownership by the department does not negatively influence the individual faculty member's motivation or vested interests in participating in the curriculum. It may be that schools need to have one departmental configuration for business purposes and another to meet the needs of the academic mission.

Curriculum content also will be better aligned with population health needs. This will make medical schools more in keeping with their social contract. Although not all medical schools are positioned to meet all the learning needs for future physicians, each should develop its curriculum premised on its mission. This might well help to balance training of varying types of physicians (e.g., research oriented, rural practitioners).

As noted in previous reports, doctors must promote health, prevent and treat diseases, and rehabilitate the disabled in a compassionate, ethical way (Gastel & Rogers, 1989; Walton, 1994). But society also expects that doctors be better providers of primary care; communicators; information specialists; practitioners of applied economics, sociology, epidemiology, and behavior medicine; health team managers; and advocates of communities. Core curriculum content will need to address these topics. For example, dissatisfaction of patients and the public is due more to poor communication than to any other professional deficiency. Courses will need to be designed or integrated into current courses/clerkships to accomplish this. The Association of American Medical Colleges Medical School Objectives Program (MSOP) identifies many of these "streamer" skills considered critical to future physicians regardless of future discipline.

Another area needing reconsideration is the science curriculum, the heart of any medical school curriculum. Science will need to be more purposefully streamlined throughout the curriculum and not emphasized only in the preclinical years. The need for this has already been somewhat realized given some schools are offering more basic science courses or electives in the fourth-year. But more attention needs to be paid to reinforcing the sciences throughout the curriculum.

Where the curriculum takes place will continue to undergo change. Although many schools have increased exposure to the ambulatory setting, many still rely on the inpatient setting. The hospital is well suited for some aspects of medical education, but it is increasingly a poor site for general clinical education (Gastel & Rogers, 1989). Contemporary doctors cannot be educated in university or community hospitals alone. These often concentrate on tertiary levels of care and involve patients characterized by rare diseases and expensive treatments. Instead, medical students must be taught in environments wherein most patients exist in order to bridge the gap between what they need to learn and the medical practice environment. Whereas hospital based education is undeniably important to postgraduate education, it seldom provides experiences appropriate to student level learning objectives.

An integrated curriculum will require centralized budgeting and financial support. Staff and other resources will be needed to manage the curriculum once departmental control of the curriculum is removed. Curriculum deans will need to be well informed of curriculum details because they will need to be centrally managed: collecting, maintaining, and making quickly and widely available information on what is taught, when, by whom, and how. Cross-referencing the content by discipline will be critical as well as deciding who needs access to what information. Curriculum deans also will need to set up centralized progressive performance data warehouses so student progress can be monitored systematically and contextually. Feedback loops will need to be built to inform the centralized curriculum group on the value and quality of various parts of the curriculum. These types of information management efforts are critical to maintaining the "big picture" of the curriculum and to keeping the curriculum decision makers well informed as well as the other faculty members and students.

Technology will play a major role in future curriculum planning, decision making, and operations. It has barely touched the surface of its potential, and has yet to permeate fully the ways medical schools teach and medical students learn. But we are at the edge of major changes ahead. Future curriculum committees will shift their focus from content to how students learn. This trend already has emerged to some extent, but most schools still place students in traditional passive roles as receptacles for information supplied by professors during various parts of the curriculum. Curriculum developments such as problem-based learning and evidenced-based learning rest on the foundation on what has been coined as "resource-based learning," which is the basis for student achievement of information literacy (Gastel & Rogers, 1989). For example, for students to engage in a problem-based learning tutorial session, they will need to identify what they already know, what else they need to know to solve the patient problem, how to access the information needed efficiently, and finally how to interpret and apply it. In 1970, Alvin Toffler used the phrase "information overload" in his book, *Future Shock* (Breivik, 1998). Almost 30 years later, we truly understand its meaning and the consequential need for faculty and students to possess abilities, to access, evaluate, organize, and present information from all the real-world sources existing in today's society. Learning tools such as books, journals, television, online databases, worldwide experts, government agencies, the Internet, and CD-ROMS are key resources. Moreover, time is quickly approaching when people will not have to go to the resources; the resources will come to them. Learners will have "just-in-time" information access, meaning they will be able to query information resources available when a need to know or teachable moment arises. Faculty will need to alter their approaches to curriculum planning to respond to changes in how students learn.

Education technology opens the door to more independent learning as well as collaborative learning via computers. Education can take place anywhere in the world rather than be limited to those students and faculty members on campus, giving way to possibilities for distance learning curriculum or a worldwide medical school curriculum designed to augment patient care experiences.

Education technology is valuable if used correctly (i.e., when the content is difficult to explain without pictures or video). Technology should be introduced into the curriculum with care. Currently, several computer programs simply offer a different medium of information dissemination, which could just as well have been provided in paper form at less expense. This implies that faculty will need new skills in developing curriculum to make optimal use of the new educational technology. Too often today, Web-based programs and computer-assisted learning modules are developed that serve more as eye candy than a way to meet learners' needs. Faculty will need access to technology experts as well as instructional design specialists to increase the likelihood of a more favorable outcome.

Change is constant and likely will be more dramatic in the future. Carefully planned pilot studies funded to test curriculum evolvements are needed before large-scale change occurs. Leadership in medical schools must require the same culture of excellence and evidence in education as they already do in clinical and research arenas. Within an educationally supportive culture, curriculum development can transform from a fundamentally political, mechanistic, and single-discipline operation to a creative operation of designing adventures in learning that makes use of expert teams from multiple disciplines. Medical schools continue to be challenged to create multidisciplinary courses and courses addressing skills not previously taught in medical schools. The need for a methodic and collaborative strategy, facilitated by the faculty, learners, and practitioners, and provided with sufficient resources for developing and implementing curriculum, will remain critical to the success of these efforts.

REFERENCES

Breivik, P. S. (1998). *Student learning in the information age.* Phoenix, AZ: Oryx.

Cafferella, R. S. (1994). *Planning programs for adult learners.* San Francisco: Jossey-Bass.

DaRosa, D., Dunnington, G., Stearns, J., Ferenchick, G., Bowen, J., & Simpson, D. (1997). Ambulatory teaching "Lite": Less clinic time, more educationally fulfilling. *Academic Medicine, 72*(5), 358-361.

Dunnington, G. L. (1998). *Surgeons as educators: A syllabus.* Chicago: American College of Surgeons.

Ferenchick, G., Simpson, D. E., Blackman, J., DaRosa, D. A., & Dunnington, G. L. (1997). Strategies for efficient and effective teaching in the ambulatory setting. *Academic Medicine, 72,* 277-280.

Galpin, T. J. (1996). *The human side of change.* San Francisco: Jossey-Bass.

Gastel, B., & Rogers, D. E. (Eds.), (1989). Clinical education and the doctor of tomorrow. *Proceedings of the Josiah Macy Jr. Foundation.* National Seminar on Medical Education, New York.

Knowles, M. (1990). *The adult learning: A neglected species.* Houston, TX: Golf.

Mager, R. F. (1997). *Preparing instructional objectives*. Atlanta, GA: Center for Effective Performance.

Walton, H. J. (1994). The changing medical profession: Recommendations of the World Summit on Medical Education. *Journal of the College of Physicians and Surgeons of Pakistan, 4*(2), 39-46.

CHAPTER SEVEN

Adapting Teaching to the Learning Environment

Gary L. Dunnington
Southern Illinois University School of Medicine

The pupils . . . are not to converse with the patients or nurses. During operations and while on the wards, they are to abstain from conversation with each other; in all cases in which it will be proper for the pupil to make any personal examination of the patient, such as feeling the pulse, examining a tumor, etc., an intimation to that effect will be given them by the physician or surgeon. It must be obvious that great inconveniences must arise if such examinations were commonly made by the pupils. (Jackson & Warren, 1824)

The preceding is an excerpt from the ruling of the managers of the Massachusetts General Hospital in May of 1824. Although medical education had moved from the proprietary medical schools involving classroom learning only to the hospital environment, the typical experience designed to complement the theoretical learning was an experience of observation only. By the end of the 18th century, many were becoming highly critical of this theoretical learning. Fortunately, by the early 19th century, the pendulum had swung so that Osler at Hopkins and physicians elsewhere recognized the hospital wards, the clinics, and the operating room as laboratories extraordinaire and the ideal active learning environment for medical students and residents. Although emphasis has shifted over the years among these three key learning environments because of changes in medical practice, the bedside, the clinic, and the operating room still are recognized as the critical learning environments for clerkship and residency education. The future, however, may diminish the significance of bedside teaching as hospitals increasingly become populated with only critically ill patients or early postoperative patients, providing

69

less than ideal circumstances for meaningful teaching. This change will continue to enhance the importance of teaching in the ambulatory setting as patients continue to have more and more of their care delivered in this setting.

Although a well-rounded learning experience involves participation in all of the key learning environments, the concept of site-specific teaching has emerged as important in establishing the learning objectives for each setting. For example, the clinic likely is the most useful site for teaching and learning in the area of focused history and physical examination skills, development of differential diagnoses, cost-effective diagnostic workup, selection of management options, and medical practice issues. The inpatient bedside is the best environment for teaching the concept of evaluation of the patient as a whole, postoperative care, and issues in critical care. The operating room is ideally suited for discussion of anatomy, pathology, pathophysiology, and certainly surgical technique. This concept of site-specific teaching should be used by faculty in the development of specific learning goals and objectives for students and residents in the three environments.

TEACHING AT THE BEDSIDE

Sylvius was probably the first to champion the technique of bedside teaching in medical education. After his appointment to the Chair of Medicine at Leiden, he was the most famous clinical teacher of the 17th century. In 1664, Sylvius wrote, "My method . . . is to lead my students by the hand to the practice of medicine, taking them every day to see patients in the public hospital, that they hear the patients symptoms and see their physical findings" (Bettman, 1956, p. 151). A student described his method of bedside teaching:

> When he came with his pupils to the patient and began to teach, he appeared completely in the dark as to the causes of the nature of the affection the patient was suffering from, and at first expressed no opinion upon the case; he then began by questions put to different members of his audience to fish out everything and finally united the facts discovered in this manner into a complete picture of the disease in such a way that the students received the impression that they themselves made the diagnosis and had not learnt it from him. (Puschmann, 1891)

Bedside teaching in some medical schools has become increasingly infrequent over the past few years. Linfors and Neelson (1980, p. 1233) stated that a sort of "clinical entropy is dispersing learners from the bedside." They suggested possible reasons such as an unwarranted concern for bedside teaching as interfering with patient privacy, subspecialization, and a rise in laboratory research among full-time faculty, making them less clinically experienced (thin-ice syndrome). Others have suggested that with the tremendous technological advances and the availability of abundant diagnostic studies at our disposal, there is a perception that the repertoire of physical examination skills once appreciated at the bedside are no longer of critical importance.

In contrast to these reasons for less bedside teaching, the importance of bedside teaching cannot be overemphasized for student and house staff training. It is in this learning environment that the patient can be seen as an individual with whom medical decisions are made rather than to whom procedures and tests are applied. This humanizes and personalizes medical care. As well, the presence of the patient makes the learning process more participatory. A bedside teaching session is the ultimate in problem-oriented learning experiences. Edwards (1990) emphasized the active nature of bedside rounds in her discussion on the use of visual images. She described the use of the patient as the classic visual image and contrasted this with more contemporary images used such as electrocardiograms (ECGs), computerized tomography (CT) scans, magnetic resonance images (MRIs), and other radiographic studies.

Kosslyn (1980) published a theory that explains how adults represent and access information from visual mental images. The theory suggests that images are first generated as skeletal images that can be elaborated by using verbal information to generate new parts or combine additional parts with a skeletal image. The patient's body is an image, that the students and residents use to process information. Experienced physicians often organize the information about a disease process around the image of the patient they once treated when they were students or houseofficers. Edwards (1990) suggested that the classic use of images is qualitative and personal, as contrasted with the contemporary use of images, which is quantitative and impersonal. Ideally, faculty should combine classic and contemporary visual images for effective clinical teaching. In addition, bedside teaching offers the ultimate manifestation of the physician as teacher rather than lecturer, discussant, or consultant. This role modeling is critical in the student's professional development of attitudes.

Finally, bedside teaching provides an opportunity for direct observation of clinical skills. This is the only way in which evaluation of interviewing, physical examination, and psychomotor skills can be assessed accurately and feedback provided immediately. More than 40 years ago, Francis Peabody (1927, p. 877) warned medical educators that the burgeoning volume of scientific knowledge to be learned would take precedence over the teaching of clinical skills and reminded his colleagues that "the practice of medicine in its broadest sense includes the whole relationship of a physician with his patients." The term "clinical skills deficiency syndrome" (Dunnington, Reisner, Witzke, & Fulginiti, 1992, pp. 110-114) has been used to describe a deterioration of history taking, physical examination, and patient physician interaction skills from early years of medical school to clerkship and residency experiences in the absence of frequent observation and feedback. Bedside teaching provides an ideal learning environment in which to reinforce these critical clinical skills.

Tips for Teaching at the Bedside

The following teaching tips are offered to enhance the quality of bedside rounds.

- *Bedside rounds should occur at the bedside.* Although faculty often are more comfortable "walking the corridors" or conducting what they describe as bedside teaching rounds in a nearby classroom, doing them at the bedside provides the patient as a focus for the discussion.

- *Avoid business (minor patient care decisions) on bedside teaching rounds.* The most effective teaching rounds are those in which the principal goal is learning rather than conducting the work of the wards. For chief residents, grappling with this issue, morning rounds may be quick and efficient, with the focus on getting the work done as long as junior house staff and students realize that during afternoon rounds the pace will slow on one or two patients with a focus on critical learning issues.

- *Focus the teaching agenda on data generated by or about the patient.* The patient often is unnecessary for the frequent discussions about etiology, natural history, relative value of various diagnostic tests, and medical and surgical options. These discussions may occur best in the hallway, or better still, in the radiology department or classroom. The bedside discussion should focus on the details of the history, the pathophysiology of the elicited history, and the pertinent findings on the physical examination. In this discussion, the patient is a critical player.

- *The session should be orderly with decorum and punctuality.* Both the attending and the students should be punctual with a designated start and stop time, with strict adherence. The professionalism of the session should convince the patient that, although house staff and students are involved in their care, the attending is clearly in charge. Attention should be paid to positioning of learners around the bedside, with the teacher at the head of the bed next to the patient and the students and residents around the foot of the bed.

- *Conduct bedside rounds with respect for patients' comfort and dignity.* In this sense, bedside rounds are an opportunity for role modeling of appropriate physician-patient interaction skills. The attending should demonstrate attention to patient comfort, privacy, and modesty. The attending should ensure that students avoid impersonal terms that would only perplex the patient, and that complex issues are explained in understandable terms. Patient acceptance and valuing of the benefit of bedside teaching rounds can be enhanced when the attending offers the patient and family the opportunity to ask questions about the diagnosis or care at the conclusion of the bedside teaching session.

- *Prepare the patient and student for the experience.* Someone should contact the patient before the teaching rounds to ensure the patient's willingness to cooperate with the experience. Sessions should begin outside the patient's room, with an explanation of the objectives to students and residents, a statement of how long the session will last, what will be discussed, and what should be reserved for later discussion after the patient encounter.

- *Segment the presentation for active involvement of all learners with higher level questioning.* A very useful technique is to ask the student or resident responsible for the patient to give the initial part of the history or present illness at the bedside. The other students can be subsequently asked to address additional questions to the patient to complete their perspective of the patient's problem. Similarly, segmenting the presentation allows for higher level questioning with such queries as "What if dysphagia were present without weight loss as opposed to with weight loss?" These types of "what if" questions promote the development of critical thinking skills over lower level questions that ask for factual recall only.

- *Make teaching multilevel when appropriate.* It is a difficult challenge to conduct effective teaching rounds when the learners range from third-year medical students to senior residents and fellows in their fifth-, sixth-, or seventh-year of training. If possible, it is easier and probably of greater learning value periodically to conduct bedside rounds with students separate from rounds with house staff. If multilevel rounds are practiced, the student focus should be on history, physical examination, and differential diagnosis. Diagnostic workup and evaluation issues can be addressed with intern and junior resident participation, whereas treatment and appropriate surgical management of potential complications can be addressed to chief residents.

- *Use bedside rounds to teach clinical assessment skills.* Studies (Dunnington et al., 1992; McGlynn, Sayre, & Kennedy, 1978; Stillman, May, Meyer, Rutala, Veach, et al., 1981) have shown an incidence of errors ranging from 32% to 42% when medical students are directly observed performing complete physical examinations. Aloia and Jonas (1976) showed that house staff demonstrate a decreasing incidence of errors on examination with each year of training, but that the number of errors remains significant even in the latter years of training. Faculty often make errant assumptions about the abilities of their trainees in this critical area, and bedside rounds provide the ideal setting in which to focus on these deficiencies.

- *Use every opportunity to provide feedback.* Bedside teaching provides the ultimate opportunity for taking advantage of the teachable moment. No more effective feedback could be described than that given at the bedside in a demonstration of the proper way to palpate a liver edge when a student has just demonstrated an incorrect method.

The art of teaching at the bedside is one well worth pursuing by young academic physicians. As Linfors and Neelson (1980, p. 1233) suggested, bedside teaching will "discourage passivity, dogmatism and a narrow, barren view of medicine."

TEACHING IN THE AMBULATORY CARE SETTING

There are significant differences between the learning environment of bedside rounds and that of the ambulatory care setting. Inpatient teaching places an emphasis on depth of knowledge, whereas the outpatient setting emphasizes breadth of knowledge with a large number of varied cases. The emphasis is on rapid diagnosis and efficient management of a number of problems. The inpatient setting is a group process with one attending and often a host of students and residents, whereas the outpatient setting involves a one-on-one teaching-learning process. Whereas a resident or student can prepare for attending rounds, no specific learner preparation is possible for outpatient teaching, thus making it more spontaneous. Whereas the inpatient encounter is prolonged over a course of time, the outpatient setting involves short encounters. Finally, in the inpatient setting there is often a limited amount of input on management from the patient. The outpatient, however, is much more in control and autonomous, requiring a different approach on the part of the treating physician. The ambulatory setting, however, has emerged as a critically important learning environment for students and house staff. In surgical specialties, between 50% and 85% of patient problems encountered in the ambulatory setting would never be encountered by the learner participating only in inpatient experiences (Dunnington, 1990).

A number of barriers to effective teaching in the ambulatory setting have been cited. For faculty, there often are inadequate rewards for outpatient education, a perceived patient dissatisfaction with student and resident involvement, and surgical specialization, all of which make it difficult to teach in the general clinic setting. Administratively, there are the significant cost of teaching in the clinic, space requirements, service structures that often fail to accommodate students' and residents' clinic participation, the frequent problem of too many learners, and new government requirements for faculty documentation. These issues have been addressed carefully in the ambulatory care literature over the past several years.

The first major priority of a faculty group is to establish clear goals in the outpatient experience for medical students and residents. Tables 7.1 and 7.2 give an example of goals developed during a faculty development workshop in a department of surgery for the surgical residency experience and the medical student experience in the outpatient clinic.

TABLE 7.1
Surgical Residency

Goals of the Outpatient Experiences
• Cost effective diagnostic evaluation
• Patient selection for outpatient surgery
• Surgical risk assessment
• Postoperative surveillance
• Communication to referring physicians
• Patient education and counseling skills
• Surgical complications

TABLE 7.2
Surgical Clerkship

Goals of the Outpatient Experiences
• Skills for a focused history
• Physical examination skills
• Patient-physician interaction skills
• Focus on surgical diseases commonly seen in primary care practice
• Follow-up, surveillance, and the understanding of the disability after surgical intervention
• Minor technical skills appropriate for primary care physicians
• Cost-effective diagnostic workup
• Principles of appropriate triage

The second important task for the clerkship director or program director is to select appropriate ambulatory care sites for effective teaching and learning. Smith and Irby (1997) suggested criteria for selecting such sites. The sites should offer an appropriate case mix, enthusiastic and committed preceptors, accommodating clinical facilities, and structures that promote communication and continuity.

There are a number of suggestions in the literature for creative methods to enhance ambulatory clinic teaching without adding significantly to the time or costs of the actual clinic. A recent article entitled Ambulatory Teaching "Lite": Less Clinic Time, More Educationally Fulfilling (DaRosa, Dunnington, Stearns, Ferenchick, Bowen, & Simpson, 1997) makes several suggestions for such creative methods to enhance teaching. These activities can be conducted before or after the clinic to enhance the learning experience. A case of the week may offer pearls of wisdom on a common diagnosis or a diagnosis that may result in significant morbidity or mortality if not identified. Exit rounds at the end of a busy clinic may allow reflection on critical learning issues. Morning and afternoon rounds, simulating the inpatient environment, may either preview key learning issues identified in upcoming clinic visits or review key diagnostic and management issues seen during the clinic experience. An ambulatory care journal club is a useful learning technique and may be conducted on a Website or with a listserve for distance learning at outlying ambulatory sites. Independent learning modules can prepare students for their learning experience and avoid redundant explanation of basic principles, such as students reviewing an independent learning module on breast imaging including mammography and ultrasound before attending a breast clinic. Standardized patients offer opportunities to provide uniform experiences on critical diagnoses. A virtual clinic may be established with a group of such patients to ensure uniform experience of medical students when time is limited for specialty clinics. Home visits may provide significant educational enrichment in helping the student or resident see the patient as an ambulatory patient whose illness must be addressed in the patient's own environment.

In addition to the complex administrative issues in designing meaningful ambulatory experiences, a number of suggestions can be made to enhance the effectiveness of faculty teaching in this environment.

Tips For Teaching in the Ambulatory Care Setting

Orientation and objectives should be provided as for any other learning experience.

Table 7.3 provides suggestions for both general and site--specific orientation for learners in ambulatory care settings. Clear objectives for the students' ambulatory experience will allow them to monitor their own experience to ensure that objectives are being met.

- *Ensure patient comfort and cooperation with the teaching and learning process.* The literature suggests that patients are very satisfied with participation of students and residents in their physician encounter in the ambulatory setting. O'Malley, Omori, Landry, Jackson, and Kroenke (1997) recently published the first prospective study of a group of patients in a general medicine clinic, measuring patient satisfaction using a Medical Outcomes Study Questionnaire. They found that 99% of patients rated their encounter as good, very good, or excellent, and that 95% would be willing or probably willing to see a trainee-staff team in the future. Patients in this study cited benefits of such an encounter as greater provider interaction, enhanced education, and overall improved level of care. Patients should clearly understand the role of the learner in their care and must sense that the attending physician is in a significant supervisory role.
- *Assess the learners' needs before patient assignment.* Whitman suggested that knowledge is assessed by questioning, clinical skills by direct observation, and attitudes by professional intimacy. It is particularly important for the student early in his or her clinical

experience to be assigned patients with good communication skills prototypical presentations, and manageable complexity, as well as patients that specifically meet curriculum objectives (Smith & Irby, 1997).

- *Include learner involvement in patients without a diagnosis.* This is critical for both students and house staff because current practice patterns often preclude learner involvement in the diagnostic phase, as patients present to the hospital with complete diagnostic workups and definitive diagnoses. Learners benefit significantly more from evaluating a patient presenting with "dysphagia" than being sent to evaluate a patient with esophageal cancer.

- *Use the clinic setting to teach the concept of focused history and examination.* This is particularly important for medical students because their introduction to clinical medicine course often has emphasized the complete history and physical examination. For example, for a patient presenting with a lump in the breast, the student must understand what is included in a focused history and examination or efficient medical practice.

Focus on a limited teaching agenda by capturing the "teachable moment." Faculty often are frustrated because of their perceived need to "teach it all" in each encounter with a student or resident. A more effective approach would be to make one or two key points at each encounter, with the focus on learner needs rather than the case itself. The teachable moment

- is discovered during observation of a clinical skill deficiency, a misguided focus noted on chart review, or knowledge deficits uncovered during higher level questioning (Lesky & Borkan, 1990).

TABLE 7.3
Orientation for Learners in Ambulatory Care Settings

General Orientation	Site Specific
• Course syllabus, objectives, expectations	• Introduction of team members
• Medical chart organization and review techniques	• Overview of site operations
• Videotapes of focused history and physical exams	• Description of practice population
• Prescription writing	• Available community resources
• Clinic professional behavior	• Unique practice guidelines
• Dictation, charting skills	• Expectation for learners' role

- *Use higher level questions to promote development of critical thinking skills*. Studies of medical faculty in teaching settings indicate that most questions are low-level questions that require factual recall. Critical thinking skills are best developed by questions that require synthesis, evaluation, comparison, and analysis.
- *Include practice issues in clinic discussion*. With the advent of managed care, it has become increasingly important to incorporate practice issues into educational experiences. This discussion would include practices to enhance physician referral, precertification for surgical patients, efficient clinical operations, and participation in health care teams.
- *Teach good physician-patient interaction skills*. Multiple short encounters with a large number of patients offer unique opportunities to role model professionalism in patient interaction. Learners benefit from opportunities to discuss physician approaches to issues such as presenting a diagnosis of cancer or results of a positive human immunodeficiency virus (HIV) test.
- *Teach patient education skills*. Learners must understand the concept that the most compliant patient is a well-informed patient. Furthermore, spending time providing education to patients also can be an effective way to teach key concepts to student learners simultaneously.

One of the most useful strategies for effective teaching in the ambulatory setting was originally described by Neher, Gordon, Meyer, and Stevens, (1992) as microskills of teaching or "the one-minute preceptor." These five microskills provide a useful methodology for interacting with a student or resident presenting an ambulatory case to a preceptor:

- Obtain a commitment: "What do you think is going on?"
- Probe for supporting evidence: "What supports your diagnosis?"
- Teach general rules; make one or two key points.
- Reinforce what was right with specific and positive feedback.
- Correct mistakes identified in knowledge base or clinical skills

TEACHING IN THE OPERATING ROOM

Of the teaching environments used by medical teachers, the least is published about effective teaching in the operating room. However, there are at least three fundamental components of operating room teaching:

- instruction in operative technique
- training in the overall conduct of the operation
- discussion of the overall care of the patient's problem.

Most published work focuses on the teaching and learning of technical and procedural skills. This section focuses on the appropriate content for operating room teaching and teaching behaviors that contribute to student and resident learning. Dunnington, DaRosa, and Kolm (1993) conducted a needs assessment to identify important content areas and teaching behaviors from the perspective of the learner. They have used this information to provide an evaluation instrument for assessment of teaching performance in the operating room. The needs assessment was conducted through a survey of third- and fourth-year medical students as well as surgical residents from two institutions. Learners were asked to provide their perspective on content and teaching behavior with a frame of reference method that asked them to judge content coverage and teaching behavior of their "best" as well as a hypothetical "ideal" surgical teacher. Table 7.4 describes the highest rated content areas in priority order by house staff and students. House staff and medical students agreed on the importance of discussing normal and abnormal anatomic findings during a surgical procedure, thus illustrating the site-specific nature of the operating room as a teaching environment. House staff placed increased emphasis on the technical aspects of operating room teaching.

The second part of this study asked participants to render opinions regarding the frequency of 27 teaching behaviors that characterize the operating room teaching of their selected "best" teacher and "ideal" teacher.

TABLE 7.4
Needs Assessment for Operating Room Teaching
Highest Rated Content Areas

By Students	By House Staff
• Normal anatomy	• Operative technique
• Abnormal anatomic findings	• Normal anatomy in operative field
• Potential postoperative complications	• Abnormal anatomic findings
• Follow-up plan	• Potential postoperative complications
• Natural history with/or without surgical intervention	• Pathophysiology
• Pathophysiology	• Expected outcome (symptoms relief, recurrence, survival)
• Etiology	• Follow-up plan
• Expected outcome	• Alternative operative approaches
• Nonsurgical treatment options	• Etiology
• Operative technique	• Natural history with/or without surgical intervention
• Alternative operative approaches	• Nonsurgical treatment options

Table 7.5 shows the highest rated teaching behaviors in order of priority by students and house staff, respectively. Later, both students and house staff emphasized the importance of a calm and approachable attending demeanor. The rating of teaching behaviors by students reinforces work in the literature emphasizing the powerful role of clinical preceptor as a role model. The importance of specific feedback delivered without belittling also is evident, with the most useful feedback provided soon after the operative procedure. Both students and house staff emphasize the importance of a calm and approachable demeanor. Ensuring a supportive learning environment is one of the underlying principles of adult learning, and this is further enhanced with faculty attitudes of tolerance and flexibility, which encourage critical thinking.

This work resulted in a valid and reliable evaluation instrument (alpha coefficient of 0.93) that can be used in an effort to improve faculty teaching in the operating room. This instrument is most effective if completed by a trained nurse or senior resident immediately after the operative event. The form then can be returned to the faculty member, providing effective feedback on the content and effectiveness of his or her teaching.

Tips for Teaching in the Operating Room

As with the previous two environments, this section also offers the recommendations for improvement of individual faculty teaching in the environment of the operating room.

TABLE 7.5
Needs Assessment for Operating Room Teaching
Highest Rated Teaching Behaviors

By Students	By House Staff
• Demonstrates respect for patient	• Answers questions clearly
• Role models good interaction with operating room staff	• Confident in role as surgeon and teacher
• Allows learners to "feel" pathology	• Provides feedback without belittling
• Answers questions clearly	• Remains calm and courteous
• Provides feedback without belittling	• Exhibits fairness toward house officers, no favorites
• Remains calm, courteous	• Role models good interaction with operating room staff
• Teaches with enthusiasm	• Explains reasons for his or her actions/decisions
• Provides multilevel operating room teaching	• Allows learners to "feel" pathology
• Ensures good view of operative field	• Demonstrates respect for patient
• Exhibits fairness toward students, no favorites	• Teaches with enthusiasm

- *Insist on preoperative preparation of all learners.* Learning in the operating room should be an active experience that can occur only with learner preparation.

- *Role model good interaction with operating room staff.* This is increasingly important because changing health care delivery patterns place added value on physicians' ability to work collaboratively in teams with other health care personnel.

- *Ensure a supportive learning environment.* A calm, courteous, and approachable demeanor on the part of the surgeon significantly promotes such an atmosphere. The attending surgeon also should ensure considerate treatment of learners by all nursing staff. This stimulates active involvement by all in the teaching-learning process.

- *Establish priorities in the content of operating room teaching.* The previously noted study of student and resident content needs should assist in making the content more appropriate for all levels of learners in the operating room. As with teaching in the ambulatory clinic, there often is not time to "teach it all." Therefore, the focus should be on those issues best taught and illustrated by the living, breathing, pulsating visual aids of the operating room.

- *Promote active learning experiences.* Make sure all learners have an adequate view of the operative procedure and find ways for students to use their hands such as following or cutting suture, opening the surgical specimen on the back table, and participating in wound closure.

- *Provide multilevel teaching.* As with bedside rounds, the challenge is to make the experience meaningful for a group of participants ranging from third-year medical students to senior fellows.

- *Answer questions clearly and precisely.* Some faculty are more comfortable delaying questions until after the operative event, but failure to respond altogether to student and house staff questions inhibits intellectual curiosity and the development of critical thinking skills.

- *Conduct house staff teaching commensurate with level of training.* The goal of all teaching experiences is to move the learner from the position of dependence on the faculty to one of independence. Recognizing this graduation in maturity, Table 7.6 provides suggestions for appropriate issues for teaching at the intern, junior resident, and chief resident levels.

- *Provide specific feedback for performance.* Effective feedback is specific and focused on the behavior rather than the individual, avoids belittling, and is given promptly after the educational encounter.

TABLE 7.6
House Staff Teaching Issues

The Intern
• Suture placement
• Knot tying
• Use of instruments
• Handling of tissue
• Surgical anatomy

The Junior Resident
• Operative report dictation
• Abdominal exploration
• Stapling techniques
• Communication with operating room staff
• Surgical diary (log of complex or infrequently performed procedures)

The Chief Resident
• Overall organization of the operation
• Economy of motion, effort
• First assistant skills
• Crisis management
• Interaction with anesthesiologist

- *Approach operating room teaching with enthusiasm.* Be creative in methods to enhance teaching in the operating room.

REFERENCES

Aloia, J. F., & Jonas, E. (1976). Skills in history-taking and physical examination. *Journal of Medical Education, 51,* 410-415.

Bettman, B. (1956). *A pictorial history of medicine, 151.* Springfield, IL: C.C. Thomas.

DaRosa, D., Dunnington, G., Stearns, J., Ferenchick, G., Bowen, J., & Simpson, D. (1997). Ambulatory teaching "Lite": Less clinic time, more educationally fulfilling. *Academic Medicine, 72*(5), 358-361.

Dunnington, G.. L. (1990). The outpatient clinic as a critical setting for surgical clerkship teaching. *Teaching and Learning in Medicine: An International Journal, 2*(4), 212-214.

Dunnington, G.. L., Reisner, E., Witzke, D., & Fulginiti, J. (1992). Teaching and evaluation of physical examination skills on the surgical clerkship. *Teaching and Learning in Medicine: An International Journal, 4*(2), 110-114.

Dunnington, G. L., DaRosa, D., & Kolm P. (1993). Development of a model for evaluating teaching in the operating room. *Current Surgery, 50,* 7.

Edwards, J. C. (1990, May) Ideas for medical education: Using classic and contemporary visual images in clinical teaching. *Academic Medicine, 65*(5), 297-298.

Jackson, J. & Warren, J. C. (1824). File, "Medical Education," Massachusetts General Hospital Archives.

Kosslyn, S. M. (1980). *Image and mind.* Cambridge, MA: Harvard University Press.

Lesky, L. G., & Borkan, S. C. (1990). Strategies to improve teaching in the ambulatory medicine setting. *Archives Internal Medicine, 150,* 2133-2137.

Linfors, E. W., & Neelson, F. A. (1980). The case for bedside rounds. *New England Journal of Medicine, 303*(21), 1233.

Massachusetts General Hospital. (1824, May). statement written by James Jackson & John C. Warren, File, "Medical Education," Massachusetts General Hospital Archives.

McGlynn, T. J., Sayre, A., & Kennedy, D. (1978). Physical diagnosis course: A question of emphasis. *Journal of Family Practice, 6*, 565-571.

Neher, J. O., Gordon, K. C., Meyer, B., & Stevens, N. (1992). A five-step "microskills" model of clinical teaching. *Journal American Board Family Practice, 5*, 419-424.

O'Malley P. G., Omori, D. M., Landry F. J., Jackson J., & Kroenke, K. (1997). A prospective study to assess the effect of ambulatory teaching on patient satisfaction. *Academic Medicine, 72*(11), 1015-1017.

Peabody, F. W. (1927). The care of the patient. *Journal of the American Medical Association, 88*, 877.

Puschmann, T. (1891). *A history of medical education from the most remote to the most recent times.* London, England: H K Lewis.

Smith, C. S., & Irby, D. M. (1997). The roles of experience and reflection in ambulatory care education. *Academic Medicine, 72*(1), 32-35.

Stillman, P. L., May, J. R., Meyer, D. M., Rutala, P. J., Veach, T. L., & Montgomery, A. B. (1981). A collaborative effort to study methods of teaching physical examination skills. *Journal of Medical Education, 56*, 301-306.

Whitman, N. (1990). Creative Medical Teaching. [Monograph]. *Department of Family and Preventive Medicine, 139-142.* Salt Lake City, UT.

CHAPTER EIGHT

Large Group Teaching

Ajit K. Sachdeva

MCP Hahnemann School of Medicine

Teaching large groups of individuals presents special challenges and opportunities in medical and surgical education. Although the definition of a large group in the context of education is somewhat arbitrary, educational researchers have frequently categorized a group of 100 or more students as large, whereas, the students themselves have felt that a group becomes large when it includes 75 or more individuals (Litke, 1995). Faculty members often have biases against large group teaching because many of them believe that increase in class size leads to decrease in student learning and satisfaction, that large classes cannot be taught as effectively as small classes, and that student ratings of instructors are lower in large classes (Litke, 1995). Furthermore, several specific challenges have been identified with this form of teaching and learning (Christensen, 1994; Herr, 1989).

Pedagogical challenges for teachers include difficulties in delivering the message effectively, using media appropriately, dealing with poor student attention, monitoring student progress and providing feedback, and tailoring student tasks to meet individual learning needs. Teachers sometimes are unable physically to reach some sections of a large classroom and may be inclined to avoid educational strategies that work well with smaller groups but become increasingly complex and difficult to implement with a large group.

Managerial challenges include logistical difficulties in conducting activities that typically require small group interactions, high noise levels during student activities, difficulty in attending to all the students, problems in enforcing rules, and practical difficulties involved with reviewing and correcting assignments given to large numbers of students. Affective challenges include impersonal interactions with students, as well as difficulties in learning student names, establishing good rapport

85

with students, assessing the individual interests and needs of students, and working with students who require special attention.

Additional challenges are associated with teaching large groups of students located at different sites and linked through videoconferencing or by asynchronous transfer mode (ATM) systems. These and other problems may have a negative impact on the effectiveness of the large group teaching session and require special skills on the part of a teacher to ensure successful outcomes. In addition, decisions regarding whether or not to implement large group activities have been influenced by the wider acceptance of the principles of adult education, which underscore the importance of a learner-centered approach to education (Knowles, 1990). When these principles are used to design contemporary educational programs, small group teaching often is favored over teaching in large groups, even though the principles can be applied successfully in the large group settings as well.

Despite the current emphasis on small group teaching in medical and surgical education and the aforementioned traditional challenges, large group teaching has a place in contemporary models of adult education. Large group teaching can be highly effective when used skillfully to address certain learning objectives, and faculty members should be able to overcome common problems attributed to such teaching through appropriate training and practice. Students can learn successfully in large groups and can have positive attitudes regarding this format of teaching and learning. The critical issue is the quality of instruction and not the size of the class as an isolated factor. Considerable numbers of students actually like learning in large groups and enjoy the opportunities for exchange of varied experiences, opinions, and viewpoints available in such environments (Litke, 1995). Advantages of teaching in large groups include the efficient use of scarce faculty resources, especially the time of renowned and experienced individuals, and reduction of cost. In addition, this approach can help with the standardization of teaching (Chism, 1989).

Strategies to make large group teaching sessions more effective, along with a number of creative approaches to make such teaching more innovative, are outlined in the following sections of this chapter. The suggestions made in these sections need to be adapted to the specific teaching and learning environments of the teacher as well as the teacher's individual style. Throughout the text of the chapter, the word "student" is used in a generic sense and encompasses adult learners of all types: medical students, residents, fellows, and practicing physicians. The word "teacher" is used synonymously with "faculty member."

PLANNING AND PREPARING FOR A
LARGE GROUP TEACHING SESSION

In planning for a large group teaching session, the faculty member needs to determine how such a session will fit into the overall educational program. A large group teaching session may be particularly well suited for addressing specific educational objectives that require the use of scarce faculty resources, especially those in areas of special expertise and those of interest and importance to large numbers of students. Another situation that may be ideal for large group sessions is the presentation of standardized curricular material to large bodies of students (especially students located at different sites). This can help to ensure that the same material is addressed in an identical fashion for larger numbers of students. Large group sessions also can be effective for presentation of topics or sessions that do not need extensive, ongoing, close interaction between the students themselves to achieve the desired results. Moreover, large group teaching can be included to complement small group teaching activities, which may be conducted either before or after the large group session.

Faculty members planning a large group session should be cognizant of several potential pitfalls. A critical step during the early stages of planning for a large group session involves thorough analysis of the learning needs of the student group. This is especially important because the large group environment makes it more difficult for the teacher to assess the individual needs of students during the course of the session.

Faculty members have reported that misjudging the specific needs of a group of learners is a common cause of failure in teaching (Pinsky & Irby, 1997). This can be precluded through a series of proactive steps. The composition and background of the students should be carefully assessed and information obtained pertaining to the following items: other related educational activities in the curriculum, student performance on relevant tests, student feedback from previous sessions, and faculty input regarding appropriateness of content for the learners. These data should form the basis for the development of specific goals and objectives for the large group session.

Another common problem is that teachers often are overly ambitious when making decisions regarding the amount of content to be presented, as they feel obliged to "cover the ground." Overzealous inclusion of material should be diligently avoided because this allows fewer options for interaction and makes the session less effective. Realistic teaching objectives need to be established for the session, which should be structured on the basis of these objectives. The strong tendency on the part of teachers to resort to the lecture-type format for teaching large groups needs to be resisted. Such passive learning experiences are not very effective and do not provide students appropriate opportunities to develop as adult learners or to explore adequately their own strengths and weaknesses. The teacher should make special efforts to include interactive discussions and regular student activities throughout the course of the large group teaching session.

Each teaching session needs to have three separate but linked components: the opening, the body, and the closure (Claus, Hendricson, Kleffner, Scheid, Titus, et al., 1996; Workbook of Continuing Education Course, 1998). The opening should include review of the objectives for the session from the standpoint of what measurable behaviors the students will be able to demonstrate at the completion of the session. The objectives established by the faculty member before the session may be modified on the basis of additional information from student input in order to address the learning needs of students better. Discussion of the specific learning objectives in the beginning helps to establish the framework for the session and focuses the attention of students on the important items. A brief description of the format of the session during the opening also helps students to comprehend fully their respective roles for the session and establishes basic ground rules, such as whether they may interrupt the teacher to ask questions. In addition, the teacher should explain in advance how the material to be presented during the session is linked to the existing knowledge and skills of the students. This helps to anchor the new information to previously established knowledge structures of the students, and thus facilitates the learning process.

The body of the presentation should be appropriately structured for the teaching and learning process to proceed in a logical fashion, building from one item to the next in sequential progression. Cause-and-effect relationships should be clearly described, comparisons and contrasts between items discussed, and examples, analogies, and metaphors used to explain the key elements and to build the higher order thinking skills of the students. Use of personal references relating to one's own experiences establishes the teacher's credibility with the student group and helps to build stronger bonds between the teacher and the students. The students need to be aware of the knowledge and expertise of the teacher, without being overwhelmed by the complexity of the material presented.

Effective questioning should be used to build interaction and to enhance the cognitive abilities of students. Principles underlying the process of effective questioning have been defined, and should be followed to ensure the desired outcomes (Sachdeva, 1996b). Use of varied questions anchored to the taxonomy of thinking skills can be very effective in developing higher order skills, such as those of application, analysis, synthesis, and evaluation. Certain questions, known as pivotal questions, can be built into the teaching plan before commencement of the session and used to steer the direction of the subsequent discussion. Questions that are not preplanned but surface as a result of interaction are known as emerging questions. Both types of questions should be used effectively throughout the teaching session. Questions should be phrased well and adapted to the needs of the learners. Interposition of sufficient wait time (approximately five-s) after each question is important, because this simple step gives the students time to think, can result in a productive exchange with students, and encourages higher order responses from them.

The body of the teaching session has to be crafted and managed skillfully because this is the time when students in large groups have a tendency to let their minds wander and allow their attention to stray from the principal focus of the session. If the session is longer than one half hour, well-defined student activities should be prospectively built into the teaching plan. Such activities can keep the students involved and contribute directly to achieving the learning objectives. For example, specific questions may be posed to the entire student group to facilitate interactive discussion. Students can be asked to share their responses with the entire group or to discuss the item with a colleague sitting next to them. The latter strategy validates the students' own concepts, encourages everyone to get involved, and can be used to have students apply the information. The students might be asked to analyze data and subsequently present their results to the entire group, or they may be asked to work in small groups and then reassemble for a summary discussion at the end. Other components of the teaching session also can be structured in such a way as to create variety and stimulate attention. Changes in the sensory channels being used by the student, the learning environment, and levels of mental activity can be used individually or in combination to maintain attentiveness. For example, the teacher might proceed from a primarily aural channel to adding a visual channel with slides, switch from one visual medium to another (e.g., slides to a chalkboard), or use a prop for demonstration. These changes are even more effective when combined with a change in the level of mental activity (e.g., by turning off the slides and initiating interactive discussion).

Audiovisual aids, when appropriately selected and effectively used, can enhance large group teaching. Such aids help to focus the attention of students on the key points, reinforce concepts, illustrate specific items, stimulate interest, add variety, and keep the teacher on track. However, poorly designed or ineffectively used audiovisual aids can very easily destroy an otherwise good teaching session. First and foremost, the teacher needs to determine whether any kind of audiovisual support is needed and how it will add specifically to the teaching session. An axiom worth remembering is that the teacher is the best audiovisual medium; all other aids are supplementary!

If audiovisual support is needed in large group settings, 35-mm slides work very well in most situations. Slides may be prepared with ease using computer software that is readily available (e.g., Microsoft PowerPointR) and are convenient to use.

For the greatest impact, slides must be specifically designed for the session, and their preparation should follow a number of well-recognized principles. Each slide should have a title that captures the attention of the students; the material on the slides should be grammatically parallel; and only essential information should be included. Slides must not be cluttered with too much information. Five to seven lines of written text in bullet or itemized form generally is quite effective. Selection of the appropriate font also is important: Serif fonts are easy to read, particularly if there are a significant number of words on a slide, whereas sans serif fonts are easy to read only when the number of words is limited and the letters are large. Pictures can be effectively incorporated into the slides to support the verbal presentation. If dual projection is available, a picture on one slide could be used to complement the writing on the adjacent slide. Dual projection should not be used merely to present twice as much written text.

Although faculty members vary in their preferences for various types of slides, color slides can be very helpful in stimulating interest and introducing variety. The author has found the following guidelines to be useful: no more than three or four colors should be used on a slide; white or yellow writing on a blue background generally projects well even when the room is adequately lit for note taking; and red words and letters are hard to read, may interfere with pointing when a laser pointer (with a red beam) is used, and can present additional problems for red and green color-blind students, if present in the audience.

A useful rule of thumb for the use of slides in large group teaching is to allow an average of three- to five-minutes to discuss the material from each slide during the session. This allows the teacher to delve into the material in some depth and also facilitates interaction with the students. Contemporary technology allows teachers to use computer-aided projection for large group teaching. This approach can introduce dynamism, and the technology may be used interactively by the teacher. However, the potential risk of technical problems with computer systems is real, and a backup plan should be readily available in case problems arise.

Overhead transparencies may be used in large group teaching, but generally are more useful for smaller groups. They provide greater flexibility for the teacher because one can readily omit some of the transparencies based on the assessment of needs of the group during the course of teaching. Use of transparencies requires a little more physical movement on the part of the teacher, which can create some animation and visual variety. Overhead transparencies can be used without lowering the lights, which makes maintenance of contact with the students easier. If such transparencies are used during interactive discussions to record input and develop ideas, care must be taken to ensure that the writing is legible. The teacher may want to prepare good-quality color transparencies similar in appearance to slides, in advance of the session. If the group is very large, overhead transparencies may become difficult to read, and they also convey a message of informality, which may not be appropriate for certain large group teaching sessions.

Another very effective audiovisual method is projection of videotapes on multiple monitors or on a large screen. Videotapes can be used to demonstrate certain images, activities, and interactions, and vignettes portrayed in "trigger tapes" can be used to generate analysis and discussion. The audiovisual equipment should be thoroughly checked, and the teacher needs to familiarize him- or herself with the controls of the lectern before the session. If there is opportunity, a trial run, which includes projection of the entire set of slides, transparencies, or videotapes, should be conducted before the session.

Another form of visual aid, paper handouts, can be used in a variety of different ways for large group teaching. The handouts may provide a brief outline or various topics to be addressed during the session and allow students to write notes in the spaces below various headings. The handouts can be used in a more interactive fashion by having the students work, either alone or in small groups, to carry out a task based on a handout. Such exercises can be conducted during the body of the session to allow students to use their preexisting knowledge, and skills, and information learned during the earlier part of the session, or the exercise may be conducted at the beginning of the session to bring pertinent existing knowledge to the fore or; stimulate awareness of the relevance of the session.

Handouts also can be very useful in providing students with text relating to difficult terminology used during the course of the session. If the goal of the handout is to provide supplementary written material for students to use later, the handout should not be distributed to the students in the beginning of the session because it tends to take their attention away from the teacher. Such handouts should be made available to students at the conclusion of the session along with instructions regarding their use, including advice on how to link the material in the handout with the information covered during the session.

There is a natural tendency for students to become more attentive toward the end of the time allotted for the large group session. This opportunity should be seized to highlight the critical elements and to summarize the important items addressed during the session. Also, topics to be discussed in the future might be previewed for appropriate linkage of the material. Adequate time must be built into the session for students to ask questions pertaining to the material covered during the session. Follow-up to determine the effectiveness of the large group teaching session may be accomplished through subsequent testing, performance of specific tasks based on the information learned, or self-directed assessment.

CONDUCTING LARGE GROUP TEACHING SESSIONS

To ensure maximum impact, large group teaching should be conducted by adapting principles of effective teaching to the teacher's style and the learning needs of the student group (Carruthers, 1988; Claus, Hendricson, Kleffner, Scheid, Titus, et al., 1996; Cooper, 1989; Gelula, 1997; Herbert, 1988; Laidlaw, 1988; Sachdeva, 1996b; Workbook of Continuing Education Course, 1998). The learning environment, or physical room arrangement, for large group sessions generally involves a classroom-style or theater-style setting. Quite often, the seats are fixed, and the physical layout does not provide the teacher adequate options to create the ideal learning environment. However, even in these situations, certain steps may be taken to improve the teaching and learning process. If the room is much larger than the size of the student group and students are scattered throughout, they should be asked to move to one section of the room, for example, to one side of the aisle. Also, students sitting in the back of the room should be asked to move to the front. These maneuvers help to congregate students in one section of the room and allow the teacher to direct his or her attention to the entire student body. If the layout of the room permits movement of chairs, they should be turned so that the students can face one another. Such an arrangement facilitates interaction between students, allowing them to function more effectively in smaller groups, which may then be created to accomplish certain tasks.

In addition to the physical arrangements of the learning environment, faculty must monitor and manage the learning climate, or the affective component involving interactions between teacher and students. The learning climate should balance some level of tension (which keeps the students attentive) and a warm and supportive ambiance (in which the students feel free to participate without fear or hesitation). Maintaining such a balance with large groups requires more effort than with small groups because of the larger number of students and their individual needs.

However, even with large groups, the teacher can create a conducive learning climate through the skillful application of various verbal and nonverbal behaviors. The teacher should build a bond with the audience as soon as possible by pausing for a moment and making eye contact with a few students in the beginning of the session. A brief dialogue that reflects the teacher's interest in the students may be initiated. For example, a question about an in-house call during the previous night or a patient seen recently by a student, or a statement about an item of common interest can break the ice quite easily and effectively. Also, a smile at the beginning of the session projects warmth and helps to build a bridge with the student group. The teacher must clearly convey his or her interest in the students, enthusiasm for the session, and desire to communicate with the group.

Effective nonverbal behaviors should be used throughout the course of the session. These should include sufficient eye contact, appropriate facial expressions, poise and confidence, purposeful body movements, and use of hands and arms to emphasize specific points. In a large group, the teacher frequently is unable to make eye contact with each member of the audience over the course of the session. Specific individuals should be selected in turn from different sections of the room and eye contact made with them individually. When eye contact is made with a single individual, several people around that person also feel that the teacher is addressing them. Thus, the impact of this action extends to a larger segment of the student body around each individual.

Eye contact should be made for three- to five-seconds or until such time that the student appears to acknowledge the contact through appropriate facial expressions or a nod. Then the faculty member can move to another student. All segments of the student group should be addressed in this fashion during the session. Another effective approach involves moving physically closer to one section of the student group while maintaining eye contact with and addressing another section. This keeps students in both sections connected with the teacher. Purposeless nonverbal actions such as pacing across the room or fidgeting with a pointer or remote control cord are distracting and should be avoided, as should extraneous noises resulting from certain behaviors, such as jingling of coins.

If the teacher needs to stand behind a lectern during a formal session, he or she still can maintain contact with a large group by moving a little to the left or right of the lectern or by leaning over in one direction or the other but maintaining effective eye contact during this movement. A lavaliere microphone can allow the teacher to move away from the lectern and into the student group, which helps the teacher to connect further with the students. The teacher can move back to the lectern or to a table in the front of the room to refer to notes as necessary. Use of the various audiovisual controls and devices should not limit the movement and physical actions of the teacher. When the pointer or remote control is not being actively used, it should be placed on the lectern to allow unrestricted movement about the room. The teacher should take special care not to speak facing the screen with the back toward the audience. Effective pointing to specific areas on a slide with a light or laser pointer can help to enhance the effectiveness of the discussion and presentation.

Nonpurposeful movements of the light or laser beam across the screen or the room can be very distracting and must be avoided.

Effective verbal behavior typically exhibits the following characteristics. The voice of the teacher must project adequately to be heard across all sections of the room, and the words need to be enunciated clearly and pronounced properly. This is especially important in large group settings, as there may be interference with the clarity because of the size or acoustical properties of the room. The tempo of the delivery needs to be paced appropriately so that it allows comprehension but maintains the listener's attention. A comfortable delivery rate of approximately 120 words per minute should be used as a baseline for the presentation. This contrasts with a more rapid rate of delivery during one-on-one conversations in which approximately 200 words per minute are spoken. The pace should be set appropriately to avoid the need to rush toward the end of the session. The voice needs to convey vitality, and monotonous delivery should be avoided by introducing appropriate variation in volume, pitch, and tempo. Changes in tempo, especially when coupled with a change in the volume or pitch of the voice, can be very effective in highlighting key points and can be matched to the meaning of the message. The voice also can be modulated and used as a means to maintain contact with students in various parts of the room. By speaking more loudly when addressing a student in the back of the room and more softly (though still audible to all) when addressing a student in the front of the room, the teacher is able to command the attention of the entire group, connecting with distant students with higher volume and students nearby with close personal contact. Additional variation in the voice can be accomplished by interjection of pauses throughout the course of a presentation. Pauses of three- to five-seconds should be included at appropriate times to add emphasis, impact, or variety. Longer pauses may be needed after assignment of tasks.

One particularly effective technique for emphasizing an important point combines a pause with eye contact. This is done by establishing and sustaining eye contact with an individual while verbally making the essential point and then pausing, while continuing to maintain eye contact with the same individual. Other important verbal behaviors include the use simple language even while explaining complex items. Distractive and extraneous verbal habits such as "ums" and "ahs" and repetitive and meaningless habitual expressions such as "okay" and "you know" should be replaced by effective pauses.

The teacher may need to modify the content during the course of the session on the basis of responses to the questions. If students are unable to answer a question, the teacher should start with a simpler concept and build further. Students may benefit by the addition of statements that provide guidance as to the progress of the session. For example, several summary statements at the end of each section may help to bring the content to closure, emphasize key points covered, and link these points to the next section. A transition statement such as "Now let us proceed to" helps to bridge one section of the presentation with the next and prepares students for the next concept. Repetition is a key feature of effective teaching in any learning environment because it plays an important role in reinforcing important concepts and items. In the large group environment, repetition becomes even more crucial because a student may have missed an important point and not had the opportunity to ask that it be presented again.

The verbal and nonverbal behaviors of the students also are important for teachers to monitor in large group sessions. Teachers should use this information as a basis for making decisions regarding the progress of the session. Cues from the facial expressions or activities of the students should be used as feedback for the teacher to decide whether to maintain the set course or change it to meet the needs of the particular student group. For example, if the majority of the students look confused, the teacher should go back to ascertain their baseline knowledge before proceeding further. Verbal and nonverbal behaviors also can be used to gauge the group's general interest and energy levels to determine whether the methods being used are engaging and whether a brief break or student activity may need to be interposed. Some students in a large group might get distracted and begin talking with their peers adjacent to them. Such behavior should not be tolerated. The teacher should intervene, selecting from a variety of available options, and the students subsequently engaged in productive discussions. Disruptive students should be reminded about being courteous to their peers, and may need to be dealt with firmly. An occasional student who gets out of hand might even need to be counseled individually after the session.

INCLUSION OF LARGE GROUP TEACHING SESSIONS IN EDUCATIONAL MODELS FOR THE 21ST CENTURY

Large group teaching is likely to continue playing an important role in the educational models of the future. Decreases in funding for medical and health sciences education will make the efficient use of faculty members' time even more important. Through large group sessions, expert faculty members would be able to continue to reach large numbers of students, allowing parsimonious use of resources.

Effectively planned and skillfully conducted large group sessions can be successfully included in contemporary educational models, and the challenges generally associated with such teaching overcome using the strategies outlined in the previous sections. Inclusion of even simple activities in large group teaching, such as engaging students in filling out sections of incomplete handouts, can generate sufficient interest to increase student satisfaction (Butler, 1992). This underscores the positive impact of student activities. Several creative approaches have been used to enhance the teaching of students in large groups (Duncan-Hewitt, 1996; Schwartz, 1989; Stein, Neill, & Houston, 1990), and a variety of such options may be used to make large group teaching more interactive. For example, a debate may be added to facilitate dialogue between the students, or students may be asked to discuss an item among themselves, with a few students selected to present the results of the discussions. Such strategies get everyone involved, and the silence becomes less a problem because everyone feels compelled to participate actively, in a way similar to the process that characterizes small groups interactions. The large student group may be divided and sent to other rooms in smaller groups to perform certain tasks or to address specific issues (with or without preparatory reading), and then asked to return to share the results with the rest of the large group members.

Problem-based learning may be conducted in larger groups with some modifications in the traditional problem-based learning format (Barrows, Myers, Williams, & Moticka, 1986). The teacher can use an interactive approach to address the important steps of the clinical reasoning process. The learning issues generated can then be used to direct self-study between the large group sessions similar to small group problem-based learning. However, the teacher needs to play a more active role in managing the large group session as compared with the tutor in small group problem-based learning.

Another student activity that can be incorporated into large group sessions is role play. For example, role-play scenarios can be completed by the students in smaller groups followed by debriefing in the large group to highlight key psychosocial issues (Mann, Sachdeva, Nieman, Nielan, Rovito, et al. 1996). Additionally, computer-based simulations or standardized patients can be used to generate discussions in large groups.

Advances in technology should make options for interactive teaching across sites through asynchronous transfer mode (ATM) links more routinely available. Consequently, faculty members will most likely need to learn how to use such technology for maximum impact. However, teachers should not become slaves to exciting new technology, which should be used only as a tool to support the teaching process. With training of faculty members in the principles of adult education and effective teaching, more innovation in large group teaching is likely to occur in the future. The author believes that improvements in large group teaching will result from more transfer of the approaches traditionally used in small group teaching to the large group environment through creative approaches and strategies similar to those outlined earlier. The push toward accountability and the increasing support for reward and recognition of teachers and educators should catalyze changes that are necessary to improve traditional forms of passive large group teaching, which are still being conducted by many faculty members.

The greater emphasis on student-directed learning has resulted in increasing numbers of students asking teachers to design and conduct large group teaching sessions based on the learning needs identified by the students themselves. Although the general principles of effective large group teaching covered in the previous sections apply to these sessions as well, certain additional steps are necessary to ensure the desired outcomes. Students should be asked to meet with the teacher before the session to share their perceived learning needs. This may be accomplished through a meeting that involves the entire student group or a few representatives who can convey the needs of the entire student body. Thus, the specific learning objectives for the proposed session may be defined in order to meet the needs of students adequately. Input from students can be used to design the format of the session as well. The teacher may consider suggesting selected readings for the students before the proposed session, which can help to make the learning process more participatory and interactive. Students therefore should play a more active and collaborative role during both the design and implementation of such a student-directed session to achieve the optimum results.

TRAINING OF FACULTY IN EFFECTIVE LARGE GROUP PRESENTATIONS

The variety of options for training faculty members in effective large group teaching includes courses and workshops, peer coaching, mentoring and consultations (Wilkerson & Irby, 1998). Videotaping and supportive critiquing are very effective techniques for modifying teaching behaviors. Faculty members may be individually videotaped and their performance critiqued, highlighting the effective approaches and behaviors as well as those that require change. Specific items that need improvement can be addressed and the faculty members asked to practice and return for repeat videotaping and additional feedback. Thus, over a certain period, various elements can be addressed sequentially and the overall presentation enhanced, building from one session to the next. One such workshop has been used successfully to enhance the teaching skills of faculty members from various health care disciplines (Workbook of Continuing Education Course, 1998). Additional specific attention can be directed to certain areas that need improvement through the technique of microteaching , in which the individual faculty member works with an expert to practice a component of a teaching skill to improve it over time (Van Ort, Woodtli, & Hazzard, 1991; Workbook of Continuing Education Course, 1998). Opportunities for one-on-one observation and feedback also may be offered in the context of the faculty member's own teaching environment. Teaching sessions in real environments can be videotaped and critiqued later by an expert working closely with the teacher. Depending on the needs of the individual teacher and the resources available, any and all of these faculty development techniques may be very helpful. To achieve the desired outcomes, all feedback used to improve faculty teaching should be supportive and follow established principles for sharing feedback effectively (Sachdeva, 1996a).

CONCLUSION

Large group teaching will continue to play an important role in medical and surgical education. Although this format of teaching presents certain challenges, it can be conducted effectively to achieve the optimum outcomes. Careful planning, including the establishment of realistic objectives, development of a logical structure, and preparation of well-designed audiovisual materials, coupled with the use of effective teaching techniques such as management of the learning environment and climate, use of appropriate verbal and nonverbal behaviors, and inclusion of effective questioning should lead to positive outcomes. Special efforts to ensure that students learn actively in large group teaching sessions include the use of small group exercises within the group, problem-based learning, computer-based simulations, standardized patients, debates, and role play. Such creative approaches can be successfully incorporated into the large group teaching environment. Faculty members need to be appropriately trained to ensure that this form of teaching and learning is used effectively in educational models for the 21st century.

REFERENCES

Barrows, H. S., Myers, A., Williams, R. G., & Moticka, E. J. (1986). Large group problem-based learning: A possible solution for the "2 sigma problem." *Medical Teacher, 8*(4), 325-331.

Butler, J. A. (1992). Use of teaching methods within the lecture format. *Medical Teacher, 14*(1), 11-25.

Carruthers, D. B. (1988). Twelve mistakes made by university lecturers. *Medical Teacher, 10*(2), 165-167.

Chism, N. V. (1989). Large enrollment classes: Necessary evil or not necessarily evil? *Notes on Teaching, 5*. Columbus, OH: Ohio State University.

Christensen, T. (1994). Large classes and their influence on language teaching. *Journal of Hokusei Junior College, 30*, 121-129.

Claus, J. M., Hendricson, B. D., Kleffner, J. H., Scheid, R. C., Titus, H. W., & Winter, M. G. (1996). Designing effective lectures. *Journal of Dental Education, 60*(1), 6-11.

Cooper, S. S. (1989). Teaching tips: Some lecturing do's and don'ts. *Journal of Continuing Education in Nursing, 20*(3), 140-141.

Duncan-Hewitt, W. C. (1996). A focus on process improves problem-based learning outcomes in large classes. *American Journal of Pharmaceutical Education, 60*, 408-416.

Gelula, M. H. (1997). Effective lecture presentation skills. *Surgical Neurology, 47*, 201-204.

Herbert, W. N. P. (1988). On improving the lecture. *Obstetrics and Gynecology, 72*(6),937-939.

Herr, K. U. (1989). *Improving teaching and learning in large classes: A practical manual.* Fort Collins, CO: Colorado State University.

Knowles, M. (1990). *The adult learner: A neglected species.* Houston, TX: Gulf Publishing Company.

Laidlaw, J. M. (1988). Twelve tips for lecturers. *Medical Teacher, 10*(1), 13-17.

Litke, R. A. (1995). Learning lessons from students: What they like most and least about large classes. *Journal on Excellence in College Teaching, 6*(2), 113-129.

Mann, B. D., Sachdeva, A. K., Nieman, L. Z., Nielan, B. A., Rovito, M. A., & Damsker, J. I. (1996). Teaching medical students by role-playing: A model for integrating psychosocial issues with disease management. *Journal of Cancer Education, 11*(2) 65-72.

Pinsky, L. E., & Irby, D. M. (1997). "If at first you don't succeed": Using failure to improve teaching. *Academic Medicine, 72*, 973-976.

Sachdeva, A. K. (1996a). Use of effective feedback to facilitate adult learning. *Journal of Cancer Education, 11*, 106-118.

Sachdeva, A. K. (1996b). Use of effective questioning to enhance the cognitive abilities of students. *Journal of Cancer Education, 11*, 17-24.

Schwartz, P. L. (1989). Active, small group learning with a large group in a lecture theatre: A practical example. *Medical Teacher, 11*(1), 81-86.

Stein, M., Neill, P., & Houston, S. (1990). Case discussion in clinical pharmacology: Application of small group teaching methods to a large group. *Medical Teacher, 12*(2), 193-196.

Van Ort, S., Woodtli, A., & Hazzard, M. E. (1991). Microteaching: Developing tomorrow's teachers. *Nurse Educator, 16*(1) 30-33.

Wilkerson, L., & Irby, D. M. (1998). Strategies for improving teaching practices: A comprehensive approach to faculty development. *Academic Medicine, 73,* 387-396.

Workbook of Continuing Education Course. (1998). *Effective teaching: Improving your skills.* Philadelphia: Allegheny University of the Health Sciences.

CHAPTER NINE

Small Group Teaching[*]

Richard G. Tiberius
University of Toronto

Although the current movement toward small group teaching in medical schools has generally been met with enthusiasm by clinician-teachers, many are troubled by the burden of learning a new form of teaching. Moreover, clinician-teachers seldom have a clear idea of how to become better at teaching. Few have had teacher training as part of their education. Even among schools that enjoy strong medical education programs, systematic training of teachers is rare. This chapter attempts to anticipate and answer questions that the clinician-teacher may ask about how to become a teacher of small groups: Do I need any instruction, or do I already know enough about small group teaching and learning from my experience as a student? Do I need formal instruction, or can I pick up the ability to lead small groups by doing it? If I do need formal instruction, can I get it by viewing videotapes or by reading? Do I have to engage in workshops or training sessions?

INFORMAL KNOWLEDGE:
HOW MUCH DO I ALREADY KNOW?

The good news is that you already possess more knowledge about small groups than you will ever acquire by formal study. The knowledge you possess is called "informal knowledge" (Bereiter & Scardamalia, 1993). Informal knowledge is the vast store of background information learned from a lifetime of experience with

---

[*] Some of the ideas in this article were developed during the planning of many workshops on small groups with my colleague, Jane Tipping.

groups: learning groups, peer groups, even family. Although you are largely unaware of this knowledge, it is critically important to successful group leadership. The problem with this knowledge is that it is specific to particular contexts or "situated," to use the language of the cognitive theorists (Brown, Collins, & Duguid, 1989). For example, the rules for successful interaction in a purely social group are different from the rules for successful interaction in an educational group. Even in educational groups, the rules for successful interaction vary depending on the discipline, the institutional culture, and the culture of the participants. Teachers who are used to the structured environment of the lecture hall may be shocked by the casual intimacy of small group interaction.

Can such informal knowledge of groups be gained by deliberate action? Although the usual method of acquiring informal knowledge about group process is by immersion in group interaction over a long period of time, it is possible to increase the amount of learning that one derives from everyday group situations. The difficulty of learning from everyday life experience is that the patterns of our actions are invisible as we perform them (Erickson, 1990). Teachers are too preoccupied with both leading the group and acting as resource persons to reflect on group process. A useful strategy, therefore, is to structure the group meetings so that during some of the time you are released from the constant pressure of leading. One such structure gives learners the leadership functions temporarily. Another engages the learners in exercises or requires them to make presentations. Such student-led periods can provide the teacher with excellent opportunities to observe and learn about their students. Student-led periods also can provide the students with valuable practice in leadership skills, especially if their leadership is informed by guidelines for group interaction (see Tiberius, 1990, pp. 66-69, for a description of such guidelines).

A more systematic approach to discovering what is happening in the group wherein you are participating requires that you assume the posture of a qualitative researcher, employing the skills of "participant observation." It is beyond the scope of this article to present a detailed guide to participant observation, but a few pointers will convey the flavor. Begin with general observations of the group atmosphere and move toward analysis of specific details. Cycle between observation, reflection, conceptualization, and further observation. For example, you might observe how the group organizes itself, solves problems, or deals with disruptions, and then analyze specific moves that initiated organization or problem solving. You might note key events in the group's development, and then find out what these events mean to the members of the group. You might test your concepts by applying them or checking them out with the group. Gradually, you build an insider's view of the group (Jorgensen, 1989).

FORMAL KNOWLEDGE OR TEXTBOOK KNOWLEDGE: WHAT CAN YOU LEARN FROM READING BOOKS OR WATCHING VIDEOTAPES?

What can books and videotapes provide that we cannot learn by our own observations? Recently, a number of works on small group teaching have been written specifically for medical educators, (Walton, 1997; Westberg & Jason, 1996; Whitman & Schwenk, 1983). These writings pass on the collected wisdom from hundreds of researchers who have observed small groups over the past 50 years. A few examples can be mentioned. First, these writings provide a rationale for using small groups in terms of enhancing both the effectiveness of learning and the motivation for learning. Talking and listening are among the most powerful ways that students can become actively engaged in learning, and active involvement motivates students and helps them to learn effectively (Bonwell & Eison, 1991). Interaction helps the thinking process by facilitating connections between the material and the learners' most salient ideas and thoughts (Simpson & Galbo, 1987).

Second, literature provides the teacher with benchmarks of the "well-functioning" group and primary functions of the small group leader. For example, the effective group is characterized by an informal atmosphere, lots of discussion pertinent to the topic, a sharing of participation, freedom to disagree, and a sense of awareness of the group process. A teacher who knows the characteristics of a well-functioning group has a standard against which to evaluate his or her own performance as well as the performance of the group. The primary functions of a small group leader include setting goals, maintaining discussion and adherence to the topic, and summarizing and dealing with disruptions.

The literature also is a good source of useful concepts such as Bales' (1950) classic distinction between "task" functions of the group and "process" or "interpersonal" functions. Task functions are those that accomplish the group goals such as discussing the topic or asking and answering questions. "Interpersonal" functions determine the way the members of the group interact. Understanding this distinction is essential if the small group leader is to learn to recognize interpersonal problems when they arise and to deal with them by pausing in pursuit of the task to attend to the interpersonal dynamics. Another important concept is the stages of development of the typical group. The teacher who knows about the developmental stages of a group might appreciate that a new member entering the group partway through its development could cause the group to revert temporarily to an earlier stage. Such teachers are more likely to be patient with the power struggles in the group if they understand that normal group development includes such phases.

If you choose to read about small groups, you should do so while you are teaching one, if you can. Factual information and concepts are much more likely to affect practice if they are learned in the context of practice.

STRATEGIC KNOWLEDGE (SKILLS): WHAT MUST BE LEARNED BY PRACTICE WITH FEEDBACK?

The informal and formal knowledge discussed in the preceding sections constitutes information *about* small groups. Such information can lead to an understanding of small groups, but not to the skill of leading them. Learning *how to* teach in small groups means learning skills, and the gold standard for the teaching of skills is "practice with feedback." Moreover, the closer the practice situation is to the authentic context (i.e., the context in which the skill will be used), the more likely the skill will transfer to that situation (Brown, Collins & Duguid, 1989).

Self-regulatory Strategies: Knowing How To Use Your Knowledge.

Bereiter and Scardamalia (1993) describe self-regulatory knowledge as "knowledge that controls the application of other knowledge" (p. 60). Self-regulatory strategies are vital to teachers of small groups. When disruptive behaviors push your button, you may respond with trigger reflexes that are not helpful to the learning. For example, when a group member challenges your authority, if you respond by counting to 10 and then gently attempting to clarify the challenger's point of view, you are using a self-regulatory strategy. Parker Palmer (1998) described self-regulatory strategies for dealing with the "student from hell," the one student in a class who fails to respond to your efforts. Other examples of situations requiring self-regulation come to mind easily. One is the teacher who was aware that a particular student made him angry, but was unable to do anything about it. Another is the teacher who discovered, while viewing a videotape of his teaching, that he talked most of the time, but was unaware of it.

Developing self-regulatory behavior requires reflection on one's actions (Schön, 1987). Essentially, you must become aware of your automatic responses to events to be able to substitute more desirable responses. The author and his colleagues have developed a workshop in which participants observe a role play and then disclose what they thought and felt as well as what actions they would have taken had they been in the position of teacher (Tiberius, Tipping, & Silver, 1998). They guide the discussion to help members become more aware of the vital role their feelings play in the unwitting selection of the strategies they used. Awareness of one's own feelings is the first step toward control.

Heuristic Strategies

Heuristic strategies consist of the so-called "tricks of the trade," the useful moves that, under most conditions, will help the group to achieve its learning objectives. Heuristic strategies include clarifying the topic, setting ground rules and keeping the group on track. Heuristics also consist of remedies for the common presenting problems of the group such as disruptive students, unclear objectives, and lack of interest. The most common requests for help by teachers of small groups are for such strategies. There is a book devoted entirely to presenting remedies for problems that arise in the small group (Tiberius, 1990), and another dealing specifically with small group teaching in the medical context (Westberg & Jason, 1996). Useful strategies for small group teachers have been in the published literature for decades (Abercrombie, 1971; Dimock, 1973; McGregor, 1967; McKeachie & Kulik, 1975; McLeish, Matheson, & Park, 1973; Miles, 1959; Mill, 1980; Rudduck, 1978).

At the very least, trainees should acquire skills that would enable them to carry out the basic functions of a small group leader, such as summarizing or keeping the group on track, and they should acquire a repertoire of strategies to handle problems that arise frequently. A number of highly popular and effective techniques involve the use of role play to focus on specific strategies. The likelihood that teachers actually will use a strategy rises sharply with practice. Indeed, rehearsing the words themselves is an important aspect of the training in that it puts these helpful phrases readily at the teacher's command. Without such practice, attempts to address a problem may backfire because of inappropriate language.

Diagnostic Strategies: Knowing When To Do What.

In this chapter the word "diagnosis" means the exploratory process by which the group leader can discover what is happening in the group, a broader usage than usual in a medical context. Diagnostic strategies can provide information necessary to an accurate perception of the group. Such information is essential in choosing the right teaching strategy to use at the right time. A misreading of the group that leads to an application of the wrong remedy may worsen the situation, even if the remedy were executed perfectly. To mistake an angry student for a shy one or a reflective group for a bored one can lead to remedies that worsen the dysfunctional situation.

Donald Schön (1987), in *Educating the Reflective Practitioner*, has distinguished three kinds of diagnostic processes used by teachers and other practitioners. The first is an exploratory process, a kind of playful probing, to *see what follows*, without trying to discriminate between hypotheses or predictions. The second is a process he calls *move-testing experiment*, a more deliberate action to test or try something out. The third process, *hypothesis testing,* is the experimental process used by researchers (Schön, 1987, p. 71). This latter process is seldom used to diagnose groups because in small groups there usually are too many confounding changes taking place at once to enable the teacher to isolate the effects of a particular move.

An exploratory process can be almost any action driven by a curiosity to find out what might happen rather than by a desire to test a particular move. For example, a discussion leader who senses that the discussion is stagnating might engage in one of the following two exploratory processes: call for a 10-minute break and ask members to take different seats after the break or draw a picture of the ideas on a flip chart.

Exploratory activities can provide the leader with a feel for the group and may lead to discovery of something new. Experienced group leaders, when they feel relaxed, engage in such activities regularly.

Move-testing experiments are more deliberate. For example, a discussion leader who hypothesizes that a group's silence resulted from inhibition might break the group into pairs for a while to test whether they say more when they can talk more privately. The discussion leader who hypothesizes that a group's silence results from failure to recognize a dilemma might try to sharpen the dilemma and put it to the group again. To test the hypothesis that the group has wandered, a discussion leader might want to summarize the goals and current progress of the group to see if that will rejuvenate the group discussion. It should be noted that these move-testing procedures are actions. The leader is simply doing something and observing the reactions of members. He or she is not asking members to describe how they think or feel.

It is worthwhile to invest time in creating a safe psychological climate in the group. A safe group climate fosters the kind of disclosure and openness that encourages frank and timely feedback.

IMPRESSIONISTIC KNOWLEDGE: FEELINGS AND IMPRESSIONS

Feelings are important in educational groups, not only because they influence perceptions, actions, and the climate of the group, but also because strong feelings tend to make events more memorable (Bereiter & Scardamalia, 1993). For the purposes of small group teaching, the most important function of impressionistic knowledge is that it provides the basis for intuition because intuition guides the group leader's decisions and actions.

One of the most powerful procedures for acquiring feelings and impressions is role reversal, a group training exercise in which the members switch roles partway through the exercise. In a typical procedure, one member takes the role of defending an unpopular view while the others are severely critical. After conflicts and difficulties emerge, the scenario is halted and the protagonists are asked to change seats and roles. Again, after difficulties emerge, the role players are interviewed for their insights into the feelings of the other. Such exercises almost never fail to bring out the fact that misperceptions of the feelings of others often result from an inability to reverse roles, to put oneself in the place of the other.

WHAT TRAINING WILL SMALL GROUP TEACHERS NEED IN THE FUTURE?

The use of small group teaching clearly is increasing in higher education. Its popularity is driven by current concepts of learning as an active process (Bonwell & Eison, 1991) that is inherently relational (DeVito, 1986) and social (Tiberius & Billson, 1991). The trend is reinforced in medical education by the increasing popularity of problem-based learning. The author's prediction is that, in medical schools, the need for small group teachers soon will outstrip the supply, and heavily time-pressured medical faculty are an inelastic teaching resource. The ensuing crisis will precipitate either a return to the dominance of large group teaching or to a reduction of the role of teachers in the learning group. The latter presents an exciting opportunity for small group teachers. Students could take over the leadership functions in their own small group learning. The model for doing so already exists in the rapidly growing literature on cooperative learning, as noted by Westberg and Jason (1996, p. xvi). For an excellent review of the collaborative approach applied to higher education see Millis and Cottell (1998).

What small group teaching skills will medical teachers of the future be learning? If the author's prediction comes true, they will be learning techniques that engage learners by involving them in activities rather than by heavy reliance on the teacher. Cooperative learning strategies and other active methods of learning are ideally suited to produce high learner engagement with low teacher involvement (Bonwell & Eison, 1991). The author and his colleague, Ivan Silver, have been conducting training sessions to help workshop leaders use cooperative and active learning techniques. They have been surprised by the popularity of their workshops. They review some widely known techniques such as brainstorming, buzz groups, and role-enactment, as well as problem-based and case-based learning. They also introduce techniques that are often new to our colleagues such as "think-pair-share," "helping trios," and some educational games developed by the author's colleague (Silver, 1998a; Silver, 1998b).

The "think-pair-share" procedure was developed by Frank Lyman (Millis, 1995). During the first phase of a "think-pair-share" procedure, all of the participants are engaged in thinking about a problem or question presented by the teacher. After a few minutes, participants are invited to form pairs and share the problem with their partners. During the third phase, learners can share their thoughts with larger groups or the entire workshop. This procedure not only provides a lot of floor time for everyone, but it also provides an easy route into sharing for shy or more pensive members. It gives them time to formulate their thoughts by trying them out in pairs before going public.

"Helping trios" is a particularly useful procedure for interpersonal skills training (e.g., in teaching and medical interviewing). It increases the active engagement of participants to 100%. The group divides into teams of three. One member of the team performs a procedure (e.g., giving feedback to the other) while the third observes. A checklist often aids observers. After the performance, all three participants give feedback to one another. Each player appreciates aspects of the performance that are invisible to the others. After one iteration, performers switch roles and play it again. After three turns, everyone has taken each role, and all of the triads join in a general discussion of the problems and issues involved in the targeted performance.

If, as the author has predicted, teachers of small groups substantially shift their techniques toward those that engage learners by involving them in cooperative and self-directed activities, the teachers will become facilitators of learning in two senses. They will help students learn and develop learning skills, and their students will become active, cooperative, and self-directed learners.

REFERENCES

Abercrombie, M. L. J. (1971). *Aims and techniques of group teaching.* Guildford, Surrey, England: Society for Research into Higher Education.

Bales, R. F. (1950). *Interaction process analysis.* Cambridge: Addison Wesley.

Bereiter, C., & Scardamalia, M. (1993). *Surpassing ourselves: An inquiry into the nature and implications of expertise.* Chicago: Open Court.

Bonwell, C., & Eison, J. (1991). Active learning: Creating excitement in the classroom. *ASHE-ERIC Higher Education Report No 1,* Washington, DC: The George Washington University.

Brown, J. S., Collins, A., & Duguid, P. (1989). Situated cognition and the culture of learning. *Educational Researcher, 1,* (pp. 32-42).

DeVito, J. A. (1986). Teaching as relational development. In J. M. Civikly (Ed.), *Communicating in college classrooms: New directions for teaching and learning 26,* (pp. 51-60). San Francisco: Jossey-Bass.

Dimock, H. G. (1973). *Designing and facilitating training programs.* Guelph, Ontario: Centre for Human Resources Development.

Erickson, F. (1990). Qualitative methods. *Research in Teaching and Learning, 2,* (pp. 81-86).

Jorgensen, D. L. (1989). *Participant observation: A methodology for human studies.* Newbury Park, CA: Sage.

McGregor, D. (1967). *The professional manager.* New York: McGraw-Hill.

McKeachie, W. J., & Kulik, J. A. (1975). Effective college teaching. In F. N. Kerlinger (Ed.), *Review of research in education, 3,* (pp. 67-86). Itasca, IL: Peacock.

McLeish, J., Matheson, W., & Park, J. (1973). *The psychology of the learning group.* London: Hutchinson University Library.

Miles, M. B. (1959). *Learning to work in groups: A program guide for educational leaders.* New York: Teachers College, Columbia University.

Mill, C. R. (1980). *Activities for trainers: 50 useful designs.* San Diego, CA: University Associates.

Millis, B. J. (1995). Introducing faculty to cooperative learning. In W. A. Wright (Ed.), *Teaching improvement practices: Successful strategies for higher education,* p. 5. Bolton, MA: Anker.

Millis, B. J., & Cottell, P. G. (1998). *Cooperative learning for higher education faculty.* Phoenix, AZ: Oryx Press.

Palmer, P. J. (1998). *The courage to teach: Exploring the inner landscape of a teacher's life.* San Francisco: Jossey-Bass.

Rudduck, J. (1978). *Learning through small group discussion: A study of seminar work in higher education.* Guildford, Surrey, England: Society for Research into Higher Education.

Schön D. (1987). *Educating the reflective practitioner.* San Francisco: Jossey-Bass.

Silver, I. (1998a). *Stand up and be counted: Educational game.* Unpublished manuscript, Faculty of Medicine, University of Toronto.

Silver, I. (1998b). *Do you have any fives?: Educational game.* Unpublished manuscript, Faculty of Medicine, University of Toronto.

Simpson, R. J., & Galbo, J. J. (1987). Interaction and learning: Theorizing on the art of teaching. *Interchange, 17*(4), 37-51.

Tiberius, R. G. (1990). *Small group teaching: A trouble-shooting guide.* Toronto: OISE/U of T Press.

Tiberius, R. G., & Billson, J. M. (1991). The social context of teaching and learning. In R. J. Menges & M. Svinicki (Eds.), *College teaching: From theory to practice, New directions for Teaching and Learning, 45.* (pp. 67-86). San Francisco: Jossey Bass.

Tiberius, R. G., Tipping, J., & Silver, I. (1998). *Materials to accompany a workshop on small group teaching.* Unpublished manuscript, University of Toronto Faculty of Medicine.

Walton, H. (1997). *Small group methods in medical teaching.* Medical Education Booklet No. 1. Edinburgh: World Federation for Medical Education.

Westberg, J. & Jason, H. (1996). *Fostering learning in small groups: A practical guide.* New York: Springer.

Whitman, N. A., & Schwenk, T. L. (1983). *A handbook for group discussion leaders: Alternatives to lecturing medical students to death.* Salt Lake City, UT: University of Utah, School of Medicine.

CHAPTER TEN

Feedback for Medical Education

Eileen E. Reynolds
Jack Ende
University of Pennsylvania Health System
Presbyterian Medical Center

Feedback is essential for learning medicine. It should happen all the time. It seems simple that the more experienced should inform the less experienced about what has been done well, or what might be done better the next time. It seems simple that the feedback should be frequent, objective, expected, and timely. It seems simple that students should get such feedback frequently from teachers, and that medical educators should be well practiced at giving it. However, feedback remains a significant challenge in medical education.

This chapter reviews the recent literature on feedback in medical education, proposes a structure by which feedback can be incorporated into medical education in clinical disciplines, and then discusses the essential elements of "good" feedback. The chapter also discusses the use of practice profiles, or report cards, in graduate and undergraduate education as a means of providing feedback in a highly objective, structured manner, modeled on methods of feedback used for practicing physicians by health systems and managed care organizations.

CURRENT LITERATURE

Medical students expect feedback, especially during their clinical clerkships. (Bing-You & Stratos, 1995; Gil, Heins, & Jones, 1984). However, they receive less than they think they need, both from faculty and from house staff. Residents also expect feedback, but few are satisfied with the amount they receive or its quality. In one study from a large academic center, only eight percent of the residents reported being "very satisfied" with the feedback process on the annual program evaluation, whereas 80% reported infrequently or never receiving corrective feedback (Isaacson, Posk, Liaker, & Halperin, 1995).

Why do students and residents sense that they receive inadequate feedback? There are several explanations. Both receivers and givers may be at fault. Students may deny feedback, particularly if the information is critical in a negative sense. Feedback can be difficult to hear. Medical students rely heavily on letters of recommendation from attendings, so students can take even constructive comments as harsh personal judgments (even when they are not). Most students (and residents) have no training in seeking out feedback and in interpreting it, although some programs have experimented with training programs designed to make students into expert feedback getters and takers.

In addition to being hard to receive, feedback may be hard to give, or to give well. Most faculty are not practiced at giving feedback; most have never had special training. Many attendings spend only one month per year on the ward service, and so may not have the time to give learners midmonth and end-of-month input. With the increasing number of ambulatory rotations during the third and fourth years of medical school, students often work with many preceptors during even a single week, so meaningful, ongoing feedback is rare, and responsibility for giving it often is diffused. Residents, too, spend an increasing amount of time in the ambulatory setting, but feedback often is infrequent for them as well. When residents do have the chance to work closely with attendings, the attendings often fail to give corrective feedback directly about the cases they are observing or precepting, preferring instead to use indirect corrective strategies to maintain resident autonomy and self-esteem (Ende, Pomerantz, & Erickson, 1995).

Faculty development programs can address these issues related to feedback, among other teaching skills. These programs teach the fundamentals of how to give feedback, and have faculty role play and work with videotaping to improve skills (Edwards & Marier, 1988; Skeff, 1998; Skeff, Stratos, & Mygdal, DeWalt, Manfred, et al., 1997).

However, although programs instructing teachers to give feedback have proliferated, few investigators have looked closely at what the content of the feedback should be. Several authors have proposed simplified schemes, based on the business and educational literature, about how feedback should be given, (Ende, 1993; Hewson & Little, 1996; Westberg & Jason, 1993), but only recently has any research validated hypotheses about what feedback should cover and how it should be offered.

One recent article attempted to validate prior models of giving feedback. Hewson and Little (1998) asked participants in a week-long, intensive faculty development course to write down incidents of helpful and unhelpful feedback they had been given by colleagues during the course. The study found that the helpful and unhelpful techniques were very similar to those proposed previously in the literature.

It was found that feedback is enhanced by a good interpersonal relationship, by a neutral or appropriate location, by approaching common or mutually agreed on goals, by reflecting on observed behaviors, by being nonjudgmental, and by offering feedback in the right quantity. These characteristics now identified experimentally closely mirror the techniques initially recommended in the medical literature in the 1980s, and taught in special courses for faculty and residents.

CHARACTERISTICS OF EFFECTIVE FEEDBACK

Before giving feedback, thought needs to go into its content, and into the principles that shape its delivery. Hewson and Little's (1998) work confirmed the basic principles described earlier regarding the guidelines for feedback discussions. The most important principles in giving feedback are as follows:

- *Feedback should represent shared goals that are meaningful and important for a student and faculty member.* These goals need to be agreed on in advance by both parties. If feedback is focused on areas with which the student is unconcerned, it will be ignored. Likewise, if the faculty member is unaware of the student's goals, opportunities for feedback will be missed.

- *Feedback should be expected by the learner and well-timed.* If it is expected that feedback will be part of the fabric of teaching and day-to-day interactions, it can take place in unscheduled but convenient moments that are close temporally to important incidents that require comment, either positive or negative.

- *Feedback should be based on firsthand data.* Those giving feedback need to comment directly on experiences that are observed. Feedback can be helpful only if the faculty member or feedback-giver has significant hands on experience with the actions of the trainee and reports on those behaviors. Whereas a summative evaluation of a student's or resident's progress may include comments made by others, feedback should be based directly on observed behaviors.

- *Feedback should be regulated in quantity.* Frequent small portions of feedback are preferable to infrequent, long sessions that deal with many issues. Smaller amounts often fit into unscheduled time, and so can be less threatening to the student. Limited amounts will be better remembered, less overwhelming, and more likely to lead to behavioral change. An example would be comments focused on a student's presentation to only the history or only the physical examination: "Today let's focus on the history of the present illness. In deciding what to put into the history of present illness (HPI), think about the differential diagnosis of right lower quadrant pain, and include information on your patient's pattern of pain, last menstrual period, and previous surgical history," rather than "Include more information in the HPI, such as menstrual history. Be more complete with past surgical history. Don't forget to include all the vital signs in your history. All women with pelvic pain need to have a pelvic examination performed, and also a pregnancy test checked."

- *Feedback should deal with specific performances, not generalizations.* Students need specific information on what they should improve or continue. For example, it is much more helpful to a student to be told "Your social history of the pancreatitis showed your understanding of pathophysiology and allowed us to focus more on biliary tract disease and less on alcoholism," than to be told "Your history-taking is excellent and complete."

- *Feedback should be phrased in descriptive, nonevaluative language.* An example might be "Rob, patients and staff expect to see their doctors looking professional, wearing clean white coats," not "Rob, you look unprofessional."

- *Feedback should deal with decisions and actions rather than assumed intentions or interpretations.* Do not think for the student. Deal with what has been observed directly, rather than assume that you understand the motives. For example, it would be better to say, "When you take the history, you should include a sexual history. Take it as a part of your routine history on every patient," rather than "Even though you assumed that a sexual history wouldn't be pertinent in this case, you still should have elicited one because it can relate to the etiology of rectal cancer."

A STRATEGY FOR INCORPORATING FEEDBACK INTO TEACHING

A personal system that encourages feedback, and that you institute in each teaching situation will help. A recommended strategy for making feedback part of your regular routine in teaching follows.

Setting the Stage:
The first step in giving effective feedback is to think about setting the stage to allow your learners to expect and receive feedback.

- *Create an environment conducive to feedback and discussion.* Make members of your group feel comfortable participating in discussions, and in advancing their own theories and ideas. Value the contributions of learners at every level. Avoid lecturing. Rather, open discussion with provocative questions. Show support for the answers you get, and voice your positive regard for group members.

- *Determine the learner's goals at the beginning of the rotation/experience.* Sit down with each team member or class member at the beginning of your time together. Discuss what the student plans to get out of the experience, and add to the student's goals. Consider having the student or resident put the goals in writing, so you can refer to them later on in the rotation.
- *Establish the expectation that feedback will be given throughout the rotation/experience, both informally and in scheduled, formal sessions.* Let the students and residents know that you would like to give them appropriate, even frequent, feedback based on your observations of their work. Schedule time for the middle of the rotation during which you will meet with each trainee and provide feedback, and then again for the end of the rotation. Also, let the students and residents know that you hope to work closely with them and provide feedback informally, not just during your scheduled times.
- *Invite the learner's feedback on your own performance.* Most learners will be uncomfortable commenting on the teacher's actions, but one option is to teach everyone on your team about giving feedback, and then have them practice it on each other, and on you. Inviting feedback on your own actions reinforces the view that feedback is to be desired and not feared.

Conducting the Feedback Session:

After setting the stage, the next step is to make sure that you give feedback frequently. These suggestions for scheduled sessions apply as well for feedback delivered as part of daily rounds or during moments in the office.

- *First, invite the learner's self-assessment,* both positive and negative. Having the learner refer back to goals you set together and commenting on his or her progress toward those goals is a constructive way to begin a feedback session.
- *Provide your feedback.* Remember feedback should be positive as well as negative, limited in amount, and linked to mutually agreed on goals. Expand the goals as necessary, particularly during midcourse or end-of-course feedback sessions.
- *Check for understanding throughout the discussion.* Ask the trainee to tell you what you just said in his or her own words. Make sure that he or she understands what you meant.
- *Help the learner turn negative feedback into constructive challenges.* Offer specific suggestions for ways to improve on negative points. Avoid lecturing. Make an action plan, with steps agreed on by both of you that address your constructive comments.

Follow-up:

After each session, make sure that you follow up with the learner.

- *Meet again during your time together.* Ensure that the learner has been following a plan, and that you have arranged a way to monitor his or her progress where appropriate.
- Ask for feedback on our own performance, *again.*

Using Modern Tools of Physician Assessment in Educational Settings

Traditional feedback, as shown in the preceding discussion, remains essential to the education of physicians. However, once out in practice, physicians no longer receive considered, constructive feedback of the one-on-one variety. Practicing physicians now receive practice profiles, or "report cards."

In clinical practice, report cards usually are formulated by insurance companies attempting to measure quality of care, by health systems, or even by the government. Report cards from insurance companies usually include ratings of patient satisfaction, comprehensiveness of care, accessibility, and, occasionally, clinical outcomes. Physician income, incentives, and even inclusion on managed care referral lists rely on satisfactory performance as rated on these measures.

Practice profiles usually are derived from chart audits, although in the future they will derive more and more frequently from electronic databases. Physicians must submit charts for audit annually. Then they receive a standardized report of their results compared with those of other practices and with national standards such as Health Employers Data Information Set (HEDIS) guidelines. There are many problems with these report cards: They sometimes are based on incomplete information; attempts to risk-adjust scores generally raise concerns of accuracy and reliability; and patient satisfaction information often is based on imperfect survey methods and low response rates.

However, practice profiles represent feedback in a very pure form. Practice profiles are expected by physicians (although not always welcomed!). They are based on data drawn directly from the physician's practice. The feedback is limited in quantity and focuses on specific goals and behaviors: Is there an immunization record? How many women had mammograms? What is the average glycohemoglobin?

What is the role of practice profiles in the training of residents and students? There is a small but growing literature about the use of profiling in medical education. Two studies looked at the results of giving feedback from chart audits to residents about their use of laboratory tests (Martin, Marshall, Lawrence, & Dzauv, 1980) and at the use of feedback on charting in an emergency room setting (Harchelroad, Martin, Kremen, & Murray, 1984). Both studies found that behavior changed with the feedback. A more recent study evaluated the effect of feedback to medical house staff on chart documentation and quality of care in the outpatient setting (Opila, 1997). Using a report based on HEDIS 3.0 requirements, the investigator gave periodic feedback to house staff and found that although the quality of care did not improve with the feedback (at least as they could measure it), chart documentation did improve.

However, expecting that report cards or similar instruments will change outcomes during a short clinical experience and brief period of feedback may be missing the point. For students and residents, equally pertinent outcomes are how they perceive the process; whether they appreciate that it has changed their learning, practice, or attitudes; and how it prepares them for a practice environment wherein objective profiling will be the rule, not the exception. In the authors' experience, insurance-company-modeled report cards have had a positive effect upon the practices of our primary care residents (Reynolds, Shea, Alexander, Shah, & Ende, unpublished data). The residents welcome the feedback, consider it essential to their education, and feel that it is the most reliable, objective measure of their clinical performance. They have not found the report cards to foster competition, and have not been concerned about their program director's using the information for evaluative purposes. Moreover, the authors believe the residents will be better prepared to practice in systems that rely upon outcome-based assessment.

Practice profiling of this sort should be introduced in educational settings with several caveats in mind. Students and residents have a very limited clinical experience. Report cards that are generated often will be based on small numbers of patients, limiting their generalizability. An alternative to individual report cards is group reports, in which all residents in a certain practice or residency or all students on a rotation are rated together. Using report cards requires significant resources. Charts must be reviewed, and then the data must be turned into reports, charts, or graphs. Programs may not have the person-power, time, or money to accomplish the task.

Finally, care must be taken, especially with students, to make sure that the report cards do not turn into tools for evaluation, instead of being used purely for feedback. The data simply are not robust enough to allow comparison between students, or to formulate decisions about students' overall performance. Practice profiles are, however, a powerful tool for getting the learners to examine their practice patterns and performance. The authors believe that practice profiling in medical education settings is worth the effort and may, in fact, represent a significant step forward in delivering feedback.

Feedback, be it traditional or based on practice profiling, remains central to the clinical education of students and residents. It will always involve the traditional one-on-one direct feedback that must be practiced, and hopefully will follow the aforementioned guidelines. However, as medical students move to the outpatient setting, and as the practice environment becomes more and more electronically based, teachers will want to begin to use newer tools to assist them in making their feedback objective and performance based.

REFERENCES

Bing-You, R. G., & Stratos, G. A. (1995). Medical students' needs for feedback from residents during the clinical clerkship year. *Teaching and Learning in Medicine: An International Journal, 7,* 172-176.

Edwards, J. C., & Marier, R. L. (Eds.), (1988). *Clinical teaching for medical residents: roles, techniques, and programs.* New York: Springer.

Ende, J. (1993). Feedback in clinical medical education. *Journal of the American Medical Association, 250,* 777-781.

Ende, J., Pomerantz, A., & Erickson, F. (1995). Preceptors' strategies for correcting residents in an ambulatory care medicine setting: A qualitative analysis. *Academic Medicine, 70,* 224-229.

Gil, D. H., Heins, M., & Jones, P. B. (1984). Perceptions of medical school faculty members and students on clinical clerkship feedback. *Journal of Medical Education, 59,* 856-864.

Harchelroad, F. P., Martin, M. L., Kremen, R. M., & Murray, K.W. (1984). Emergency department daily record review: A quality assurance system in a teaching hospital. *Quality Revue Bulletin, 14,* 45-49.

Hewson, M., & Little, M. (1996). Giving feedback effectively. *Medical Encounter, 12,* 2-4.

Hewson, M. G., & Little, M. L. (1998). Giving feedback in medical education: Verification of recommended techniques. *Journal of General Internal Medicine, 13,* 111-116.

Isaacson, J. H., Posk, L. K., Liaker, D. G., & Halperin, A. K. (1995). Resident perceptions of the evaluation process. *Journal of General Internal Medicine, 10,* S89.

Martin, A. R., Marshall, A. W., Lawrence, A. T., & Dzauv, B. E. (1980). A trial of two strategies to modify the test-ordering behavior of medical residents. *New England Journal of Medicine, 303,* 1330-1336.

Opila, D. A. (1997). The impact of feedback to medical housestaff on chart documentation and quality of care in the outpatient setting. *Journal of General Internal Medicine, 12,* 352-356.

Reynolds, E. E., Shea, J. A., Ende, J., Alexander, P., & Shah, S. Unpublished data.

Skeff, K. M. (1998). Enhancing teaching effectiveness and vitality in the ambulatory setting. *Journal of General Internal Medicine, 3,* S26-S33.

Skeff, K. M., Stratos, G. A., Mygdal, W., DeWitt, T. A., Manfred, L., Quirk, M., Roberts, K., Greenberg, L., & Bland, C. J. (1997). Faculty development. A resource for clinical teachers. *Journal of General Internal Medicine, 12,* S56-S63.

Westberg, J., & Jason, H. (1993). Providing constructive feedback In *Collaborate clinical education: The foundation of effective health care.* New York: Springer. 297-334.

CHAPTER ELEVEN

Instructional Technology in Medical Education

Kenneth B. Williamson
Indiana University Medical School

The field of medical education has long engaged in a love-hate relationship with computers. It is suspected that anyone with more than a few years of experience in medical education has heard--if not held--the belief that "computers are another passing fad," one that will go the way of other teaching advances such as radio, film, and television (Cuban, 1986). This does not seem to be the case, however. The call for integrating computers into the curriculum has been heard for decades (Hoffer, Barnett, Farquhar, & Prather, 1975), and continues today (Association of American Medical Colleges [AAMC], 1984; Association of American Medical Colleges, 1992). Despite warnings of unfulfilled and overexuberant expectations (Friedman, 1996, Stolurow, 1982), the use of technology in medical education continues to grow.

For example, a search of MEDLINE from 1990 to 1998 with "Computer-Assisted Instruction as the major focus returned 1,150 citations.[1] A review of the AAMC Innovations in Medical Education (IME) exhibits from 1989 to 1997 showed that exhibits featuring technology accounted for one fourth of all exhibits (368 of 1,444) during that time. Recent AAMC programs have hosted small-group discussions, miniworkshops, Research in Medical Education (RIME) abstracts sessions, and a special interest group that all focused on computer technology in medical education. The 1998 Liaison Committee on Medical Education (LCME) survey (1996-1997) showed that approximately 85% of the 125 accredited medical

---

[1] Accessed June 9, 1998 through Internet Grateful Med - http://igm.nlm.nih.gov

schools in the United States ostensibly use computer technology in the curriculum. All but three have Web sites (Medical Schools of the United States and Canada, 1998).

The magnitude of this activity attests to a strong and continuing interest in computers, yet the goal of integrating them into the curriculum remains unmet (Association of American Medical Colleges, 1992; Koschmann, 1995). Given so many applications and the recognized need for the technology, why do schools continue to brook this delay? Many factors might explain the problem, not the least of which include cost, poor design, and lack of faculty incentives. This chapter explores these issues by examining the scope of computer applications in medical education and the challenges that developers face in achieving their goal.

Scope of Instructional Technology

What is instructional technology? The term means different things to different people. To some people it refers to any machine, device, or innovation used to facilitate instruction (Cuban, 1986). Chalkboards, slide rules, and film projectors fit this definition. More recently, the term refers to the use of computers to deliver instruction. Now with the relative ubiquity of computers, the growing influence of communications, and the fact that information technology pervades most aspects of Western civilization, the appropriateness of the term "instructional technology" depends on the context.

Context Matters

To illustrate, consider a widely available program, DxR (Diagnostic Reasoning: 1998), that aims to teach clinical problem solving in a way akin to problem-based learning. The program presents a complex clinical case that the learner must "workup" by asking questions, performing simulated physical examinations, ordering laboratory tests, evaluating x-ray images, and heart and breath sounds, and generally exploring information relevant to a patient encounter. At each step in the process, the learner must generate and refine a differential diagnosis until committing to a final diagnosis. The program provides feedback on the diagnosis and records the "solution path" to a file for later review by the instructor. Most people would consider this program a good example of instructional technology.

Now imagine that the same learner sees actual patients in a clinic and must write a history and physical (H&P) on each. The student uses a computer in the student room to do the work. He opens a standard case template with a Web browser to enter the notes. The writeup is saved to a file, printed on a nearby printer, and turned in to the nurse instructor as one in a number of weekly assignments. In this case, the computer functions as a typewriter. Does its use constitute instructional technology?

Further imagine that the system forwarded the student's H&P to his mentor by way of e-mail. The mentor reviews the case at a later time, makes comments, suggests readings, and then e-mails the H&P with comments back to the student. At the same time, the case along with the mentor's comments is transferred into a database of cases that allows cases to be searched, downloaded, and made into instructional materials. Does this use constitute instructional technology?

In each example, case information is manipulated by a person using a computer. Although the goal of each action differs--solve a problem, write a report, communicate with a mentor--the technology provides the means to accomplish a task that has an educational aim. Within this context, each of these applications constitutes instructional technology.

Evolution of Educational Computing

Early instructional uses of computers generally fell into one of three basic categories: computer-assisted instruction (CAI), computer-based testing (CBT), and computer-managed instruction (CMI), that is, teaching, testing, and record-keeping applications, respectively.

Computer-Assisted Instruction (CAI)

Computer-assisted instruction refers to programs that deliver didactic presentations in a predefined sequence. The Medical Subject Heading index (MESH) used by MEDLINE defines CAI as "a self-learning technique, usually online, involving interaction of the student with programmed instructional materials." Examples of computer-delivered programmed instruction span decades of literature, beginning with mainframes, through micro-computers, to the Internet.

The key terms "programmed instruction" and "self-learning" denote the class. These programs were designed to provide one-on-one instruction using the computer to deliver a branching presentation sequence. Many developers have written programs, called authoring tools,[2] that make creating computerized programmed instruction relatively easy for those who are content experts but not programmers. History shows, however, that computerized programmed instruction, although often effective, rapidly becomes deadly boring despite interesting content, sound effects, and attention-grabbing images (Instructional Transactions in CBI, 1994).

---

[2] A review of authoring tools, including the vast array of materials created with them, goes well beyond the scope of this chapter. See the Cognitive Science branch of NLM Web site reviews of these tools at http://wwwcgsb.nlm.nih.gov/coursedb/

Computer-Based Testing (CBT)

As with CAI, developers have created software tools to facilitate common evaluation tasks. Applications of CBT use the computer to support item writing, item banking, test construction, administration and scoring, test and item analysis, and report generation (Linn, 1989).

Computer-based testing programs have proved their use in formative and summative venues along a range of applications from experimental tests to nationally standardized exams. Fortunately current CBT software is relatively inexpensive compared with its mainframe ancestors and is readily usable on a small scale with modern desktop technology.

Computer-Managed Instruction (CMI)

Computer-managed instruction refers to computer programs that organize material, monitor students' progress, help identify learning problems and prescribe interventions, generate reports, and analyze curricular content. As an instructional innovation, these programs traditionally serve administrative purposes and have little direct effect on student learning (Kulick, 1994).

In many areas of education including the health sciences, computer-managed instruction has evolved into sophisticated database systems designed to support curriculum delivery, student progress tracking, program certification and educational outcomes research.

Simulations

These programs create a representation of events that can range in breadth from discrete physiologic processes to full-blown, context-rich "microworlds." Simulations afford a learner the ability to explore systems, ask "what if" questions, and discover how the systems work. They also vary greatly in complexity (Friedman, 1995) and production cost.

Intelligent-Tutoring Systems(ITS)

A fully attentive, dedicated teacher defines the gold standard for instructional delivery. In this context, expertise connotes a person fluent with the concepts of a domain, and cognizant of common misconceptions, who can pose meaningful questions and explain difficult constructs in terms to which learners can connect.

Advances from the field of artificial intelligence attempt to program the computer to perform these very skills (Sleeman & Brown, 1982). Intelligent-tutoring systems programs (also known as intelligent CAI) are far more complex than branching programmed instruction. For example, one strategy, termed "Coaching," programs the computer to "watch" the learner and suggest paths or options during the interaction.

BEYOND SELF-INSTRUCTION: THE IMPACT OF COMMUNICATIONS TECHNOLOGY

The preceding applications cast computers in the role of an instructional delivery vehicle or a record keeper. Communications technology expands that role. Developments in audio- and video-related technologies combined with the Internet afford users interaction from different places, at different times, and with varying degrees of realism.

Almost everyone has seen a videoconference setup that uses television cameras and monitors to link distant rooms together and allow participants to see and hear one another in real time. Simpler technologies exist that allow users at a workstation to interact similarly over the Internet--at the cost of reduced resolution and speed. Electronic mail can serve as a speedier form of the traditional correspondence course, and the World Wide Web provides easy access to educational materials from almost anywhere (MacKenzie & Greenes, 1997).

When communications technology supports instruction, that use is often referred to as "distance education." Moore & Kearsley (1996, p. 2) defined "distance education" as "planned learning that normally occurs in a different place from teaching and as a result requires special techniques of course design, special instructional technologies, special methods of communication by electronic and other technologies, as well as special organizational and administrative arrangements." This definition would characterize telemedicine by substituting the doctor-patient context for teacher-student in the preceding discussion. Certainly the technologies are similar.

What then is the broader context that communications technology offers? Videoconferencing with students still has the look and feel of traditional education--only at a distance rather than in the lecture hall or clinic. Koschmann (1996) described an emerging paradigm based on an appreciation of the social factors that influence learning. Termed "computer-supported collaborative learning" (CSCL), these approaches use communications and computer technology to provide a context within which participants can engage in coordinated problem solving efforts. Whether delivering didactics or facilitating collaboration, communications technology used to support educational aims fits within the scope of instructional technology.

WHAT'S IN A NAME

Note that the different categories of instructional technology described in the preceding discussion are not mutually exclusive. Multiple functions can exist in a single system. Imagine an instructional program in the area of fluid and electrolyte balance that begins with a classic rule-example-practice sequence (Merrill, 1994). The program might present a general introduction to the concept of hyponatremia (rule), provide some prerequisite information, and then describe several cases that illustrate how the condition may present (example). The learner then practices solving routine hyponatremia cases, with the computer providing corrective feedback (practice). Afterward, the learner explores a "computerized patient" that presents with fluid and electrolyte disorders (simulation) and must experiment with various fluid orders to explore how the body's systems behave. Finally, the program administers a test to assess what the student learned (CBT), the results of which are automatically transferred into the student's progress record (CMI) and e-mailed to the student's preceptor, who comments on the performance through return e-mail (distance education).

The way an author chooses to characterize (i.e., name his or her program) depends on the content material, the presentation sequence, the pedagogical intent, and the particular technology used. A program can be denoted as case-based, inquiry-based, problem-based, assessment, didactic, or exploratory depending on what information is available as well as when and how the user interacts with it. Computers can be programmed to administer, adapt, aid, assist, assess, bridge, coach, engage, evaluate, instruct, integrate, interact, manage, mediate, present, simulate, test, and/or tutor a learner depending on what the author wants to accomplish.

The learner can interact with the program through any combination of text, graphics, images, sound, video, and touch. By way of that interaction, the learner can access, author, calculate, interpret, compare, contrast, classify, synthesize, integrate, explain, predict, explore, identify, define, recognize, remember, solve, and so on through a range of observable or inferable behaviors depending on the tasks imposed by the program designer.

During this interaction, the sensory information presented by the computer, often referred to as media, conveys the content of the domain under instruction. When several media are included in a single presentation, particularly sound and video, the term multimedia typically is used. Unfortunately, most people confuse content and media in an instructional program. With all due respect to Marshall McLuhan, the medium is not the message; it is what carries the message. Clark (1983) argued that the characteristics of the message determine learning, not the vehicle that delivers it. Interestingly, the computer's ability to present media in ways that parallel human cognition may further confound this distinction (Mishra, Spiro, & Feltovich, 1996).

COMPUTER APPLICATIONS IN MEDICAL EDUCATION

Computers have become a common appliance in medical schools, not as ubiquitous as beepers or telephones, but readily available to those who seek them out. More than 75% of medial schools report using computers in the curriculum (LCME Annual Medical School questionnaire, 1996-1997). Whereas this section cites mere handsful of these applications, the quantity found in the literature casts doubt on any assertion that little software is available.

Annotated Atlases and Electronic Texts

Computerized image atlases and electronic textbooks comprise a widely developed resource for courses such as gross anatomy (Animated Dissection of Anatomy for Medicine [ADAM], 1998); Interactive Atlas of Human Anatomy, 1998); Seymour, Messer, Thomas, & Pages, 1997 neuro anatomy (Johnson, Wynne, & Alves, 1994; Pearson, Barnett & Matthews, 1997; Webber, Osborn, Stensaas, Burrows, Wald, et. al., 1995 pathology (Trelstad, 1998), histology (Keyboard Histology Resources, 1998), physiology (Lilienfeld & Broering, 1994), and surgery (Jameson, Hobsley, Buckton, & O'Hanlon, 1995). The text-editing and graphics abilities of the computer provide a simple means for adding legends and overlays to images. Hypertext functions allow students to link to definitions, elaborative text, and references, and to browse topics from multiple perspectives. Although these applications have an intuitive appeal to many technophiles, they are sometimes criticized as expensive substitutes for a textbook. Some developers have argued that enough are available that no more need to be made. Criticisms aside, however, atlases and electronic texts are relatively easy to develop, and they afford search, navigation, and self-testing abilities that books cannot provide.

Programmed Instruction and Tutorials

The computer can provide substantial pedagogy along with images. Content authors have developed instruction on many visual topics by linking instructional text to images and by programming a logical (e.g., simple to complex) presentation sequence. Recent examples include instructional programs in gross anatomy (Brinkley, Sundsten, Eno, & Rosse, 1998; Nieder & Nagy, 1997), clinical chemistry (Hooper, Price, Cheesmar, & O'Connor, 1995), pathology (Borowsky & Gray, 1997; Gray & Sowter, 1995), radiology (Cooper & McCandless, 1996), microbiology (Inglis, Kwok-Chan, & Fu, 1995), fluid balance (Stewart, 1995), histology (Downing, 1995), and fiberoptic intubation (Katz, Sorten, Popitz, & Pearlman, 1997). Such programs also have been used effectively in clinical training as preoperative tutorials (Hong, Regehr, & Reznick, 1996).

Programmed instruction with images can be rapidly developed by using authoring tools. For example the Virgil Project (Borowsky & Gray, 1997) used medical students to develop lessons under faculty supervision. In a short time, the computer-based materials completely supplanted the slide carousels with handouts used in the second-year pathology course.

A preprogrammed sequence does not require a computer, however. Downing (1995) created a multimedia histology laboratory manual that uses a textbook and bar-code reader. The computer merely reads the codes and displays images.

With the increasing popularity of World Wide Web browser technology, many authors have created content browsers that allow learners to peruse content of their own choosing. Content browsers typically are less structured than programmed instruction and may include topic presentations, case presentations, or a mix of both. Current examples of content browsers include those for pathology (Cooper & McCandless, 1996), emergency medicine (Savitt & Steele, 1997) and dermatology (Bittorf, Diepgen, & Krejci-Papa, 1995). Simple case browsers reside on the Internet in areas such as nuclear medicine (Wallis, Miller, Miller, & Vreeland, 1995), emergency medicine (University of Texas, 1999) and radiology (McEnery, Roth, & Walkup, 1996). One also can find "integrated systems" (Ivanovic, Koethe, & Krogull, 1997; Khonsari & Fabri, 1997) that provide materials linked across disciplines, disease processes, and time.

Simulations

Simulations used in medical education typically present biologic processes (e.g., muscle [Maw, Greig, & Frank, 1996] and respiratory [Kaye, Metaxas, & Primiano, 1995] physiology) or clinical experiences. Computer-based clinical simulations have evolved from text-oriented presentations to multimedia-based systems over the past two decades. Such systems can be quite complex and multidimensional in scope (Friedman, 1995; Meller, 1997; Mihalas, Lungeanu, Kigyosi, & Vernic, 1995). For example, case simulations such as DxR and PlanAlyzer represent elaborate case constructions designed to teach clinical reasoning. Less complex designs such as Short Rounds present cases as a simulated medical record.[3]

Despite advances in authoring procedures (Berger & Boxwala, 1995), complex case simulations are expensive and time consuming to produce (Meller, 1997). Researchers at Stanford University (Felciano & Dev, 1994) are attempting to overcome this problem by building simulators that take input from existing patient records, thereby shortening case development time.

Even multimedia simulations suffer from low fidelity (i.e., realism of the encounter). Wofford and Wofford (1997) argued that any case simulation will always be only a partial representation of an actual patient encounter. Developments in virtual reality (VR) promise to improve the fidelity limitations. Hoffman and Vu

---

[3] Many examples of case presenters reside on the World Wide Web. For a listing of some of these resources, see http://www.siumed.edu/sig/new/ aamc97/cases.html, accessed June 15, 1998.

(1997, p. 1076) defined VR as "a highly interactive and dynamic form of simulation in which a computer generated world . . . can be entered and . . . explored using visual, aural, and haptic (touching) senses." These systems convey to the learner a sense of presence through high resolution, stereoscopic display, and real-time interactivity with the environment.

Developments in image guided surgery have contributed to VR's emergence in medical and surgical education. The image display and manipulation tools used in this discipline, along with ready access to high-quality video, prompted developers to apply VR to simulate exploring body spaces (Weidemann, Hohn, Hiltner, Tochtermann, Tresp, et. al, 1997), arthroscopy (Muller, Soldner, Bauer, & Ziegler, 1995), laparoscopy (Ota, Keller, Lea, Saito, & Loftin, 1995), and endoscopy (Dumay & Jense, 1995; Noar, 1995). However, the challenges inherent in developing realistic patient and sensory models render surgical simulation a complex and difficult goal to attain.

For example, realistic representation of hands-on experience tends to defy most computer simulations, whereas the use of physical models for procedural training is commonplace (Norman & Wilkins, 1996). Combining these technologies into mannequin-based[4] simulators such as SAM (Tome & Fletcher, 1996) and HARVEY has enabled more realistic tactile response.

Recent advances in tactile feedback address the fidelity issue in limited ways. Haptic technology refers to computer input devices that allow the user to sense shape, texture and other tactile cues through touch. An interesting example is the endoscopic sinus surgery simulator (Edmond, Heskamp, Sluis, Stredney, Sessanna, et al., 1997) that allows trainees to progress through increasingly complex skill levels in a realistic virtual environment. The "novice" model trains basic instrument and navigation skills, the intermediate model adds complexity and other sensory cues, and the "expert" model requires unassisted performance. Each model presents realistic and progressively more complex tactile cues. Many developers are exploring this technology.

Computerized Testing

Few would deny that computer technology affords testing capabilities that conventional tests cannot match (Linn, 1989). Graphics and images are simple to display and much easier to create and edit on computer than with film or paper. Sound and video stimuli are awkward at best to present in conventional ways. Technology's ability to deliver complex branching presentations, measure item response times, and immediately score and report results makes the limits of paper and pencil tests acutely clear.

---

[4] Readers can find an illuminating description of mannequin-based anesthesiology simulators at the Washington University Anesthesiology site (*http://medinfo.wustl.edu/~anesthes/* A list of other simulators resides at http://weber.u.washington.edu/~anesoft/index. html

HOW HAS THIS TECHNOLOGY BEEN
USED IN MEDICAL EDUCATION?

The most common use of computerized testing is in formative testing, that is, practice tests and self-quizzes. According to AAMC data (LCME Annual Medical School questionnaire, 1996-1997), 82% of schools provide banks of multiple-choice or other item formats for student self-evaluation. Examples of practice tests can be found easily at conference exhibits (Downing, 1995; Fawcett & Vincent, 1997; Frisby, Jensh, & Braster, 1998) and on the Web (Rathe, Cornwall, & Lin, 1997). Others have developed similar instruments for course and clerkship evaluation (Winter & Jones, 1997; Deretchin, Wheeler, & Jefferson, 1997).

The most notable new development in this area is computerized adaptive testing (CAT), a strategy based on advances in test development, psychometrics, computer technology, and 30 years of research (Wainer, 1990). The technique allows the computer to adapt the test to the learner by dynamically choosing test items more closely matched in difficulty to the ability of the examinee, thereby improving test efficiency over conventional tests.

Recently, CAT achieved prominence in our field when the National Board of Medical Examiners adopted the technology for the United States Medical Licensing Examination (USMLE). In addition to the aforementioned advantages, this move benefits students by making the examination more convenient, timely, and accessible (why CBT is being used). It also increases the urgency for schools to integrate computerized testing into their curricula.

Computers can facilitate evaluation in more ways than improving multiple-choice tests. New developments use simulation and testing technology together for assessing performance (Downs, Friedman, Marasigan, & Gartner, 1997). Some developers use complex case simulations to assess diagnostic and patient management skills that cannot be evaluated through either conventional or adaptive testing (Orr & Clyman, 1997; Woolridge, 1995; Costello, Mann, & Dane, 1997).

CURRICULUM INFORMATION SYSTEMS

Straightforward CMI continues to prove useful for many schools. Systems such as McMaster's (DeGara, Baillie, Thomas, Cougler, & Birch, 1997). Surgical residency tracking database are familiar to most program directors. Web technology also has made its mark: student "home pages" (Binder, Manheim, & McAuley, 1997) containing syllabi, schedules, calendars, handbooks, instructional materials, and links to other important, even cross-institutional (LectureLinks) sites have become almost routine on the Internet.

Other developers apply database technology more broadly to curriculum design. Curriculum information systems (CIS) have evolved largely to help schools facilitate curriculum reform, in part related to LCME accreditation requirements.[5] Attendees at the 1994 Innovations in Medical Education (IME) exhibits had the opportunity to view several approaches to curriculum database design (Conlon, Asman, Werner, & Hoe, 1994; Eisner, 1994; Mann & Nowacek, 1994; Mattern, Anderson, Wagner, Fisher-Neenan, & Dabney, 1994; Rawitch, 1994). Each design provided tools for documenting, analyzing, summarizing, searching, and/or displaying curriculum content in various ways. Friedman and Nowacek (1995) distinguished among designs on the basis of whose needs the system was optimized to serve: administration, faculty, or students. They argued that no single system can serve the purposes of each group effectively. Mattern, in collaboration with the AAMC, developed the first "national" curriculum database that will allow direct comparisons among medical school curricula over time (Salas & Anderson, 1997).

CHALLENGES TO DEVELOPING AND IMPLEMENTING INSTRUCTIONAL TECHNOLOGY

Given the breadth and apparent availability of instructional technology, why have schools seemingly failed to integrate it into the curriculum? The following section explores some of the issues.

Hardware Costs and the Obsolescence Problem

Schools have long known of the need to provide accessible computer technology to students, yet it appears that schools cannot or will not provide sufficient access. One important reason concerns cost: Computers are expensive to purchase, to maintain, and to support well. Traditionally, education has ranked lower in priority than other activities in medicine, particularly in the light of shrinking research funding and the realities of managed care. However, without sufficient access to and support for computers, students cannot use them effectively.

On the surface, the cost point might be disputed: A basic computer costs less than $3,000, not much in the grand scheme of things. This represents a mere fraction of the total cost of ownership, however. Software can cost from 10% to more than 100% of the workstation price. Workstations require periodic upgrades, such as new software, memory, hard drive, and the occasional keyboard replacement to remain useful. This can add 10% to 20% of the purchase cost per year.

Novice users require initial training and intermittent support to use the technology effectively. One full-time employee for each 100 clients appears to be the rule of thumb. The cost of network support, printers, accessories, and supplies can match the workstation cost each year, making the total cost of owning a $3,000 workstation $10,000 to $12,000 over its life span (Weissman, 1990).

---

[5] Al Salas, AAMC, personal communication.

Technology currently advances at a rate that roughly doubles processing power each year (Moore's law). New software that requires new processors follow soon thereafter (Parkinson's law). This progress leads to a "buyers dilemma": whether to get a deal on soon-to-be underpowered hardware, to pay more for "state of the art," or to wait for the new models to arrive in the next few months. As a result, administrators have become frustrated with the unexpected continuing costs and the struggle to fund the technology that students need.

Some schools have considered leasing computer equipment, shifting the costs to the operating budget,[6] and thus paying the leasing company to handle the problem. About 20% of schools have shifted some of the costs to students by requiring a computer purchase when entering the school (LCME Annual Medical School questionnaire, 1996-1997; McAuley, 1998). Some find this solution objectionable, arguing that the infrastructure is the schools' responsibility.

A further complication involves setting standards. Schools must consolidate purchases to realize economies of scale. Whereas desktop computers suit home or laboratory use, laptops afford portability, and less obtrusive palmtops find favor during clinical rotations (Rathe, 1988). Managing these change-overs effectively requires creative and persistent administrative support. New more powerful machines should go to the users who need faster processors, moving lower power machines to less intensive users. Students should shift to portability when they reach their clinical years. As machines approach the end of their life cycle, medical schools should donate them to K-12 schools that do not have sufficient hardware, an ideal that recalls the "trickle-down" economics of the 1980's.

Infrastructure and Access Issues

Infrastructure connotes the basic facilities and equipment needed for a functioning organization. For computing, infrastructure refers to the availability of key services, the reliability of those services, and the extent to which the services have support staff. Many schools do not or cannot maintain the workstations and network, nor can they provide sufficient training, troubleshooting, and technical help for users to work effectively.

Fortunately for medical education, the economics of telemedicine may ameliorate this problem. The infrastructure needed to support telemedicine can sustain all but the most esoteric instructional applications. As medical centers develop telemedicine capabilities, the infrastructure they create will leverage technology into the curriculum (Clark, 1992).

---

[6] Robert Rubeck, University of Kentucky, personal communication.

Development Costs

Assuming that students have access to machines, they also need access to relevant software. If no acceptable materials are available, instructors will have to develop them. This is an expensive activity. Developer workstations often require additional memory, power, input, and display capabilities as well as specialized and expensive software (Hardin & Reis, 1997).

The production of quality instructional materials requires specialized skills including not only the skills of a content expert, but often those of a programmer, medical illustrator, graphic artist, video editor, and instructional designer, plus special equipment and production arrangements depending on the scale of the project (Mooney & Bligh, 1997).

Few researchers report data on development costs (Keane, Norman, & Vickers, 1991), although strategies for effectively managing those costs have appeared (Cimino, Reichel, & Serrano, 1995). However you view it, the required mix of skills and advanced technology multiplies the cost of software development.

Copyright and the Quest For Funding

Some schools attempt to recover their development costs by selling their materials. Most educators have seen developers promoting their software at meetings, through consortia[7] or commercial publishers,[8] all with varying degrees of success. It generally is felt that no one will become rich selling instructional software. Those that do well have managed to expand beyond the medical school market.

Barter would seem a practical approach for schools. Given the high cost of development, sharing software through consortia arrangements appears to be a reasonable solution. However, this approach also has met with mixed results. Copyright concerns and the ensuing contract delays make much of the software too expensive or obsolete by the time it becomes available.

The Generalizability Problem or the "Not Invented Here" Syndrome

A further impediment to sharing revolves around the extent to which instructional materials developed in one context can be generalized to another. One would think

---

[7] Links to instructional technology consortia in the health sciences include the following:
- Informatics in Medical Education and Development (IMED): *http://meded.com.com.uci. edu/IMED/(IME1994)*
- Health Sciences Library Consortium (HSLC): *http://hslc.org/*
- North East Medical School Consortium (NEMSC) (IME1990), now defunct: *http://camis.stanford.edu/projects/triad.html*

[8] See IME exhibits for lists of commercial publishers.

that an effective teaching program would be useful to students at any school regardless where it was developed. With many schools developing materials for different parts of the curriculum, broad coverage would eventually be obtained. Again, reality falls short of the ideal.

At trade shows and developer meetings, one can overhear comments such as this: "That's interesting, but it's not the way I teach it," or "That program covers too much/too little. It's okay for residents/nursing students, but not for my course," or "I cover the topics in a different order and this will confuse my students," and so on through a litany of criticisms.

Frequently termed the "not invented here" (NIH) syndrome, this phenomenon refers to the tendency of people not to support innovations they have not had a hand in creating. The NIH Syndrome may be more a symptom than a cause, however. Cuban and Tyack (1995) argued that many technology initiatives do not succeed because developers fail to accommodate the expectations and needs of faculty (i.e., the grammar of school). As frustrating as NIH may be to technophiles, the phenomenon illustrates the complexity of integrating technology into the curriculum. It is as much a social challenge as a technological one.

Lack of Institutional Incentives

It is generally believed that faculty are not rewarded for their efforts in developing instructional materials. Except for a few "leading-edge institutions," software authoring ranks lower than research or other scholarly activity for promotional reviews (Bader, 1993). This perception stems from the fact that instructional materials do not receive the same level of peer review as other types of scholarly publications. Although software evaluation protocols exist (Glenn, 1996; Huber & Giuse, 1995; Posel, 1993) as well as collaborative efforts to accomplish peer review (AV-Line; Task Force on Medical Education Software Resources), software development ranks on a par with teaching at best. Clearly, software authoring is a labor of love.

The Effectiveness Question

Try a simple experiment. At your next conference, ask any program author whether he or she has been asked, "How do you know that students learn from your programs? Is it really any better than traditional instruction?" Most will take a deep breath, maybe roll their eyes, and agree. The author calls this the ubiquitous effectiveness question. It is asked not only by skeptical faculty, but also by administrators who must find ways to fund development. They ask this question with good reason: Technology is expensive, and the investment must be worth the cost.

Fortunately, plenty of evidence suggests that it works. Decades of research on instructional technology shows that it helps students learn. Kulik (1994, p. 26) stated: "Meta-analysts have demonstrated repeatedly that programs of computer-based instruction usually have positive effects on student learning. This conclusion has emerged from too many separate meta-analyses to be considered controversial."

Kulik's conclusion does not mean that all effectiveness studies show positive results. Simply providing technology to students does not necessarily help them learn. Clark (1992) argued that the instructional design of the material (i.e., the instructional methods embedded in the program and whether those methods are appropriate for the objectives and the students) has far more impact on learning than the fact that the computer delivers it.

Poorly designed, implemented, or supported technology has no effect at best. However, well-designed, integrated, and supported material does help learning, sometimes despite students' perceptions to the contrary (Richardson, 1997).

Computer Literacy

An artisan's fluency with the tools largely determines the quality of the work. In the same way, learners must achieve some fluency with a computer to realize its benefit. This holds true for teaching programs, authoring tools, productivity packages, collaborative learning systems--any computer tool. In a small group learning venue, for example, each participant needs to use the tools well enough to interact effectively. Most schools address this need by providing a facility where students, faculty, and staff can learn to use technology. Typical sessions include reading and sending e-mail, browsing the Web, searching the medical literature, creating a slide presentation, or using any number of other applications. Schools that develop instructional technology typically have staff who teach faculty to use authoring tools and other resources.

There is one often overlooked point about computer literacy, however. It does not simply mean teaching people to use the tools, but also concerns design--the tools need to be easier to use. For example, an elaborate clinical simulation makes an ineffective teaching tool when the only people who can use it are the programmers who developed it. In the same way, collaborative tools must facilitate interactions among people. The tools cannot require so much effort to learn or use that potential collaborators reject them. Norman (1993, p. 2) argued that technology should conform to people, not the other way around. On his Web page he stated:

> In this new age of portable, powerful, fully communicating tools, it is ever more important to develop a humane technology, one that takes into account the needs and capabilities of people. The technical problems are relatively easy. It is the people part that is hard: The social, psychological, cultural, and political problems are the ones that are the most difficult--and the most essential--to address.

This point should hit home for developers. We must concern ourselves as much with how students and faculty use our programs as with what information we put into them.

CONCLUSION

The preceding review cuts a rather broad swath through the literature on instructional technology in medical education. In the process it is hoped that it provides insight into the problems that medical schools face. One should infer from this that schools need to create certain conditions for initiatives with technology to succeed (Cuban, 1986). As we move into the 21st century, the author believes we need to focus on three main areas: infrastructure, incentives, and student engagement.

First, schools must develop adequate infrastructure to support educational technology. This means several things. It means that they must provide sufficient, conveniently accessible workstations that are kept current in form and function as technology evolves. The networks that connect workstations must support useful services and be reliably maintained. A computer crash during a presentation would rankle any clinical professor. Finally, there must be sufficient people support. When things do go wrong, competent help must be readily available.

Second, faculty must invest in the technology. They must see how it will benefit them and their students, and they must have a hand in selecting or developing it. Resources must be provided to help faculty author materials or modify existing materials to meet their needs. Technology initiatives must have administrative support. Faculty must be encouraged to develop materials, and incentives must accrue to those who do. This holds true particularly for junior faculty with regard to promotion. However, initiatives cannot convey the sense of a "top-down directive." That perception creates resistance. Instead, "grass-roots" initiatives should be supported.

Finally, students must see the advantage of using the technology, that it helps them learn, gives them access to information they need, or makes it possible to do what they require. Instructional technology must be well integrated into courses. More than simply corresponding to course objectives, the materials should be "required," and students should know that they will be tested over the content. Supplemental software for students to use "if they want to" rarely sees the light of the CRT.

Overall, the use of technology must become part of the culture of things. Faculty, students, administrators, and staff must be encouraged to change their focus away from the computer per se, that is, the appliance, and toward what the appliance can help one do. These are the problems the author believes must be adequately addressed for medical schools to truly integrate technology into the curricula.

REFERENCES

A.D.A.M. Interactive Anatomy. (1998). http://www.adam.com/

Association of American Medical Colleges. (1984). *Physicians for the twenty-first century*. The GPEP Report, Report of the Panel on the General Professional Education of the Physician and College Preparation for Medicine.

Association of American Medical Colleges. (1992). *ACME-TRI Report. Educating medical students: Assessing change in medical education--the road to implementation.* Washington, DC.

AV-Line. http://www.nlm.nih.gov/pubs/factsheet/online databases.html#avline.

Bader, S. A. (1993). Are computer-based educational materials recognized as publications? An analysis of promotion documents at American medical colleges. *Proceedings of the Annual Symposium on Computer Applications, Medical Care,* pp. 747-751.

Berger, R. G., & Boxwala, A. (1995). Multimedia medical case authorship and simulator program. *Medinfo, 8,* Pt 2:1693.

Binder, L., Manheim, M., & McAuley, R. (1997). The student affairs home page at the UIC College of Medicine at Chicago, 53. *Annual Meeting, Association of American Medical Colleges,* Washington DC: AAMC.

Bittorf, A., Diepgen, T. L., & Krejci-Papa, N. C. (1995). Development of a dermatological image atlas with worldwide access for the continuing education of physicians. *Journal of Telemedicine Telecare, 1,* 45-53.

Borowsky, A., & Gray, G. (1997). Virgil pathology lessons: Over 50 HyperCard stacks with photos and animations fill a CD for second-year pathology students. *Proceedings Slice of Life.* Chicago: The Virgil Project. http://www.mc.Vanderbilt.Edu/adl/virgildescription.html

Brinkley, J., Sundsten, J., Eno, K., & Rosse, C. (1998). *Anatomy browser for the digital anatomist.* http://www.nnlm.nlm.nig.gov/pnr/b2b/b2bbrow.html.

Cimino, C., Reichel J., & Serrano, M. (1995). Cost efficient management of educational material. *Proceedings Annual Symposium Computer Applications, Medical Care,* pp. 493-497. Bethesda, MD: American Medical Informatics Association.

Clark, R. E. (1983). Reconsidering research on learning from media. *Review of Educational Research., 53,* 445-460.

Clark, R. E. (1992). Dangers in the evaluation of instructional media. *Academic Medicine, 67,* 819-820.

Conlon, M., Asman, S., Werner, E., & Hoe, R. (1994). *A data base program for tracking medical school curricula, 62.* Annual Meeting, Association of American Medical Colleges, Washington DC.

Cooper, J. A., & McCandless, B. K. (1996). Development of cross-platform computer-based tutorial. *Canadian Journal of Surgery, 39,* 221-224.

Costello, W. J., Mann, D. D., & Dane, P. B. (1997). Computer case simulations for student evaluation in a PBL track. *Academic Medicine, 72,* 416.

Cuban, L. (1986). *Teachers and machines: The classroom use of technology since 1920.* New York: Teacher's College Press.

Cuban, L., & Tyack, D. (1995). *Tinkering toward utopia: A century of public school reform.* Cambridge, MA: Harvard University Press.

De Gara, C., Baillie, F., Thomas, E., Cougler, K., & Birch, D. (1997). *Computerizing a surgical residency,* (p. 71). Annual Meeting, Association of American Medical Colleges, Washington DC.

Deretchin, L. F., Wheeler, D. A., & Jefferson, L. S. (1997). A Web-based evaluation system. *Academic Medicine, 72,* 418-419.

Downing, S. W. (1995). A multimedia-based histology laboratory course: Elimination of the traditional microscope laboratory. *Medinfo, 8,* 1695.

Downs, S. M., Friedman, C. P., Marasigan, F., & Gartner, G. (1997). A decision analytic method for scoring performance on computer-based patient simulations. *American Medical Information Association Proceedings,* Nashville, TN.

Dumay, A. C., & Jense, G. J. (1995). Endoscopic surgery simulation in a virtual environment. *Computing Biology, 25,* 139-148.

DxR - Diagnostic Reasoning. http://www.kpub.com/catpage/catalogpageidcfindid11.htm.

Edmond, C. V., Heskamp, D., Sluis, D., Stredney, D., Sessanna, D., Wiet, G., Yagel, R., Weghorst, S., Oppenheimer, P., Miller, J., Levin, M., Rosenberg, L. (1997). ENT Endoscopic surgical training simulator. In: K. S. Morgan (Ed.), *Medicine meets virtual reality: Global healthcare grid,* (pp. 518-528). Amsterdam, The Netherlands: IOS Press.

Eisner, J. (1994). *Curriculum analysis tools (CATs) for medical education, 61.* Annual Meeting, Association of American Medical Colleges, Washington DC.

Fawcett, B., & Vincent, D. (1997). *Exam Master Corporation,* (p. 56). Annual Meeting, Association of American Medical Colleges, Washington DC.

Felciano, R. M., & Dev, P. (1994). *Multimedia clinical simulation based on patient records:* Authoring, user interface, pedagogy, (pp. 59-63). *Proceedings Annual Symposium Computer Applications.* Medical Care: American Medical Information Association.

Friedman, C. P. (1995). Anatomy of the clinical simulation. *Academic Medicine, 70,* 205-209.

Friedman, C. P. (1996). Top ten reasons the World Wide Web may fail to change medical education. *Academic Medicine, 71,* 979-981.

Friedman, C. P., & Nowacek, G. (1995). Issues and challenges in the design of curriculum information systems. *Academic Medicine, 70,* 1096-1100.

Frisby, A., Jensh, R., & Braster, C. (1998). Microscopic anatomy: Atlas CD-ROM for tutorial, course supplement and self-assessment. *Proceedings Slice of Life Workshop,* Tampa, FL.

Glenn, J. (1996). A consumer-oriented model for evaluating computer-assisted instructional materials for medical education. *Academic Medicine, 71,* 251-255.

Gray, E., & Sowter, C. (1995). The home tutor: A new tool for training in microscope skills. *Annals of Cellular Pathology, 9,* 179-189.

Hardin, P. C., & Reis, J. (1997). Interactive multimedia software design: Concepts, process, and evaluation. *Health Education Behavior, 24,* 35-53.

Hoffer, E. P, Barnett, G. O., Farquhar B. B., & Prather, P. A. (1975). Computer-aided instruction in medicine. *Annual Review of Biophysics and Bioengineering, 4*(00), 103-118.

Hoffman, H., & Vu, D. (1997). Virtual reality: teaching tool of the twenty-first century? *Academic Medicine, 72,* 1076-1081.

Hong, D., Regehr, G., & Reznick, R. K. (1996). The efficacy of a computer-assisted preoperative tutorial for clinical clerks. *Canadian Journal of Surgery, 39,* 221-224.

Hooper, J., Price, C. P., Cheesmar R., & O'Connor, J. (1995). Tutorial software for clinical chemistry incorporating interactive multimedia clinical cases. *Clinical Chemistry, 41,* 1345-1348.

Huber, J. T., & Giuse, N. B. (1995). Educational software evaluation process. *Journal of American Medical Information Association, 2*(5), 295-296.

Inglis, T. J., Kwok-Chan, L., & Fu, B. (1995). Teaching microbiology with hypertext: First steps towards a virtual. *Medical Education, 29,* 393-396.

Instructional Transactions in CBI: A Discussion and Application of Merrill's Definition. (1994). http://itech1.coe.uga.edu/itforum/paper2/paper2.html.

Ivanovic, B., Koethe, S., & Krogull, S. (1997). Computer applications in medical education. *Academic Medicine, 72,* 415-416.

Jameson, D. G., Hobsley, M., Buckton, S., & O'Hanlon, P. (1995). Broadband telemedicine: Teaching on the information superhighway. *Journal of Telemedicine Telecare, 1*(2), 111-116.

Johnson, C., Wynne, R., & Alves, T. (1994). *Silverplatter education, multimedia accelerated learning, p. 213.* Annual Meeting, Association of American Medical Colleges, Boston.

Katz, D. B., Sorten, G. D., Popitz, M., & Pearlman, J. D. (1997). The development of a multimedia teaching program for fiberoptic intubation. *Journal of Clinical Monit, 13,* 287-291.

Kaye, J., Metaxas, D., Primiano, F. P., Jr. (1995). Anatomical and physiological simulation for respiratory mechanics. *Journal of Image Guide Surgery, 1,* 164-171.

Keane, D. R., Norman, G. R., & Vickers, J. (1991). The inadequacy of recent research on computer-assisted instruction. *Academic Medicine, 66,* 444-448.

Keyboard Histology Resources. (1998). http://www.kpub.com/_catpage/ onlinecatalog prodidc findid2. html.

Khonsari, L., & Fabri, P. (1997). *Distributive integration of medical informatics into the medical curriculum,* (p. 69). Annual Meeting, Association of American Medical Colleges, Washington DC.

Koschmann, T. (1995). Medical education and computer literacy: Learning about, through, and with computers. *Academic Medicine, 70*, 68-71.

Koschmann, T. (1996). Paradigm shifts and instructional technology: An introduction. *CSCL: Theory and Practice of an Emerging Paradigm,* (pp. 1-28). Hillsdale, NJ: Erlbaum.

Kulick, J. A. (1994). Meta-analytic studies of findings on computer-based instruction, (pp. 9-33). In E. Baker, & H. O'Neil, (Eds.), *Technology assessment in education and training.* Hillsdale, NJ: Erlbaum.

LectureLinks. (1999). http://omie.med.jhmi.edu/LecutreLinks.

Linn, R. I. (1989). Current perspectives and future directions. In R.L. Linn (Ed.), *Educational Measurement,* (3rd ed., pp. 1-10). New York: Macmillan.

MacKenzie, J. D., & Greenes, R. A. (1997). The World Wide Web: Redefining medical education. *Journal of American Medical Association, 278*, 1785-1786.

Mann, D., & Nowacek, G. (1994). *Curriculum data bases With full text and images, p. 63.* Annual Meeting, Association of American Medical Colleges, Washington DC.

Mattern, W., Anderson, M., Wagner, J., Fisher-Neenan, L., & Dabney, D. (1994). *Medical school curriculum databases: Update on the AAMC prototype,* (p. 64). Annual Meeting, Association of American Medical Colleges, Washington, DC.

Maw, S., Greig, G., & Frank, J. (1996). A spinal circuitry simulator as a teaching tool for neuromuscular physiology. *American Journal of Physiology, 270*, S50-S68.

McAuley, R. J. (1998). Requiring student to have computers: Questions for consideration, *Academic Medicine, 73*, 669-673.

McEnery, K. W., Roth, S. M., & Walkup, R. V. (1996). Radiology CME on the Web using secure document transfer and internationally distributed image servers, (pp. 37-40). *Proceedings of the American Medical Informatics Association Annual Fall Symposium.*

Medical Schools of the United States and Canada. (1998). http://www.aamc.org/meded/ medschls/start.html

Meller, G. (1997). A typology of simulators for medical education, *Journal of Digital Imaging, 10,* 194-196.

Merrill, M. (1994). *Instructional design theory.* Englewood Cliffs, NJ: Educational Technology Publications.

Mihalas, G. I., Lungeanu, D., Kigyosi, A., & Vernic, C. (1995). Classification criteria for simulation programs used in medical education. *Medinfo, 8*, 1209-1213.

Mishra, P., Spiro, R. J., & Feltovich, P. J. (1996). *Cognitive aspects of electronic text processing cognitive aspects of electronic text processing,* (pp. 287-306). Norwood, NJ: Ablex.

Mooney, G. A., & Bligh, J. G. (1997). Computer-based learning materials for medical education: A model production. *Medical Education, 31*(3), 197-201.

Moore, M. G., & Kearsley, G. (1996). *Distance education* (pp. 2-18). USA: Wadsworth.

Muller, W. K., Soldner, E. H., Bauer, A., & Ziegler, R. (1995). Virtual reality in surgical arthroscopic training. *Journal of Image Guide Surgery, 1*, 288-194.

Netter Atlas. (1999). Interactive Atlas of Human Anatomy (version 2.0). *http://www.meded.pharma.us. novartis.com/anatomy/iatlas.htm.*

Nieder, G., & Nagy, F. (1998). Beyond vesalius: Using the visible human data set in the gross anatomy curriculum. *Proceedings Slice of Life,* Chicago. *http://slice.gsm.com/archives.htm.*

Noar, M. D. (1995). The next generation of endoscopy simulation: Minimally invasive surgical skills simulation. *Endoscopy, 27*, 81-85.

Norman, D. A. (1993). *Things that make us smart.* Reading, MA: Addison-Wesley. *http://www.cogsci.ucsd. edu/~norman/*

Norman, J., & Wilkins, D. (1996). Simulators for anesthesia. *Journal of Clinical Monitoring, 12,* 91-99.

Orr, N., & Clyman, S. (1997). *The National Board of Medical Examiners' (NBME) PRIMUM Case simulations: Advances and plans,* (p. 145). Annual Meeting, Association of American Medical Colleges, Washington, DC.

Ota, D., Keller, J., Lea, R., Saito, T., & Loftin, B. (1995). Virtual reality in surgical education. *Computing Biology and Medicine, 25*, 127-137.

Pearson, J., Barnett, S., & Matthews, T. (1997). Multimedia development for integrated medical neuroscience education. *Proceedings Slice of Life*, Chicago.

Posel, N. (1993). Guidelines for the evaluation of instructional software by hospital nursing departments. *Computer Nurse, 11*, 273-276.

Rathe, R. (1998). *Computer purchase requirements for medical students discussion points.* http://www.med.ufl.edu/medinfo/docs/creg.html.

Rathe, R., Cornwall, G., & Lin, F. (1997). The QuizCGI system interactive testing over the Internet. *Proceedings American Medical Informatics Association*, Nashville, TN. *http://slice. gsm. com/ archives.htm.*

Rawitch, A. (1994). *Curriculum database development,* (p. 65). Annual Meeting Association of American Medical Colleges, Washington DC.

Richardson, D. (1997). Student perceptions and learning outcomes of computer-assisted versus traditional instruction in physiology. *American Journal of Physiology, 273*, S55-S58.

Salas, A. & Anderson, M. (1997) *Task force on medical education software.* Association of American Medical Colleges. www.AAMC.org/meded/software/start.htm

Savitt, D. L., & Steele, D. W. (1997). Implementation of a hypertext-based curriculum for emergency medicine on the World Wide Web. *Academy of Emergency Medicine, 4*, 1159-1162.

Seymour, J., Messer, M., Thomas, T., & Page, G. (1997). *Innovative medical software for the professional and academic markets,* (p. 167). Annual Meeting, Association of American Medical Colleges, Washington DC.

Sleeman, D., & Brown, J. S. (1982). *Intelligent tutoring systems.* New York: Academic Press.

Stead, W. W. (1997). The evolution of the IAIMS: Lessons for the next decade. *Journal of American Medical Information Association, 4*, S4-S11.

Stewart, J. A. (1995). Balancing learner control and realism with specific instructional goals: Case studies in fluid balance for nursing students. *Medinfo, 8,* 1715.

Stolurow, K. A. (1982). A perspective on instructional uses of computing in medicine. *Journal of Medical Systems, 6*(2), 165-170.

Task Force on Medical Education Software Resources. (1999). http://www.aamc.org/meded/ software/start.htm.

Tome, J., & Fletcher, J. (1996). Virtual PBL: Full-scale human simulation technology. *Academic Medicine, 71,* 523.

Trelstad, R. *Keyboard publishing--pathology.* (1998). http://www.kbpub.com/_catpage/onlinecatalog prodidcfindid1.htm.

University of Texas Health Science Center at San Antonio's Trauma Home Page. (1999). http://rmstewart.uthscsa.edu/.

Wainer, H. (1990). *Computerized adaptive testing: A primer.* Hillsdale, NJ: Erlbaum.

Wallis, J. W., Miller, M. M., Miller, T. R., & Vreeland, T. H. (1995). An internet-based nuclear medicine teaching file. *Journal of Nuclear Medicine, 36*, 1520-1527.

Webber, J. T., Osborn, A. G., Stensaas, S. S., Burrows, P. E., Wald, K. M., Sundsten, J. W., & Pingree, J. C. (1995). The cerebral ventricles: A computer-based interactive tutorial. *Radiographics, 15*(3), 697-702.

Weidemann, J., Hohn, H. P., Hiltner, J., Tochtermann, K., Tresp, C., Bozinov, D., Venjakob, K., Freund, A., Reusch, B., & Denker, H. W. (1997). A hypermedia tutorial for cross-sectional anatomy: HyperMed. *Acta Anatomica, 158*(2), 133-142.

Weissman, R. (1990). Capital budgeting and lifecycle planning for desktop technology. *Organizing and Managing Information Resources on Campus, EDUCOM Strategies Series on Information Technology.*

Why CBT is Being Used. http://www.usmle.org/whycbt.htm.

Winter, R. J., & Jones, R. J. (1997). Clerkship evaluation by students: A standardized electronic mechanism. *Academic Medicine, 72*, 418.

Wofford, J. L., & Wofford, M. M. (1997). The multimedia computer for case simulation: Survival tool for the clinician educator. *MD Computing, 14*, 88-93.

Woolridge, N. (1995). The C-ASE Project: Computer-assisted simulated examination. *Journal of Audiovisual Media Medicine, 18*, 149-155.

CHAPTER TWELVE

Curriculum Evaluation and Curriculum Change

LuAnn Wilkerson

University of California, Los Angeles, School of Medicine

Pressures to change have never been stronger in medical education, particularly clinical education (Rabkin, 1998). Certain impending events in the real world of medicine demand attention to educational practices. In moving to increase the amount and type of ambulatory education for medical students and residents, we are relying more and more heavily on voluntary, community-based physicians as teachers. What are the cost implications or quality implications of this shift in our own institutions?

With the increasing presence of managed health care systems, we have been forced to modify traditional forms of clinical education to accommodate the fast-paced, cost-conscious environment of controlled practice settings. Do students perform as well on postclerkship standardized examinations when trained in a managed care versus a nonmanaged care setting? A renewed interest in lifelong learning has led to the replacement of more didactic curricular structures with more learner-directed, interactive formats. What skills are essential for the lifelong learning demands of medical practice? It is extremely difficult to escape the discussion of these issues today if you are a member of an academic medical center or medical school.

One of the factors that continues to restrict our ability to respond in productive ways to these pressures for change was identified in the most recent study of medical education in North America, the Educating Medical Students: Assessing Change in Medical Education-The Road to Implementation (ACME-TRI) Report (1993, p. 14): "faculty members' resistance to suggested changes because they perceive no evidence that change is either necessary or beneficial." As medical educators, we have a special responsibility and opportunity in the midst of this ferment to use our interest in education and our skills as scholars to evaluate the process and outcomes of these new educational practices not only for purposes of internal improvement, but also for the purpose of generating worthwhile knowledge about teaching and learning in medicine. Whereas full-time medical education researchers are a rare breed, the number of potential investigators among clinical faculty members is enormous.

Why are so few curricular innovations evaluated? First, a tension exists between implementing and evaluating. In the rush to meet deadlines for students and curriculum committees, we implement new educational approaches without an evaluation plan in place. Then, just before the end of the new experience, realizing that we need to collect ratings from participants, we scurry around developing a quick survey that can be filled out with a minimum of fuss and bother. When resources are limited and time is of the essence, we satisfy ourselves with measures of participant satisfaction.

Second, evaluation studies of medical education may not be viewed by our departments and institutions as worthy of the title of scholarship. In a study of faculty members in higher education and how they spend their professional time, entitled *Scholarship Reconsidered*, Boyer (1990, p. 77) concluded: "We need scholars who not only skillfully explore the frontiers of knowledge, but also integrate ideas, connect thoughts to action, and inspire students." Rice (1992) described three forms of scholarship that allow for the blending of educational and research activities: the scholarship of integration, the scholarship of application, and the scholarship of teaching. The design and evaluation of innovative curricula fall soundly within this broadened view of scholarly activities.

Third, faculty members may have limited knowledge of the medical education literature (Nelson, Clayton, & Moreno, 1990). Studies of similar innovations and instruments validated in other settings are published for the most part in one of three or four medical education journals that are not widely read. Many evaluation studies are never published, but remain internal documents unavailable to faculty members charged with the design of evaluation studies of new curricula.

Fourth, faculty members, perhaps lacking skills in conducting applied social science research, may be unaware of the range of study types that can be applied to questions about medical education. If such faculty members cannot do a randomized controlled trial, is there anything else worth considering?

Finally, there are few sources of funding for educational research, little time free of patient care and research responsibilities, and few publications that welcome articles on curricular evaluation or outcomes assessment.

Despite these barriers and given the growing commitment in our institutions to curricular change, we have a responsibility to apply the standards of disciplined inquiry to evaluate our teaching practices, learning outcomes, and the institutional features that support or hinder the process of change. This chapter considers the specific features of a program evaluation study that change it from the mere collection of opinion to disciplined inquiry and discusses how such studies can be used to promote, reinforce, and stabilize curricular change.

DISCIPLINED INQUIRY

New educational approaches are implemented in our courses and clinical clerkships with little attention given to the evaluation of their impact on students, faculty, patients, or other aspects of the curriculum (Friedman, de Bliek, Greer, Mennin, Norman, et al., 1990; Stone & Qualters, 1998). Approaching this same situation as scholars, we begin to wonder from the moment a new program is considered how we will know what difference it has made for any number of stakeholders such as students, patients, faculty members, and society at large. As educational scholars, we want answers to these questions:

1. Was the innovation implemented as planned?
2. What intended and unintended outcomes resulted from the innovation?
3. To what populations, settings, and situations can any identified effect be generalized?

In asking these questions and others like them, we have expanded the purpose of our inquiry beyond the collection of data for programmatic improvement to include the generation of knowledge useful to persons in other settings.

> Disciplined inquiry has a quality that distinguishes it from other sources of opinion and belief. The disciplined inquiry is conducted and reported in such a way that the argument can be painstakingly examined . . . Whatever the character of a study, if it is disciplined, the investigator has anticipated the traditional questions that are pertinent. He institutes control at each step of information collection and reasoning to avoid the sources of error to which these questions refer. If the errors cannot be eliminated, he takes them into account by discussing the margin for error in his conclusions. (Cronbach & Suppes, 1969, p. 15)

Five features are essential in the design of an evaluation study if it is to be considered disciplined (Shulman, 1988). The discussion of each feature includes an example from the evaluation literature in medical education.

First, the study is planned to answer specific questions. An evaluation study demands the selection of a particular set of observations in response to a clearly stated question. This question must be set before the implementation of the program to be evaluated, not attached afterward to a data set collected "just to be sure." Popham (1991) suggested that the most important questions are raised by "impending events in education," whereas Bordage, Burack, Irby, and Stritter (1998, pp. 744) argued that researchers should "raise important research questions directly in the context of medical education practice". In other words, the best questions come from being reflective and inquisitive about what we are doing as medical educators.

    More recently there has been an increased emphasis on the measure of outcomes
as a tool for program evaluation (Kassebaum, 1990; Stone & Qualters, 1998). For
example, the implementation of the New Pathway (NP) curriculum at Harvard
Medical School in 1985 for a subset of students provided an opportunity to compare
the effects on students who chose and were randomly selected for the pilot study
with those who chose but were not selected. In designing a group of studies on the
outcomes of the curricular changes during the preclinical years, Moore, Block, Style,
and Mitchell (1994) hypothesized that NP students would be more oriented to
learning for understanding, would master the same basic knowledge, and would
demonstrate more humanistic attitudes than the control group students. Having
clearly defined questions allowed the investigators to plan for the use of multiple
measures over multiple times and guided the way in which students were selected for
participation in the NP.

    Second, disciplined inquiry reflects existing literature and theory. Just as in other
types of research, a review of the literature is essential in determining the exact
questions to be asked and identifying tools already developed for doing so. Where
should one look? Few subject terms are relevant to searches of educational topics in
MEDLINE. Two major medical education journals not catalogued in MEDLINE
can be accessed through a review of Educational Resources Information Center
(ERIC), a system not often available in the medical library. Often a phone call to an
author identified in an initial search can be the most productive strategy for the
beginning educational researcher. For example, Browner, Baron, Solkowitz, Adler,
and Gullion (1994) situated their study concerning the effect of a continuing medical
education (CME) program on the management of patients' serum cholesterol levels
in the published literature on the effect of CME in changing physicians' behaviors.
From the studies reviewed, the authors identified several problems in evaluating the
efficacy of CME and designed their own study to circumvent these problems.
Previous studies also provided a context in which they interpreted the unexpected
aspects of their results.

    Third, evaluation studies require the same attention to systematic methodology as
do other forms of research. According to Shulman (1988), "method is the attribute
which distinguishes research activity from mere observation and speculation" (p. 3).
Disciplined inquiry does not require adherence to a single method, for example, the
randomized controlled trial. At a minimum, it requires the use of a representative or
purposeful sample and systematic data collection tools. Evaluation studies can draw
on the tools of the ethnographers, interviewing and observation, as in the study done
by Duek, Wilkerson, and Adinolfi (1996), or on the tools of the statistician as in the
study by Schmidt and Moust (1995) on the relationship among problem-based
learning (PBL) tutor characteristics, group functioning, study time, and achievement.
It can be prospective or retrospective, longitudinal, or cross-sectional. It can involve
the measurement of knowledge, attitudes, or skills. In other words, an educational
scholar can draw from a broad range of methods from the social and biological
sciences in creating the best design for answering a specific question.

The choice of a specific method will depend on the questions being asked, the purpose of the research, and what is already available in the published literature. If the review of the literature suggests a possible answer for the question being asked, the purpose may be confirmatory. In other words, the purpose is to discover whether a particular outcome could be expected in a different setting or with a different population. The researcher states a directional hypothesis and sets about collecting the data that allows him or her to confirm or rather fail to disconfirm that hypothesis. The methods chosen will be probably experimental with random assignment to treatments, quasi-experimental using control groups, or correlational. For example, in evaluating the outcomes of a PBL module on domestic violence, Short, Cotton, and Hodgson (1997) used a quasi-experimental, nonequivalent control group design. All second-year medical students at University of California, Los Angeles (UCLA) and a control school completed a questionnaire concerning knowledge (K) attitudes (A) beliefs (B) behaviors (B) both before and after the intervention. In addition, they randomly selected 50 from each school to interview a standardized patient after the intervention.

If a review of the literature reveals that little is known about a question being asked, that a specific hypothesis cannot be stated with confidence, or that the quantitative findings are vague or unexplained, a shift might be made into the explanatory mode, drawing methods from the qualitative domain. For example, Caplow, Donaldson, Kardash, and Hosokawa (1997) used a multiple case study design to explore first-year students' perceptions of their learning with a problem-based curriculum. From weekly journals, videotapes of PBL sessions, focus group interviews, open-ended questionnaires to students, and interviews with the PBL tutors, the authors identified three themes that affect learning.

Fourth, disciplined inquiry requires that controls for bias be instituted to increase internal validity. What other factors might account for the findings? Designing an educational research study requires careful attention to the factors that may jeopardize the ability to interpret results or to generalize to other situations. These factors constitute threats to internal validity. Quantitative and qualitative methods use different strategies for increasing the validity of their findings, tools such as the use of control groups, randomization, pre-post testing, large sample sizes, or triangulation of multiple data sources.

Although often difficult to accomplish because of the field-based nature of much medical education research and the ethics of withholding a learning experience, randomization remains the most powerful tool for increasing internal validity. For example, in investigating the effect of learners' feedback on residents' teaching skills, Bing-You, Greenberg, Wiederman, and Smith (1997) randomized residents from three programs into experimental and control group conditions. Experimental group residents received verbal comments collected by an interviewer and summary statistics on a typical rating form within three weeks of completing each of the first three rotations of the year in which they were teaching. Control groups received no feedback. Randomization may be more feasible when multiple institutions are involved or the intervention is not perceived by the subjects as depriving them of the status quo benefits.

Perhaps the most difficult step in turning evaluation into disciplined inquiry is the final one: concluding the study with the production of a written document that follows the standards for professional communication. Having survived the implementation of the innovation, the researcher breathes a sigh of relief. Even the collection of pre-post data was managed without alienating anyone. What happens next in the busy life of an academic faculty member? The data is quickly scanned. Maybe someone is enlisted to enter numerical responses, and a verbal report of the results is provided to the appropriate committee. A more careful and elaborate analysis will be performed as time permits. The data are placed away in a drawer to be analyzed when there is time. The researcher has abandoned his or her responsibility as a scholar to inform the educational practices of other colleagues.

Disciplined inquiry includes plans for analyzing and reporting data. Strategies might include using campus services for data entry, database development, statistical consultation, or identification of a graduate student from education or public health with research skills in the social sciences. Most of all, it requires scheduling protected time for writing, small blocks of time that can be squeezed into busy weeks on a regular basis, or facing a deadline for submission. Writing and presenting results is the final step in turning program evaluation into scholarly work. For example, Schwartz, Donnelly, Nash, Johnson, Young, et al. (1992) at the University of Kentucky examined the relationship between problem-based or Socratic teaching in a surgery clerkship and students' performance on an in-house modified essay examination and the Surgery subsection of the National Board of Medical Examiners, Step II. Given the relevance of the question and the findings to other surgical educators, the authors presented the paper at the Annual Meeting of the Association for Academic Surgery and subsequently submitted it for publication in a journal read almost entirely by surgeons.

CLINICAL SIGNS OF THE EVALUATION SYNDROME

Despite our best intentions, program evaluation is difficult to implement. Guba (1969) described the common "clinical signs" of evaluation failure in a classic 1969 article, The Failure of Educational Evaluation. Have you seen one or more of these symptoms in yourself or your colleagues?

- avoids evaluation whenever possible
- demonstrates signs of anxiety when faced with evaluation results
- is immobilized in the face of opportunities for evaluation
- collects data that fail to provide useful information.

The best preventive measure available to us as medical educators is the development of skills in social science research and program evaluation (Kern, Thomas, Howard, and Bass, 1998). The Association of American Medical Colleges offers a two-year fellowship in medical education research, in which participants can enhance their ability to access and review the medical education research literature, select an appropriate design for a specific question, manage the data collection and analysis processes of an educational research project, and translate educational research findings into academic presentations and publications. Programs for obtaining a master's degree in medical education with a strong emphasis on research and evaluation methods are available on a distance-education basis through the Ontario Institute for Studies in Education; the Department of Medical Education at the University of Illinois at Chicago, College of Medicine; the Division of Medical Education at the University of Southern California; and Maastricht University, Faculty of Health Sciences, The Netherlands. Numerous medical schools offer local fellowships in medical education for trainees and faculty members interested in developing their skills as educational scholars. Being prepared to ask and answer evaluation questions turns every curricular innovation into a potential opportunity for scholarship.

USING EVALUATION RESULTS IN SUPPORT OF CURRICULAR CHANGE

Evaluation data alone is insufficient to accomplish curricular change. However, evaluation data can serve several essential roles in the process of curricular change. First, it can be a useful stimulus for discussion of needed changes. Results of clinical performance examinations, United States Medical Licensing Examination (USMLE) scores, the annual Graduation Questionnaire of the Association of American Medical Colleges, or well-designed educational evaluation studies can raise awareness of needed changes when presented to members of curriculum committees, chairs of departments, faculty leaders, and administrative deans. Second, evaluation data can be used to stabilize change by documenting outcomes and answering questions about the process of implementation. Third, the publication and presentation of evaluation data to national and international colleagues can raise the visibility of the curricular change in the home institution and make it more difficult to overturn. Finally, evaluation data can provide a means of quality improvement as the faculty and students work to refine the curricular innovation. In each of these conditions, the political challenge for the evaluator is to get results into the hands of the decision makers at the right time to stimulate, stabilize, improve, or sustain curricular change. Too often, results end up in filing cabinets, uncirculated and unread. Well-timed presentations of results can stimulate questions about what has been, what is, and what still needs to be accomplished in the curriculum.

A number of explanations have been posited for the lack of meaningful change in medical education. In his article entitled, Structure and Ideology in Medical Education: An Analysis of Resistance to Change, Bloom (1988) argued that the concentration by academic medicine on a scientific mission has crowded out its social responsibility to train physicians for the society's most basic needs in the delivery of health care.

> Preparation of physicians to serve the changing health needs of the society is asserted repeatedly as the objective of medical education, but this manifest ideology of humanistic medicine is little more than a screen for the research mission which is the major concern of the institution's social structure. Education is secondary and essentially unchanging. (p. 295)

There is a historical tension among academic faculty between the dissemination of knowledge viewed as important in a particular discipline and the broader need to educate physicians who can use that knowledge to meet the health care needs of society. It is assumed that the ability to apply follows from the acquisition of knowledge.

Cantor, Cohen, Barker, Shuster, and Reynolds (1991) suggested in a review of reform initiatives in medical education that the fragmentation of the academic enterprise into discrete departments discourages all but the bold from asking how his or her particular content relates to the larger world of health care delivery. The two-plus-two structure of the preclinical and clinical educational structure and the departmental hegemony of residency training reflect the structure of most institutions, making the implementation of multidisciplinary, integrative curricula the most difficult to create or manage.

A third reason why curricular change is so difficult to accomplish is that few institutional resources are devoted to education. Efficiency rather than effectiveness drives educational decisions. There are few dollars available to fund innovation or evaluation of medical education in local institutions. Furthermore, the increasing dependence of academic medical centers on clinical practice income and research funding leave little time for faculty members to participate in the education of medical students and residents except as these are integrated with patient care or research. Even less time is available for thinking with colleagues from across an institution about the broad competencies needed by its graduates, or for developing new instructional materials and strategies. Institutional culture in academic medical centers and medical schools values research productivity over the education of future physicians.

An additional barrier is the institutional reward system that provides few incentives for faculty to make the time to participate in medical education or its improvement. In recent years, a number of institutions have developed relative value scales for teaching in an attempt to initiate program-based budgeting (Bardes & Hayes, 1995; Cantor, et al., 1991; Hilton, Fisher, Lopez, & Sanders, 1997; Johnston & Gifford, 1996; Reiser, 1995). Accountability for the educational contributions and quality of teaching of faculty members is being seen as means for sustaining the educational mission of the institution. Although such systems may strengthen the educational function on campus, there is a growing number of community physicians being recruited as teachers who have almost no access to institutional resources and rewards (Fields, Usatine, Stearns, Toffler, & Vinson, 1998). What are the characteristics of those institutions in which change has already occurred (Bussigel, Barzansky, & Grenholm, 1994; Mennin & Kalishman, 1998; Moore, 1994)?

First, there is a leader with a vision and the ability to involve others in collaboratively accomplishing that vision. Institutional leaders and opinion leaders align the institutional culture and the innovation. Their clearly articulated vision sustains the change from initial discussion through institutionalization.

Second, there are adequate institutional (and extramural) resources dedicated to the implementation and evaluation of educational programs. Of particular importance is the existence of a core of educational change agents, basic scientists, physicians, and professional educators who are skilled in facilitating the curricular change process, building consensus, navigating the political waters during the early stages of development, and evaluating curricular process and outcomes. With the help of these change agents, faculty members have ample opportunity to experiment with and learn about the proposed innovations, to participate in the design of instructional materials, and to develop the skills necessary for new teaching roles.

Third, there is broad faculty ownership of the innovation and multiple opportunities to influence the planning process. Forum for the discussion of possibilities, problems, promises, and potential are widely available.

Fourth, there are opinion leaders who provide energy and leadership for the development and initial adoption of the curricular change. These leaders are critical to the continuing renewal of intention to change.

Fifth, there are dollars to support innovation and to guarantee that faculty members have time to participate in curricular planning and implementation.

Finally, a broadened view of scholarship has permeated the organizational reward structure such that teaching and the production of innovative educational programs are seen as an important contribution to the institutional mission. These are difficult lessons to implement. They therefore will require the cooperation of visionary leaders who commit institutional resources to education and its continual improvement, the groups of faculty members who control curricular structure, and educational scholars who continue to ask and answer critical questions:

- Did we implement what we planned to implement?
- What intended and unintended outcomes resulted?
- What can be generalized from these findings to better inform educational practice in the future?

REFERENCES

ACME-TRI Report. (1993). Educating medical students: Assessing change in medical education--the road to implementation. *Academic Medicine, 68*, S1-S67.

Bardes, C. L., & Hayes, J. G. (1995). Are the teachers teaching? Measuring the educational activities of clinical faculty. *Academic Medicine, 70*, 25-28.

Bing-You, R. G., Greenberg, L. W., Wiederman, B. L., & Smith, C. S. (1997). A randomized multicenter trial to improve resident teaching with written feedback. *Teaching and Learning in Medicine: An International Journal, 9*, 10-13.

Bloom, S. W. (1988). Structure and ideology in medical education: An analysis of resistance to change. *Journal of Health and Social Behavior, 29*, 294-305.

Bordage, G., Burack, J., Irby, D., & Stritter, F. T. (1998). Education in ambulatory settings: Developing valid measures of educational outcomes, and other research priorities. *Academic Medicine, 73*, 743-750.

Boyer, E. L. (1990). *Scholarship reconsidered: Priorities of the professoriate.* Princeton: Carnegie Foundation for the Advancement of Teaching.

Browner, W. S., Baron, R. B., Solkowitz, S., Adler, L. J., & Gullion, D. S. (1994). Physician management of hypercholesterolemia: A randomized trial of continuing medical education. *Western Journal of Medicine, 161*, 572-578.

Bussigel, M. N., Barzansky, B. M., & Grenholm, G. G. *Innovation processes in medical education.* New York: Praeger.

Cantor, J. C., Cohen, A. B., Barker, S. C., Shuster, A. L., & Reynolds, R. C. (1991). Medical educators' views on medical education reform. *Journal of the American Medical Association, 285*, 1002-1006.

Caplow, J. A. H., Donaldson, J. F., Kardash, C. A., & Hosokawa, M. (1997). Learning in a problem-based medical curriculum: Students' conceptions. *Medical Education, 31*, 440-447.

Cronbach, L. J., & Suppes, P. (1969). *Research for tomorrow's schools: Disciplined inquiry for education.* New York: Macmillan.

Duek, J. E., Wilkerson, L., & Adinolfi, A. (1996). Learning issues identified by students in tutorless problem-based tutorials. *Advances in Health Sciences Education, 1*, 29-40.

Fields, S. A, Usatine, R., Stearns, J. A., Toffler, W. L., & Vinson, D. C. (1998). The use and compensation of community preceptors in U.S. medical schools. *Academic Medicine, 73*, 95-97.

Friedman, C. P., de Bliek, R., Greer, D. S., Mennin, S. P., Norman, G. R., Sheps, C. G., Swanson, D. B., & Woodward, C. A. (1990). Charting the winds of change: Evaluating innovative medical curricula. *Academic Medicine, 65*, 8-14.

Guba, E. G. (1969). The failure of educational evaluation. *Educational Technology, 9*, 29-38.

Hilton, C., Fisher W., Lopez, A., & Sanders, C. (1997). A relative-value-based system for calculating faculty productivity in teaching, research, administration, and patient care. *Academic Medicine, 72*, 787-791.

Johnston, M. A. C., & Gifford, R. H. (1996). A model for distributing teaching funds to faculty. *Academic Medicine, 1*, 138-140.

Kassebaum, D. (1990). The measure of outcomes in the assessment of educational program effectiveness. *Academic Medicine, 65*, 293-295.

Kern, D. E., Thomas, P. A., Howard, D. M., & Bass, E. B. (1998). *Curriculum development for medical education: A six-step approach.* Baltimore: The Johns Hopkins University Press.

Mennin, S. P., & Kalishman, S. (1998). Issues and strategies for reform in medical education: Lessons from eight medical schools. *Academic Medicine, 73*, S1-S90.

Moore, G. T. (1994). Strategies for change. In D. C. Tosteson, S. J. Adelstein, & S. T. Carver (Eds.), *New pathways to medical education: Learning to learn at Harvard Medical School* (pp. 30-37). Cambridge, MA: Harvard University Press.

Moore, G. T., Block, S. D., Style, C. B., & Mitchell, R. (1994). The influence of the New Pathway curriculum on Harvard medical students. *Academic Medicine, 69*, 983-989.

Nelson, M. S., Clayton, M. A., & Moreno, R. (1990). How medical school faculty regard educational research and make pedagogical decisions. *Academic Medicine, 65*, 122-126.

Popham, J. A. (1991, December). Slice of advice. *Educational Researcher, 20*, 18-19.

Rabkin, M. T. (1998). A paradigm shift in academic medicine? *Academic Medicine, 73*, 127-131.

Reiser, S. J. R. (1995). Linking excellence in teaching to departments' budgets. *Academic Medicine, 70*, 272-275.

Rice, R. E. (1992). Toward a broader conception of scholarship: The American context. In T. G. Whiston & R. L. Geiger (Eds.), *Research and higher education: The United Kingdom and the United States* (pp. 117-129). Buckingham, England: Society for Research into Higher Education and the Open University Press.

Schmidt, H. G. & Moust, J. H. C. (1995). What makes a tutor effective? A structural-equations modeling approach to learning in problem-based curricula. *Academic Medicine, 70*, 708-714.

Schwartz, R. W., Donnelly, M. B., Nash, P. P., Johnson, S. B., Young, B., White, F. M., & Griffen, Jr., W. O. (1992). Problem-based learning: An effective educational method for a surgery clerkship. *Journal of Surgical Research, 53*, 326-330.

Short, L. M., Cotton, D., & Hodgson, C. S. (1997). Evaluation of the module on domestic violence at the UCLA School of Medicine. *Academic Medicine, 72* (Suppl. 1), S75-S92.

Shulman, L. S. (1988). Disciplines of inquiry in education: An overview. In R. M. Jaeger (Ed.), *Complementary methods for research in education* (pp. 4-17). Washington, DC: American Educational Research Association.

Stone, S. L., & Qualters, D. M. (1998). Course-based assessment: Implementing outcome assessment in medical education. *Academic Medicine, 73*, 397-401.

CHAPTER THIRTEEN

Medical Faculty as Teachers: Implications for Faculty Development

Deborah E. Simpson
Medical College of Wisconsin

"Who will teach?" asked James Woolliscroft (1995). As academic physicians are buffeted by the ever-changing economic pressures of health care delivery and medical school income expectations, they are confronted with this and a number of other questions. Will clinical teachers survive as medical school faculty? If they survive, how will they distinguish themselves as educators for recognition and reward? Can faculty development play a vital role in ensuring the survival and recognition of faculty as educators? This chapter reviews several emerging trends in academic medicine specific to clinical educators and then argues that faculty development must result in products that meet both the educational needs of the individual educator and the institution.

EMERGING TRENDS IN ACADEMIC MEDICINE: ACCOUNTABILITY, ROLE DIFFERENTIATION, AND TIME CONSTRAINTS

Performance contracts, job descriptions, and posttenure review all are part of an emerging trend for accountability in academic medicine (Bland & Holloway, 1995). Concurrently, faculty roles are becoming increasingly differentiated (Bland & Simpson, 1997a). The traditional analogy of the three-legged stool (research, service, teaching) is being replaced with another object--the tricycle and its oversized front wheel--to depict better the dominance of one role. Some argue that the traditional focus on the individual and the associated issues of how to evaluate and reward individual efforts in teaching, professional service, and research will change to that of a collective unit productivity (e.g., research centers, provider groups) (Lynton, 1998). In this collective approach, performance criteria will be explicitly linked to institutional priorities.

As faculty accountability increases, roles become differentiated. As financial productivity dominates, faculty time for education is at risk. Four half-days of clinic per week belies the reality of callbacks, record-keeping, and overbooking requiring clinicians to spend two- to three- additional hours per half-clinic day. Bland and Holloway (1995) reported that although increasing patient-care responsibilities still allows clinicians "to show up and teach," increased clinical responsibilities can result in insufficient time to prepare and no additional time available for students. In one department, students' ratings concretely reflected this differentiation: no change in ratings on direct teaching items such as "asked challenging questions" or "demonstrated concern for progress/problems," but decreased student ratings on items such as "provided critiques of writeups" and "available to students."

At stake in these emerging role, fiscal, and time concepts is the vitality of the faculty. As faculty's traditional sense of autonomy is replaced by accountability for achieving department/institutional goals, physicians must ensure that their educational mission does not become the victim of these changes.

OPPORTUNITIES FOR FACULTY DEVELOPMENT: DIFFERENTIATING THE EDUCATIONAL ROLES OF THE FACULTY

What are the implications and opportunities for clinical teacher faculty development in supporting and enhancing the educational mission of medical schools in this new environment? The answers to this question begin with the step basic to all educational program development: analysis of the tasks to be performed. The faculty's educational roles and tasks and their associated knowledge, skills, and attitudes (KSAs) differ. Two primary role categories emerge: clinician educator and the clinician teacher.

Clinician Educators

Individuals who take the lead in developing course, clerkship, or residency programs need a broad-based knowledge in curriculum development, methods of instructional delivery, learner assessment, and program evaluation. Individuals who coordinate and direct these curriculum efforts will need administrative skills in management, budget allocation, negotiation, and human resources for recruitment and retention of staff and volunteer teachers. Together, these individuals are responsible for demonstrating the quality of educational program(s) for internal performance review, extramural accreditation, and student/resident recruitment. Given these educational tasks and the breadth of required educational knowledge and skills, these individuals will be referred to as "clinician educators" (CEs).

The responsibilities of CEs uniquely position them to make sustained contributions to medical education scholarship through presentations and publications as they disseminate their innovative curriculum, outcomes assessment data, and instructional strategies. Whereas these scholarly pursuits will be based on CEs daily educational responsibilities, additional skills in data collection, analysis, and reporting will be required to support dissemination.

Clinician Teachers

A different knowledge/skill set is needed if the primary responsibility of physicians is clinical service and teaching in the context of that service. These individuals, referred to as "clinician teachers" (CTs), will be evaluated in terms of clinical productivity and cost-effective teaching. Typically, the KSAs needed by CTs can be identified through the questions they ask: "What are the instructional resources that I, as a busy CT, can use in a clinical setting to increase instructional effectiveness?" "Are there new technologies that can enhance the effectiveness and efficiency of teaching with and without the patient?" "Which teaching strategies are the most effective?" "What are the criteria for evaluating medical student or resident performance at each level of training?" "What evidence can I provide to document my performance as an educator for annual performance reviews?" Thus, the educational domains of interest to CTs differ from those of the CEs whose primary responsibility is course development and/or management. A CT does not need to be facile with curriculum development or educational evaluation. Instead, the CT must effectively use the World Wide Web as an instructional tool, coordinate instructional activities among various health care providers, provide feedback, and assess learner performance in the context of a busy, financially productive clinical practice.

THE ROLE OF FACULTY DEVELOPMENT IN PROMOTING RECOGNITION AND REWARD FOR EDUCATORS

Once educational tasks are differentiated and the associated KSAs identified, one final source of information must be used if effective faculty development is to be provided. Educators, like all humans, are motivated by intrinsic and extrinsic rewards. How can faculty development build explicitly on clinicians' internal motivations to teach (and learn) in a way that provides evidence of their scholarly contributions?

As faculty role differentiation has increased, so too has the medical school's traditional reward structure begun to recognize and reward individuals whose main tricycle wheel is clinical service complemented by teaching. Although Jones reported in the late 1980s that 75% of U.S. medical schools have created clinician-educator tracks (Jones, 1987), often individuals in these tracks have been considered "second-class" citizens. The emergence of systematic approaches to documenting the quality of educational contributions through educators' portfolios (Lindemann, Beecher, Morzinski, & Simpson, 1995; Simpson, Morzinski, Beecher, & Lindemann, 1994) and dossiers has begun to challenge the exclusive conceptions of scholarship as research (Beasley, Wright, Confrancesco, Babbott, Thomas, & Bass, 1997). As the debate continues regarding what constitutes evidence of scholarly work in the arena of education, we must continue to "teach" our colleagues about reliable and valid measures of educational quality if we are to effect change in the values regarding "what counts" for promotion and tenure (Glassick, Huber, & Maeroff, 1997).

Faculty development programs must become change agents advocating the recognition and reward of education (Bland & Simpson, 1997), as they facilitate the knowledge and skills of CEs and CTs. For the tricycle to move forward, faculty development programs must use a multifaceted strategy to teach needed KSAs and advance change focused on the recognition and reward of CEs and CTs. These changes should be targeted (Bolman & Deal, 1997a) at the following:

- *individuals*: to teach participants how to collect and present evidence of their educational scholarship for high-stakes performance review

- *organizational structure formal hierarchy*: to ensure that systems are embedded in the organizational structure of medical school to support the collection and reporting of high-quality evidence (e.g., course/clerkship evaluations, clinical teaching evaluations, peer review of educational materials) to document participants' scholarly work as educators and teachers

- *formal and informal leadership*: to create opportunities for CEs and CTs to be represented in decision-making bodies and selected for positions (e.g., rank and tenure committees, departmental chairs, senior leadership) so that there is a cogent voice for educational scholarship throughout the informal as well as formal leadership structure

- *values*: to support the career development and vitality of faculty whose passions lie in clinical education, and to ensure that education is highly visible in medical ceremonies, institutional bulletins, newsletters, and college/university incentive systems and rewards.

USING FACULTY DEVELOPMENT TO (RE)IGNITE THE PASSIONS FOR EDUCATION FACULTY DEVELOPMENT: CLINICAL TEACHERS AND EDUCATORS MUST FOCUS ON THEIR HEART

Palmer, in *The Courage to Teach*, argued that good teaching cannot be reduced to technique, but emerges from the identity and integrity of the teacher (Palmer, 1998). Faculty development, to succeed, must first understand and build on the clinician's passions for education. Why do clinicians want to teach, develop, and lead educational programs? What are their underlying passions and values represented by desires to be academic physician educators? These are not simple questions, but if faculty development programs can focus on the convergence of educational scholarship, participants' educational passions and departmental/institutional priorities (Fig. 13.1), it will be possible to promote career vitality, evidence of scholarship, and institutional goals.

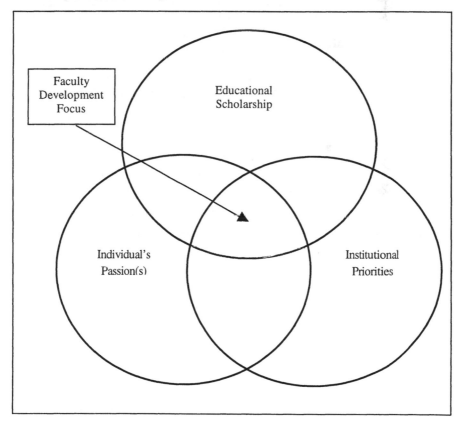

FIG. 13.1: Conceptualizing the focus of faculty development for medical educators.

More specifically, faculty development must challenge participants to identify their passion(s) as educators, and to explain how that passion can be interfaced with the educational needs and priorities of their institution. Once this convergence of personal and institutional values and priorities has been articulated, faculty development can then provide the KSAs needed to facilitate the resultant educational activities consistent with the criteria for scholarship.

Why should faculty development help clinicians crystallize their educational passion(s)? Douglas Heath (1991), in a long-term study of Haverford College graduates, found that the following three variables were critical to career success and satisfaction: (a) The individual's work must reflect his or her passion and values; (b) the employer must value and recognize the importance of the individual's work; and (c) the individual must have a perceived sense of autonomy enabling him or her to pursue actions related to that passion.

Heath's career success and satisfaction variables complement other research on career success in academic medicine (Bland, Schmitz, Stritter, Henry, & Aluise, 1990) and on physicians as learners (Slotnick, Kristjanson, Raszkowski, & Moravec, 1998), reflecting the emerging trends in faculty development activities to promote medical education. More specifically, faculty development programs should focus on (a) the KSAs that enable educators and teachers to link their passions to institutional priorities for education, (b) projects that link institutional priorities with participants' daily work as educators, and (c) the solution of real educational problems and needs that have the potential to yield scholarly projects as the mechanism whereby faculty learn critical knowledge and skills.

Do faculty development programs exist that model the linking of individual passions with institutional needs through project work teams resulting in scholarly products? A recent comprehensive review of faculty development spanning six domains associated with success in academic medicine (e.g., education, writing, research, administration, academic socialization, technology) (Bland & Simpson, 1997b) contained only two short descriptions of such programs (Roth, Werner, & Neale, 1997; Simpson & Morzinski, 1997). The remainder of this chapter briefly describes the structure and outcomes of an advanced faculty development program for clinical educators at the Medical College of Wisconsin that illustrates programmatic convergence of personal passions, institutional needs, and educational scholarship.

A MODEL FOR CLINICIAN EDUCATOR FACULTY DEVELOPMENT

On completion of a two-year comprehensive faculty development program in which family physicians obtain basic KSAs in research, administration, education, writing, and technology, participants asked, "What's next? Are we developed?" In meeting with these individuals to identify their unmet needs and to understand further the context in which they must fulfill their faculty roles, it became clear that these clinicians sought a different model of faculty development. They wanted to continue to improve their knowledge and skills as educators while working as a collaborative project group yielding scholarly products in the form of publications, instructional materials, and presentations.

A more detailed needs assessment was conducted through individual meetings with potential participants. These clinician educators sought to learn how to do qualitative educational studies so they could answer critical questions related to medical student/resident education. Concurrently, they struggled, because of their isolation, with the lack of clinician educator role models (i.e., physicians whose academic medicine careers had successfully focused on education). Through this assessment of faculty needs, a specific qualitative research question was formulated: Can one have a successful career as an educator/teacher in academic medicine? This question also met an important departmental and institutional need because family physicians have significant teaching responsibilities in all four years of their medical student curriculum in addition to resident education in five different family practice training programs.

On the basis of this assessment, a two-year advanced faculty development program for educators in the Department of Family and Community Medicine was initiated.[1] Meeting a half day per month, the six participants and two staff members undertook a qualitative research study to answer the question of academic career success as a physician educator. During the first year, they conducted a critical review of the literature regarding the careers of academic physicians as educators; designed, distributed, and analyzed the results of a postcard survey of randomly sampled members of the Society of Teachers of Family Medicine; and designed a semistructured interview protocol. During the second-year, each of the participants interviewed selected postcard respondents to explore, in-depth, their careers as academic physician educators. These interviews were audiotaped and transcribed. The participants then learned the process of qualitative data analysis using the protocols as data.

The conclusions of these studies were presented at two national meetings (Society of Teachers of Family Medicine and the Association of American Medical Colleges), and one paper was accepted for publication (Meurer, Bower, Rediske, Simpson, Lawrence, et al., 1998) with a second paper under review. Thus, participants in this advanced faculty development program were able, through collaborative work, to increase their knowledge and skills in the area of qualitative research, to answer a critical question regarding educators in academic medicine, and to advance their own scholarly records through publications and presentations.

A similar collaborative, project, work-group-based approach to faculty development also was implemented for experienced educators in general pediatrics

1 Partial Funding provided by a Faculty Development Grant in Family Medicine from the US. Department of Health and Human Services (#2 D15 PE85057)

and general internal medicine.[2] Their project focus differed as they sought to identify effective and efficient teaching strategies for primary care educators. They too began their work with a critical review of the literature on community preceptor education, instructional methods in the ambulatory setting, and the uses of technology in the ambulatory setting. At this writing, three peer-reviewed presentations have been accepted at regional and national meetings, one paper accepted (Heidenreich, Lye, Simpson, & Lourich, in press) and a second under review. During the second phase of collaboration, the group will design and implement a study to evaluate the effectiveness of each of these methods, disseminating the results of these studies through presentations and publications.

Participant attendance, satisfaction, and learning in both of these faculty development programs are high, and departments and institutions see tangible outcomes given the explicit link between projects and institutional needs. This model of faculty development, linking individuals' passions with institutional priorities through collaborative project work, yields a perceived sense of autonomy and academic productivity rewards--the key variables in Heath's satisfied and successful career equation.

SUMMARY AND CONCLUSIONS

Faculty development must respond to increasingly differentiated roles and responsibilities of clinicians as teachers and educators. When a forum is provided wherein these individuals can work collaboratively on departmentally and institutionally important projects, faculty development becomes a form of guided experiential learning that yields academic products, furthering the educational missions of our medical schools. Faculty development also must work at the organizational level advocating for education in the formal organizational structure through the informal leadership/decision-making network and visibility in the cultural and public relations vehicles of the medical school.

Who will teach? The future of medical education rests on the degree to which the vitality of our outstanding teachers and educators can be retained and maintained. Building on Heath's (1991) findings for career satisfaction, success will depend on the ability to identify and link the passions of CEs and CTs to institutional needs through collaborative project work groups operating with perceived autonomy. This approach, responsive to the emerging trends in academic medicine, enables faculty development to serve as the "big wheel" driving the education tricycle.

---

[2] Partial funding provided by a Faculty Development grant in General Internal Medicine/General Pediatrics from the U.S. Department of Health and Human Services (#1 D28 PE50072).

ACKNOWLEDGMENT

Partial funding support for the projects described in this chapter was provided through Faculty Development Grants in Family Medicine (PHS#2 D15 PE55052) and General Internal Medicine/General Pediatrics (PHS#1 D28 PE500072-02).

REFERENCES

Beasley, B. W., Wright, S. M., Confrancesco, J., Babbott, S. F., Thomas, P. A., & Bass, E. B. (1997). Promotion criteria for clinician-educators in the United States and Canada. *Journal of American Medical Association, 278*(9), 723-728.

Bland, C. J., & Holloway, R. L. (1995). A crisis of mission: Faculty roles and rewards in an era of health care reform. *Change, 28*(5), 30-35.

Bland, C. J., Schmitz, C. C., Stritter, F. T., Henry, R. C., & Aluise, J. J. (1990). *Successful faculty in academic medicine*. New York: Springer.

Bland, C. J., & Simpson, D. E. (1997a). Future faculty development in family medicine. *Family Medicine, 29*(4), 290-293.

Bland, C. J., & Simpson, D. E. (1997b). (Guest Eds.). *Family Medicine. 29*(4), 230-293.

Bolman, L. G., & Deal, T. E. (1997). *Reframing organizations: Artistry, choice, and leadership*. San Francisco: Jossey-Bass.

Glassick, C. E., Huber, M. Y., & Maeroff, G. I. (1997). *Scholarship assessed: Evaluation of the professorate*. San Francisco: Jossey-Bass.

Heath, D. (1991). *Enduring lives: Paths for maturity and success*. San Francisco: Jossey-Bass.

Heidenreich, C., Lye, P., Simpson, D., & Lovrich, M. (in press). The search for effective and efficient ambulatory teaching methods through the literature. *Pediatrics (Journal of Ambulatory Pediatric Association)*.

Jones, R. F. (1987). Clinician-educator faculty tracks in U.S. medical schools. *Journal of Medical Education, 62*, 444-447.

Lindemann, J. C., Beecher, A. C., Morzinski, J. A., & Simpson, D. E. (1995). Translating family medicine's educational expertise into academic success. *Family Medicine, 27*(30), 6-9.

Lynton, E. A. (1998). Reversing the telescope: Fitting individual tasks to common organizational ends. *AAHE Bulletin, 50*(7), 8-10.

Meurer, L. N., Bower, D. J., Rediske, V. A., Simpson, D. E., Lawrence, S. L., Wolkomir, M. S., Beacher, A. C. (1998). Career satisfaction among family physicians. *Academic Medicine, 73*(10), 570-571.

Palmer, P. J. (1998). *The courage to teach – Exploring the inner landscape of a teacher's life*. San Francisco: Jossey-Bass.

Roth, L. M., Werner, P. T., & Neale, A. V. (1997). Linking individual and organizational development through reflective faculty evaluation. *Family Medicine, 29*(4), 284.

Simpson, D. E., & Morzinski, J. A. (1997). An advanced faculty development program for academic physicians at the Medical College of Wisconsin. *Family Medicine, 29*(4), 283.

Simpson, D. E., Morzinski, J. A., Beecher, A. C., & Lindemann, J. C. (1994). Meeting the challenge to document teaching accomplishments: The educator's portfolio. *Teaching and Learning in Medicine: An International Journal, 6*(3), 203-206.

Slotnick, H. B., Kristjanson, A. F., Raszkowski, R. R., & Moravec, R. (1998). A note on mechanisms of action in physicians learning *Professions Education Researcher Quarterly, 19*(2), 5-12.

Woolliscroft, J. (1995). Who will teach? A fundamental challenge to medical education. *Academic Medicine, 70*(5), 341-342.

CHAPTER FOURTEEN

Medical Education as a Continuum

J. Roland Folse
Southern Illinois University School of Medicine

Medical education links medical science to the art of healing through a process that transforms the student into a trusted and responsible professional.

From the beginning, medical education has been an apprenticeship, a cultural rite passed on to a trusted member of the community who sought out the best remedies for treatment, sometimes by knowledge acquired from mentors and sometimes by trial and error. The outcome of this training experience was an individual whom others perceived to have special powers to heal the sick.

In the latter half of the 19th century, scientific study, experimentation, and the transmission of information through publications allowed the domain of medical education to focus on truths and put forth information that could be learned and applied. European and American medical education became centered in universities, where lectures and textbooks emphasized basic sciences and what little therapeutic medicine was known at the time. Learning the science of medicine became separated from the practice of medicine. The explosion of published information greatly accelerated medical learning, and also fostered the development of many new eclectic medical schools, particularly in North America.

By the end of the 19th century, medical education was a hodgepodge of schools, hospitals, and curricula. Gradually, as established universities provided basic science instruction and house staff training developed within hospitals, practical medical experience was brought into a controlled environment.

Throughout the 20th century, the components of medical education have remained relatively constant. The formal educational process still consists of a medical school period and a supervised practice period of residency training. Basic

161

science education still precedes clinical education, and lifelong education, in general, is left to the individual.

Why has this process of medical education remained so constant for such a long period? What have been the advantages and disadvantages of the modern system of medical education? How has this education kept up with changing times, and what can be done to make the continuum of medical education more appropriate for the future and more efficient to the learner?

This chapter addresses the individual components of this continuum, with a perspective toward how well they fit future needs.

BASIC SCIENCE EDUCATION

Rapidly expanding knowledge in the basic medical sciences has shifted the teaching emphasis from gross anatomy and physiology to molecular biology, genetics, and pharmacodynamics. Traditionally, research and the advancement of science have been the primary goals of medical school basic scientists, with the education of medical students often a secondary endeavor. The simplest form of education, requiring the least amount of faculty time, has been the lecture followed by the multiple-choice examination. Even when formal educational objectives have been established, the curriculum has been content or subject oriented. Cadaver dissections, laboratory experimentations, and other types of group interactions between faculty and students, when replaced by lectures, reduce the opportunity for faculty role modeling or mentoring and the direct observation of student performance.

On many medical school campuses, basic science education is conducted at sites separate from hospitals or other settings of clinical medicine. Students frequently dress and function more like college students than students in a professional school. The benchmark of success held by most students has been grades and passing of tests, attitudes similar to those held in undergraduate school. In addition, many schools have fostered an emphasis on the content domain by holding an National Board of Medical Examiners (NBME) test score as the pinnacle of success. Some even require a passing grade before the student can progress into the clinical sciences or graduate from medical school. Frequent multiple-choice examinations, often given weekly, have resulted in students cramming their short-term memories without allowing sufficient opportunities to assimilate what they have learned and to put the information into the context of clinical problem solving.

It is generally recognized that a strong foundation in the basic sciences is essential to becoming a good clinical scientist and practitioner. The time allocated for teaching basic sciences to medical students has not increased with the expansion of knowledge, so newer developments such as molecular biology, genetics, and immunochemistry have been added to anatomy, physiology, biochemistry, and other traditional studies.

Rapid access to new information has progressed using computer technology. The ability of students to update their knowledge database and quickly add new information has removed some of the pressure from excessive cramming of facts. Because of the accessibility of information, a paradigm shift in how we think about information storage and retrieval has simultaneously taken place. Information links have replaced stored facts, and algorithms for sorting information have replaced memorization. Because of these changes, the process of teaching and learning is changing.

The two major shortfalls of traditional basic science education, excessive emphasis on recall of factual information and inadequate opportunities to work through problems, have been addressed by problem-based learning curricula. This educational process stimulates the student to take charge of learning, emphasizes the need to identify areas of weakness, allows for small group interaction, and creates an environment conducive to inquiry synthesis of information, along with reflection. Because problem-based learning emphasizes process rather than content, some have been critical that basic science information has been inadequately assimilated. However, longitudinal studies comparing performance outcomes of students in a problem-based oriented curriculum with those from a standard curriculum show little difference when these are measured against such national standards as the United States Medical Licensing Examination (USMLE) Step examinations.

Other curricula are replacing the lecture format with small group discussions that bring together basic science faculty, clinical faculty, and students. Although this format is more time consuming for both faculty and students, the advantages are obvious. Student communication and problem-solving skills are more easily assessed, and interactions with scientists and clinicians allow students to see the relevance of the information being discussed. Solutions to patient and community health problems introduced in this format are believed to be more readily applicable in a clinical setting.

In the future, large group lectures and testing of short-term recall should be replaced by student-centered small group interactions with an opportunity for students to solve problems relevant to future practice needs. Such experiences should provide an opportunity also to develop communication, problem-solving, and professionalization skills throughout the early phase of medical school education.

BEGINNING CLINICAL SKILLS AND PATIENT MANAGEMENT

In most medical schools the third-year is the first major introduction to clinical medicine. Usually, sometime during the first two years, and frequently during the last few months of the second-year, an introduction to clinical medicine course teaches the basics of history-taking and physical examination skills.

Discipline-oriented clinical clerkships comprise most of the third-year, and these often vary in format from specialty to specialty depending on the teaching philosophy of the specialty faculty and the organization of the teaching service. Often, the organization of the clerkship closely follows the organization and rotations of the residents' services with students being assigned directly to resident teams. Residents, either by design or default, become the primary teachers on many clerkships. Teaching by residents can be somewhat erratic because many have little formal training in teaching and others look on teaching as a burden that interferes with their primary goal of advancing their own education. Despite these problems, most students praise residents and appreciate the teaching they receive. In some settings, students have successful one-on-one preceptor to preceptee relationships with faculty, particularly in primary care and outpatient environments. In these settings students may have an opportunity to experience firsthand, real-life office practice directly from a clinician faculty member without the associated interaction with residents.

In the future, residents need to become better equipped to be good teachers. The principles of adult learning including teaching skills, feedback, and evaluation should be an integral part of resident education.

Regardless of the format or the setting in which the clerkship takes place, certain educational principles must be paramount. Medical student education cannot be merely an add-on to resident education because students and residents have different learning needs. A careful needs assessment should precede all clerkship activities. Faculty must be skilled in performing frequent needs assessments and then restructuring the curriculum to meet those needs. The clerkship director and the faculty must create an environment conducive to student learning. All too often, first clinical experiences are intimidating, overwhelming, and inappropriate to the student's level of learning. An environment that fosters inquiry and discussion at a level that matches the student's background experiences leads to a more rapid clinical maturity.

Students need frequent feedback. Therefore, a system for gathering performance information from the residents and faculty must be in place so students can receive objective and critical feedback. Goals and objectives of the clerkship should be stated clearly in advance to the students, not only to guide their study and learning, but also to give fairness and relevance to the evaluation system. All too often, faculty expect students to be aware of everything there is to know about a discipline when the constraints of time and insight allow only a basic introduction.

Education should not be left to chance. The objectives of the curriculum should clearly specify levels of competency as well as the benchmarks to be measured by examinations. Different yardsticks must be used to measure knowledge and clinical skills. Objective-structured clinical evaluations or multiple-station examinations may assess clinical skills not evaluated by other knowledge-based examinations or episodic performance observations.

Changes in the health care environment have had a serious impact on clerkship education. In the past, students enjoyed the leisure of following patients in the hospital for long periods of time, which provided them an opportunity to develop clinical evaluation and communication skills through frequent interactions with the same patients. Continuity of care is lost when patients leave the hospital too soon. Students are often in competition with other health providers to evaluate patients who arrive at the hospital just in time for early morning surgery, and patients frequently are discharged home during critical phases of their recovery, thereby ending student observation.

Despite these deficiencies of the clerkship period, the third-year remains one of the most exciting, maturing, and prophetic phases in the continuum of medical education. It is a time when students begin to function as professionals. It is also a time when students sample various disciplines and make lifelong career decisions. It is a time for practicing clinical skills and learning the fundamentals of patient management. It is a time of hard work, intense study, and emotional fatigue. Too much is compressed into the third-year clerkships. Students are expected to learn fundamental clinical skills, to sample many different clinical disciplines, and to become familiar with how medicine is practiced in a real health care environment.

The focus of change for undergraduate medical education in the future will be on a better integration and amalgamation of the basic sciences and clinical medicine. The introduction of students to clinical medicine should take place far earlier in medical school. Medical school curricula should strive to integrate the basic and clinical sciences from the first day of medical school throughout its four years. Case-based small-group instruction can bring together basic science and clinical faculty, particularly during the first years of medical school.

THE TRANSITION PERIOD

The transition period from medical school to graduate specialty education may run from the end of the clerkship period in the third-year through a first preliminary residency year or internship. The fourth-year of medical school has often been characterized as an audition year because so much of the student's time and effort is devoted to selecting a career, applying for a residency, and performing numerous perfunctory tasks in order to be a competitive candidate. The task is difficult because most residency training programs have no specific prerequisite educational objectives, and each one searches through numerous candidates to select the best and the brightest. The more competitive a specialty, the more likely it is that arbitrary standards will be used for screening applicants. The USMLE test score results, the amount of prestige linked to the name of the medical school, and the letter of recommendation of the specialty department chair are often given excessive weight. Some students quickly put together research projects. Others visit prospective institutions for audition electives. Still others travel to 20 or 30 different institutions seeking interviews. While this entire job-seeking effort takes place, medical education is put on hold. Some schools have responded by making the fourth-year a nonelective year, requiring students to participate in more faculty-directed educational activities. With the recent increased interest in primary care, some schools require students to participate in outreach primary care clinics during their fourth-year. Although such experiences may be valuable, they may be less appropriate for students who already have chosen highly specialized careers. The skills learned in the primary care setting would be equally valuable for first- and second-year students.

Because most medical schools have intended to produce an undifferentiated and well-rounded graduate, the whole concept of tracking or gearing an individual student's curriculum toward prerequisite objectives defined by the specialty program have seemed foreign. Yet most medical students spend both formal and informal educational time preparing for their future residency training. Residency training, regardless of specialty, is a period of learning centered around having patient care responsibilities. It is a very important period of development for the new physician.

Prerequisite objectives for specialty residency training should provide a means for linking the fourth-year of medical school education and the internship. Residency training could be shortened and made more efficient if the fourth-year of medical school were devoted to developing and practicing clinical skills needed for becoming a responsible resident. Workforce requirements, the financing of graduate education, and changes in the delivery of health care all are factors forcing medical schools and residency training programs to coordinate the transition better between the fourth medical school year and the first-year of residency.

Residency training programs are organized around specialty rotations. These block periods allow residents to spend specific time observing, learning, and participating in patient care of a single discipline. All too frequently, the first-year resident performs many service-oriented tasks, sometimes to the detriment of learning, and often at the expense of sleep. Most residency rotations are episodic in opportunities, lack specifically defined objectives, and leave learning to chance rather than design. First-year residents, often coming from diverse medical school backgrounds, may be ill prepared for the patient care responsibilities of the first few months. Specialty programs that define prerequisite learning needs give medical students an opportunity to enter their program much better prepared for the activities and responsibilities thrust on them.

In many hospitals, service obligations drive the educational programs. Rounds, conferences, and other teaching activities are secondary to patient care needs. Yet, learning while providing service to patients is an integral part of the professionalization process. If service and education are clearly delineated by design, both can be kept in balance. If rotations are designed to meet objectives rather than time blocks, individual flexibility and innovation can be accomplished. First-year residents tracking into urology or obstetrics and gynecology may need more intensive exposure to a urologic outpatient experience than residents who will become orthopedic or vascular surgeons.

The transition period from specialty choice to specialty residency training should allow students to broaden their general medical education as well as track toward their future careers. Residency programs should clearly establish prerequisite goals so students can be provided an opportunity to prepare adequately before entering residency training. The preliminary period of residency should provide carefully supervised skill acquisition, progressive patient care responsibilities, flexibility, and learning activities based on need rather than lockstep rotations. Patient care services, although an integral part of learning on the job, should be balanced carefully with educational needs. In the future, curricular innovations that hold high educational principles will be needed to meet the challenges of a changing medical environment.

ADVANCED SPECIALTY TRAINING

As the domains of medicine have become more highly specialized, training programs have become more fragmented. The knowledge and skills necessary to become competent in a highly specialized area have been developed by adding longer periods of training. Many specialties have been reluctant to allow this differentiation to take place during the early years of residency training, fearing that graduates would have incomplete exposure to their specialty practice. Much of this dilemma arises from the need to accredit training programs and certify competence at the end of an educational period rather than recognize that the early years of residency training, although formidable, are the beginning of a training process that continues long after the completion of residency. The principles of graduate education must take precedence over the length of training. Residents must have adequate opportunity to practice skills under supervision until they are capable of performing independently. Obviously, there are different levels of skills required in any specialty, and the learner may progress through these skills at a pace different from that of other learners.

The concept of a body of knowledge of a single discipline is becoming more and more blurred as medical practice changes and new knowledge and technology redefine disciplines. Training programs must emphasize the acquisition of skills at an acceptable level of competency while the student is developing maturity to perform independently. If managed care requirements, excessive supervision, time consuming regulations, or hostile educational environments are allowed to become dominant, graduate medical education will fail in its mission to provide physicians well prepared to practice when they leave their training. If residency programs are to launch physicians who are competent for life, then all physicians must be given the tools to continue their education. An environment of inquiry, which includes research, scholarship, and easy access to new information, must be an integral part of graduate education. Environments that merely provide opportunities for rote practice do a disservice to long-term education. A stimulating faculty and an opportunity to search out and solve problems foster intellectual curiosity.

A great void exists currently in the ability of medical educators to measure clinical competency, intellectual inquiry, and honesty. Direct observation by trusted faculty proves to be the best means of judging the mature professional. It is imperative that periods of direct observation not be diluted, and that the scope of experiences not be so shortened that faculty have inadequate opportunities to judge when trainees are competent.

PROFESSIONALIZATION AND PUBLIC HEALTH AWARENESS

There is not a single purpose for the outcome of medical education. Some graduates may choose rural practice and some may choose the field of scientific research, whereas others may choose specialized, hospital-based patient care. Each individual must have an opportunity to choose an appropriate career. It is important, however, that the entire process of medical education reflect the health care needs of society. Medical education of the past half century has been greatly influenced by an explosion of scientific knowledge that has resulted in the ability to cure many diseases. Medical education has produced a medical profession that has largely set its own goals and standards. For instance, as the technology developed to implant artificial joints, it was rapidly applied to patients. Genetic engineering is making great strides to overcome inherited diseases, although this type of development has been at great cost and often with inadequate information regarding long-term outcomes. Medical education must embrace public health in its entirety and strive to use standards based on outcome results. Just as basic science must be integrated throughout clinical medicine, the principles of public health and an awareness of societal needs likewise should be a part of all aspects of medical education.

The MD degree and specialty board certification does not necessarily connote professionalism. They may provide the right to practice medicine, but if professionalism is to accompany these diplomas, an added value system must be applied. Recognition of societal needs, personal concern and empathy for individual patients, and intellectual honesty are characteristics of a professional. An educational system that selects students with high standards, emphasizes medical humanities in its medical schools and medical ethics in hospitals, and uses highly professional faculty role models will ensure that medical practice in the future will serve the needs of all of society.

EPILOGUE

The continuum of medical education begins when an individual decides to pursue a career in medicine and ends when medical practice is finally retired. Lifelong learning is the hallmark of a professional. Service to individuals and societies must be the final goal of the educational process. Evaluation and certification must ensure standards of excellence. The curriculum must be relevant to the changing needs of society and to the development of the individual professional. What one learns in formal education and training is only an introduction to the experiences gained in a professional career, which completes the educational process.

CHAPTER FIFTEEN

Residents as Teachers

Robert G. Bing-You
Maine Medical Center

Janine C. Edwards
Texas A & M University College of Medicine

A decade ago, a book entitled *Clinical Teaching for Medical Residents* (Edwards & Marier, 1988) was published, which described residents' roles as teachers, teaching techniques for residents, approaches to assessing resident teaching, and case examples of teaching improvement programs for residents. Since then, there has continued to be a steady growth of literature focusing on residents as teachers. This increased focus may, in part, result from the current requirements of both the Liaison Committee on Medical Education (1993) and the Accreditation Council for Graduate Medical Education (1996) emphasizing that residents should be given the opportunity to improve their teaching skills. Although strongly advocated by previous authors (Kassebaum, 1988; Tonesk, 1979), it is not clear to what extent residents have received preparation in this area.

As medical educators move into the 21st century, the discussion is focused on how best to improve residents' teaching skills. Although there have been few published reviews on this topic, readers are encouraged to consider two excellent resources: Edwards and Marier, 1988; Sheets, Hankin, and Schwenk, 1991. In addition to identifying this previous literature briefly, this chapter delineates more up-to-date evidence supporting important lessons learned about residents as teachers.

HOW ARE RESIDENTS VIEWED AS TEACHERS?

Barrow (1966) surveyed medical students more than 30 years ago to discover their perceptions of residents' contribution to students' education. Medical students estimated that approximately 31% of their knowledge was gained from working with interns and residents, as compared with 26% from working with attending physicians. More than three fourths of the students surveyed indicated that residents played a significant role as teachers during the clerkship year.

A study similar to Barrow's was conducted 25 years later by Bing-You and Sproul (1992). Again, students indicated that one third of their knowledge was contributed by interns and residents. Most students (a range of 58% to 84% for various clerkships) agreed that residents played a significant role as teachers. Interestingly, 93% of the students wanted to have teaching responsibilities later as residents. Similarly, 76% of the surveyed candidates to one pediatrics residency program indicated that they were "highly interested" in a residency program that helped them teach medical students (Satran & Harris, 1992).

Medical educators at Jefferson Medical College have published several studies showing that medical students' ratings of residents as teachers are statistically, positively correlated with ratings of their clerkship experiences. Ashikawa, Xu, and Veloski (1992) noted that the most important factor related to junior medical students' overall satisfaction with an otolaryngology clerkship, accounting for 20% of the variance, was their perceived experience with residents. Xu, Brigham, and Veloski, and Rodgers (1993) found that more than 500 students' overall ratings of clerkships (family practice, internal medicine, obstetrics/gynecology, pediatrics, psychiatry, and surgery) were determined by two factors related to resident teaching: resident preceptorship (e.g., "taught at the bedside, improved my physical taking") and resident mentorship (e.g., "served as role model, stimulated me to do additional reading"). Xu, Veloski, and Brigham (1995) also showed that residents' active involvement of medical students correlated positively with overall satisfaction with clerkships.

Although most residents have not received formal instruction in teaching before medical training (Apter, Metzger, & Glassroth, 1988; Brown, 1970; Satran & Harris, 1992), residents have long recognized their role as teachers of medical students and of fellow residents (Brown, 1970). Apter et al. (1988) surveyed 55 internal medicine residents at the McGaw Medical Center of Northwestern University. In this survey, 89% of the residents reported that they "enjoyed teaching," and 74% felt that students appreciated their efforts. These same residents indicated that enjoyment of teaching was positively associated with spending more than three-hours per week preparing for teaching. Bing-You and Harvey (1991), surveying 21 residents in several specialties, found that residents' desire to teach was positively correlated with enjoyment of working with students and with feeling that teaching was an important responsibility. Residents' self-perceived enjoyment of teaching was positively correlated with students' ratings of residents' overall teaching effectiveness. These latter two studies also found that residents thought their own knowledge and skills were improved by teaching others.

Although many medical students and residents perceive residents as teachers, there is a discrepancy in such perceptions. A doctoral dissertation by Wargula (1988) suggested that residents appeared to be unaware of students' expectations concerning the importance of the residents' supervisory role. In addition, students did not perceive residents actually performing characteristics of teaching functions (i.e., instruction and role modeling) as much as residents themselves perceived it.

Residents also may have varying self-perceptions of their roles. In a thoughtful qualitative study, Yedidia, Schwartz, Hirschkom, and Lipkin (1995) probed second-year residents' perceptions of differences in the learning process between the first and second years of residency, their responses to situations in which they lacked adequate clinical knowledge, and their views of their supervisory relationships with interns. These researchers found intense conflicts in residents' various roles in three categories:

1. Residents' own needs as learners frequently coincide with interns' learner needs in ways that undermine the teaching role,

2. Residents must ensure that interns get the clinical work done, sometimes at the expense of teaching and learning,

3. As clinicians, residents' first priority is to address patient care, thus making the learning needs of interns secondary.

Potential remedies for these conflicts involve equipping residents with support and training for their teaching role.

Faculty have perceived residents as having an important role as teachers. A survey by Anderson, Anderson, and Scholten (1990) of general surgery residency program directors found that 98% (n = 233) involved residents in teaching medical students. However, only 60% of program directors thought that formal instruction in teaching skills was important for residents. Almost one half of the surveyed programs offered no such preparation.

A survey of internal medicine program directors conducted by Bing-You and Tooker (1993) revealed similar findings. Whereas 84% of program directors (n = 259) felt that residents contributed to students' learning, only 52% thought that formal instruction in teaching skills was important. Furthermore, only 20% (n = 51) of the surveyed program directors offered teaching skills improvement programs.

Students' and residents' perceptions of time spent by residents teaching, approximately seven-hours per week in one study of surgical residents (Lowry, 1976), have been corroborated in time studies in different disciplines (i.e., internal medicine, pediatrics) (LaPalio, 1981; Meyers, Margolis, Sheehan, Aita, & Risser, 1974). A recent multisite study published by O'Sullivan, Weinberg, Boll, and Nelson, (1997) investigated students' educational activities during the clerkship year. Through analyzing 24-hour student logs, the authors noted that the students received a mean of 2.8-hours per day of instruction by residents. This compared with 2.1-hours of instruction per day by full-time, and 0.7-hours per day by volunteer faculty. Regarding the type of teaching, residents accounted for the majority of informal teaching (44% of total hrs. of this type), including nonclassroom interactions such as discussions in the hallway or over meals, and supervised care (56% of total hrs. of this type).

At least four observational studies have evaluated residents' teaching behaviors during work rounds in internal medicine residencies. The earliest study by Tremonti and Biddle (1982) compared resident and faculty teaching behaviors and found that residents spent more time at the bedside, rarely addressed psychosocial issues, and saw more patients in their sessions. Wilkerson, Lesky, and Medio (1986) also noted that much teaching occurred at the bedside, where residents acted as role models by interacting with patients, and verifying clinical findings. Less frequent teaching behaviors included referring to the literature, giving feedback, asking questions, and demonstrating procedures. Wray, Friedland, Ashton, Scheurich, and Zollo (1986) observed that "teaching or discussing the case" was the second most common activity on work rounds. "Talking with patient or family" occurred for an average of 12-minutes per round, which accounted for approximately one fourth of the total time. The most recent study by Ashton, Wray, Friedland, Zollo, and Scheurich (1994) attempted to investigate resident work round styles and subsequent patient outcomes. Certain work round styles (e.g., teaching about the case) actually were associated with poorer patient care (e.g., unanticipated problems) than with a "data-gathering" style (e.g., talking with the patient).

In summary, this section suggests the following potential lessons learned for the 21st century:

- Medical students continue to perceive residents as having a major role in their education, particularly during the third-year clerkship.
- Medical students' satisfaction with their clerkship experiences is correlated with their active involvement with residents.
- Residents think of themselves as teachers and enjoy this role.
- The resident's role as teacher may conflict with other roles such as clinician and learner.
- Program directors think the resident's teaching role is important, but provide little support in the way of instruction.
- Residents spend approximately one- to two-hours per day teaching.
- In internal medicine, resident teaching during work rounds focuses on bedside teaching, and specific behaviors on work rounds may have an impact on patient care.

WHAT APPROACHES TO IMPROVE RESIDENTS' TEACHING HAVE BEEN DESCRIBED?

A comprehensive review of clinical teaching improvement methods was presented by Skeff and his associates in 1988. These methods include feedback from students' ratings, peer evaluation, consultation with a professional educator, videotape review, self-evaluation, concept-based training, and multicomponent methods (seminars and workshops). The recent published reports of methods to improve resident teaching reveal wide variance in the following dimensions: instructional time, needs assessment techniques, format of programs, content areas, specialties, and postgraduate years involved.

The largest survey of teaching skills improvement programs for residents (Bing-You & Tooker, 1993) showed that instructional time varied from one- to 24-hours. Spickard, Wenger, and Corbett (1996b) characterized a three-hour session featuring two specific topics (i.e., learning climate and feedback). The annual Resident Teaching Course described by Wipf, Pinsky, and Burke (1995) is a six-hour course covering team and leadership skills, residents' roles as teachers, and microskills teaching. Other teaching skills programs are conducted over several months (Bing-You, Greenberg, 1990). Teaching skills programs are time-limited by the other priorities of residents: patient care and learning.

Regarding needs assessment, the results of studies assessing medical students' and residents' perceptions of residents as teachers can direct efforts toward promoting ways for residents to involve students actively (Xu, Veloski, & Brigham, 1995), increasing residents' desire to teach (Bing-You & Harvey, 1991), and clarifying discrepant perceptions of residents' roles (Warguyla, 1988). Besides surveying residents as to what their specific teaching skills needs are (Meleca & Schimpfhauser, 1976), other needs assessment approaches to define content areas may be used. Wilkerson, et al.'s (1986) observation of resident behavior during work rounds facilitated the development of a six-hour course on clinical teaching. Another observational study of work rounds by Arseneau (1997) focused on the question-asking behaviors of residents. Irby (1979) incorporated the use of learning and teaching style inventories into workshops. Using students' ratings, Vu, Marriott, Skeff, Stratos, and Litzelman (1997) identified areas for follow-up training of residents.

In their comprehensive survey, Bing-You and Tooker (1993) found that many content areas are included in teaching skills improvement programs for residents. In order of frequency, these were evaluation/feedback, teacher behavior, discussion leader skills, learning styles, self-assessment, lecturing skills, problem solving, learning theory, and audiovisual techniques. Several additional content areas have been identified in the broader literature. Table 15.1 lists potential content areas for resident teaching skills improvement programs. The program director is identified most frequently as the faculty member who develops and facilitates the program (Bing-You & Tooker, 1993).

TABLE 15.1. Potential Content Areas for Resident Teaching Skills Programs

Feedback	Learning theory
Evaluation	Cognitive psychology
Questioning skills	Learning styles
Problem solving	Adult learning theory
Motivating students	Self-directed learning
Teaching clinical procedures	Teaching self-assessment
Establishing and communicating goals	The problem student
One-on-one teaching	Audiovisual techniques
Group discussion skills	Team skills
Bedside teaching	Conflict resolution
Teaching on work rounds	Time management

Approaches to improve resident teaching have been described in numerous specialties, including radiology (1990), psychiatry (Doyle & Balsley, 1979; Kates & Lesser, 1985), surgery (Anderson, Anderson, & Scholten, 1990; Edwards & Marier, 1988; Sheets, Hankin, & Schwenk, 1991), pediatrics (Greenberg, Goldberg, & Jewett, 1984; Lewis & Cappelman, 1984; Johnson, Bachur, Priebe, Barnes-Ruth, Lovejoy, & Hafler, 1996), internal medicine (Bing-You & Greenberg, 1990; Bing-You & Tooker, 1993; Camp, Hoban, & Katz, 1985; Spickard, et al., 1996b; Wipf, Pinsky, & Burke. 1995), and family medicine (Susman & Gilbert, 1995). Teaching skills programs including residents from multiple specialties also have been characterized (Craig, 1988; Edwards, Kissling, Brannan, Plauche, & Marier, 1988b; Edwards & Marier, 1988; Melecca & Schimpfhauser, 1976; Pristach, Donoghue, Sarkin, Wargula, & Doerr, et al., 1991; Skeff, Stratos, Berman, & Bergen, 1992). Whether residents from different specialties have different teaching skills needs has not been clearly established. Observations of varying teaching foci (e.g., skills in surgical training [1976], self-directed learning in psychiatry; (O'Sullivan, et al., 1997) among specialties would suggest that residents' teaching needs differ.

Some programs have been open to residents from all postgraduate years (Craig, 1988), whereas many focus on improving the skills of senior residents (Camp, et al., 1985; Doyle & Balsley, 1979; Susman & Gilbert, 1995; Troupin, 1990). Incoming residents at one institution (Pristach, et al., 1991) receive instruction in large group teaching skills and bedside teaching. Johnson, et al. (1996) described a program for all pediatric residents, but content areas are specific for the year of training. Instruction in one-on-one teaching, small group discussion, and large group discussion are directed toward first-, second-, and third-year residents, respectively. However, some programs for residents, such as the Stanford Faculty Development Program (Skeff, et al., 1992) do not differentiate content areas by specialty or postgraduate year, but provide general principles of learning and teaching.

A unique method to improve senior resident teaching skills was described by Orlander, Bor, and Strunin (1994). This program uses senior residents to supervise interns undergoing a seven-station objective structured clinical examination (OSCE).

This "clinical feedback exercise" was thought to exemplify typical resident-intern interactions, and provided a structured opportunity to improve residents' feedback skills.

In view of inadequate resources, program directors' lack of support for such training (Anderson, et al., 1990; Bing-You & Tooker, 1993), and residents' time constraints, teaching skills programs may not be the only available method to improve resident teaching. Bing-You, Greenberg, Wiederman, and Smith (1997) recently described a randomized, multicenter trial addressing the impact of written learner feedback (i.e., summary of a team interview and rating forms) on resident teaching. Over a one-year period, those senior residents receiving written feedback had higher ratings for two specific teaching characteristics: establishes rapport, provides direction and feedback. Overall teaching effectiveness tended to improve for the experimental group and remained stable for the control group.

In summary, this section suggests the following potential lessons learned for the 21st century:

- There is a wide variety of resident teaching skills programs, and no standardized content or instructional method has been established.
- Teaching skills programs have been conducted in numerous specialties, and residents' teaching skills needs may vary by specialty.
- Teaching skills programs may involve residents from all postgraduate years, and content areas may need to differ by level of training.
- Multiple approaches to define content areas are available.
- Giving residents written feedback about their teaching may improve teaching.

WHAT EXISTING EVIDENCE SUPPORTS THE EFFECTIVENESS OF TEACHING SKILLS PROGRAMS FOR RESIDENTS?

Many of the studies described in the previous section assessed residents' satisfaction with participation in these programs, consistently finding that residents valued and enjoyed such instruction. Using quantitative and qualitative evaluation methods, several programs also have indicated that residents' attitudes toward teaching, confidence in their teaching, and self-perceived teaching behaviors have improved. For example, Edwards, Kissling, Plauche, and Marier (1986) found that approximately 18 months after a mandatory one half day workshop for first-year residents, residents continued to rate their teaching skills significantly higher than before the course. Residents could still recall and explain major teaching points (e.g., specifying teaching objectives, using questioning techniques).

Nine studies have attempted to assess objective changes in resident teaching behavior (i.e., other than resident selfperceptions) through either observation (direct or videotape) or learner ratings of residents' skills (Bing-You, 1990; Edwards, et al., 1988b; Edwards, et al., 1988a; Jewett, et al., 1982; Lawson & Harvill, 1980; Litzelman, Stratos, & Skeff., 1994; Snell, 1989; Spickard, et al., 1996a; White, Bassali, & Heery, 1997). These studies are summarized in Table 15.2. Similarities between these studies should be noted. For those studies detailing a statistical analysis, all except one (Jewett, et al., 1982) showed evidence of a statistically significant improvement in resident teaching behaviors, and two studies (Bing-You, 1990; Edwards, et al., 1988a) showed declines in skills over time. Postintervention assessments of residents' teaching skills have been short term (i.e., less than one-year follow-up). Except for two studies (Bing-You, 1990; Edwards, et al., 1988b), the number of residents studied has been small (range, 9 to 27). Only two studies (Edwards, et al., 1988; Jewett, et al., 1982b;) incorporated a randomized design. All of the programs used multiple educational activities, with role-modeling, skills practice, and extensive feedback used most frequently. Only one study described teaching in the context of the ambulatory setting (White, et al., 1997).

What conclusions can be drawn from these studies? These results suggest that resident teaching skills programs are effective in improving resident teaching behaviors. The ideal program (i.e., most efficient and cost effective), however, has not been clearly defined. This review provides a background for a future research agenda. Potential questions to be addressed include these: What is the long-term impact of improvement programs on resident teaching behaviors? Are programs equally effective across specialties? On what resident teaching skills should attention be focused? Do residents' teaching skills in the ambulatory setting need to be considered differently?

Recognizing that the limited number of studies precludes broad generalizations, the following lessons for the 21st century are offered:

- Teaching skills programs can improve resident teaching behaviors and perceptions.
- Multiple educational formats should be used, with particular emphasis on skills practice, role-modeling, and feedback.
- Single, time-limited (i.e., less than five-hrs.) and longer, multiple-session interventions may be effective.
- In keeping with the principles of adult learning, programs should address the context of the residents' environment (e.g., specialty, postgraduate year), the particular teaching challenges residents face (i.e., a just-in-time approach to determine practical teaching needs), and active resident participation in the program's educational activities.
- Reinforcement of improved teaching skills is important (e.g., booster sessions).

TABLE 15.2. Summary of Studies Evaluating Effectiveness
of Resident Teaching Skills Programs

Authors	No. Receiving Intervention	Intervention	Assessment Interval	Follow-Up	Change Noted
Lawson & Harvill (1980)	11	13, 1-hour sessions	Independent rating of paired, pre- and post-intervention videotapes	Immediate	Improvement in 4 skills and overall performance*
Jewett, et al. (1982)	27	Randomized; 2 one half day workshops	Ratings by faculty, peers, and students	<1 year	Instructed residents tended to be rated more often as effective
Edwards, et al. (1988a)	12	Randomized; one half day workshop	Videotape review of teaching	6-months. during and 6-months post-intervention	Increased overall teaching quality during instruction*
Edwards, et al. (1988b)	101	Mandatory, one half day workshop	Clerkship student ratings	<1 year	Increased ratings in 3 areas and overall effectiveness*
Snell (1989)	9	Five, 3-hour sessions	Ratings by instructors; ward ratings by faculty, junior residents, and students	Immediate to 5-8 months	Increased ratings in 3 areas*
Bing-You (1990)	26	8-hour instructional	Videotape review hours over 6 months	2-11 months	Increase in 3 specific skills*
Litzelman, et al. (1994)	72	Weekend retreat	Student ratings	4-months	Increase in 3 skills and overall clinical teaching
Spickard (1996)	22	3-hour workshop	Student ratings	<4-months	Improvement in 2 skills*
White (1997)	21	3.5-hour workshop	Faculty observation	3-months	Increased frequency of microskills observed

*Statistically significant findings

- Developing programs and currently conducted programs ideally should take place in the context of randomized, multicenter studies to address the many questions that remain about resident teaching skills programs.

HOW DOES THE MEDICAL EDUCATOR GET STARTED IN HELPING RESIDENTS TEACH BETTER?

It is hoped that the lessons outlined at the end of each section in this chapter will provide initial guidance for those interested in improving residents' teaching skills. Review of the many programs described, in particular those revealing positive changes in resident teaching behaviors, will provide the program planner with a multitude of options that can be tailored to his or her institutional and specialty-specific contexts. As a complementary approach to a teaching skills program, providing residents with direct feedback about their teaching (e.g., faculty observation, student ratings) may be effective. Initial efforts need not be on a grand scale, and better success may be achieved by focusing on replicating one of the time-limited programs described in the literature.

As mentioned at the beginning of this chapter, an excellent, comprehensive resource is the book entitled *Clinical Teaching for Medical Residents* (Edwards & Marier, 1988). Schwenk and Whitman (1984) also have produced a handbook to assist residents in these skills. Weinholtz and Edwards (1992) have published *Teaching During Rounds: A Handbook for Attending Physicians and Residents*. A videotape of resident teaching vignettes has been produced by Dr. Joyce Wipf and colleagues at the University of Washington School of Medicine.

Another excellent resource is the Group on Educational Affairs (GEA) Special Interest Group (SIG) for Residents' Teaching Skills. Since 1994, under the early direction of Drs. Joan Friedland (VA Medical Center, Houston, TX), Timothy Brigham (Jefferson Medical College), Linda Snell (McGill University), and Robert Bing-You (Maine Medical Center), the SIG has conducted workshops for those planning and implementing a teaching skills program. These workshops have been conducted at the annual Association of American Medical Colleges (AAMC) meeting as well as at the regional level. Besides sharing resources and approaches at these meetings, the SIG has the following ongoing projects:

- increasing awareness of the importance of residents' teaching roles
- disseminating information concerning teaching skills programs
- assisting the Organization of Resident Representatives as they define their goals
- obtaining information on existing programs, with an initial survey of all program directors.

The SIG has a home page on the Group on Educational Affairs Web site that includes a bibliography, a planning guide for beginning and implementing a program, resource contacts, and future meeting agendas. The authors close this chapter with their suggested guidelines for medical educators responsible for helping residents become better teachers:

- Secure the commitment from the program director and the necessary resources to implement a program.

- Conduct a needs assessment with residents to identify context-specific issues (i.e., needs related to the specialty, postgraduate year, or institution).

- Start with a limited activity (i.e., one format, one content area) and eventually expand to multiple educational formats, with an emphasis on skills practice.

- Reinforce teaching skills with written feedback, subsequent educational sessions or both.

REFERENCES

Accreditation Council for Graduate Medical Education. (1996). *Graduate Medical Education Directory, 1996-1997, 27*. Chicago: American Medical Association.

Anderson, K. D., Anderson, W. A., & Scholten, D. J. (1990). Surgical residents as teachers. *Current Surgery, 47*, 185-188.

Apter, A., Metzger R., & Glassroth, J. (1988). Residents' perceptions of their role as teachers. *Journal of Medical Education, 63*, 900-905.

Arseneau, R. (1997). Residents' question-asking behaviors during work rounds. *Academic Medicine, 72*, 71.

Ashikawa, H., Xu, G., & Veloski, J. J. (1992). Students' ratings of otolaryngology clerkship activities: The role of residents. *Medical Teacher, 14*, 77-81.

Ashton, C. M., Wray, N. P., Friedland, J. A., Zollo, A. J., & Scheurich, J. W. (1994). The association between residents' work-rounds styles and the process and outcome of medical care. *Journal of General Internal Medicine, 9*, 208-212.

Barrow, M. V. (1966). Medical student opinions of the house officer as a medical educator. *Journal of Medical Education, 41*, 807-810.

Bing-You, R. G. (1990). Differences in teaching skills and attitudes among residents after their formal instruction in teaching skills. *Academic Medicine, 65*, 483-484.

Bing-You, R. G., & Greenberg, L. W. (1990). Training residents in clinical teaching skills: A resident-managed program. *Medical Teacher, 12*, 305-309.

Bing-You, R. G., Greenberg, L. W., Wiederman, B. L., & Smith, C. S. (1997). A randomized multicenter trial to improve resident teaching with written feedback. *Teaching and Learning in Medicine: An International Journal, 9*, 10-13.

Bing-You, R. G., & Harvey, B. J. (1991). Factors related to residents' desire and ability to teach in the clinical setting. *Teaching and Learning in Medicine: An International Journal 3*, 95-100.

Bing-You, R. G., & Sproul, M. S. (1992). Medical students' perceptions of themselves and residents as teachers. *Medical Teacher, 14*, 133-138.

Bing-You, R. G., & Tooker, J. (1993). Teaching skills improvement programmes in U.S. internal medicine residencies. *Medical Education, 27*, 259-265.

Brown, R. S. (1970). House staff attitudes toward teaching. *Journal of Medical Education, 45*, 156-159.

Camp, M. G., Hoban, J. D., & Katz, P. (1985). A course on teaching for house officers. *Journal of Medical Education, 60*, 140-142.

Craig, J. L. (1988). Teacher training for medical faculty and residents. *Canadian Medical Association Journal, 139*, 949-952.

Doyle, B. B., & Balsley, E. (1979). Supervision of the resident as a teacher. *Journal of Medical Education, 54*, 338-339.

Edwards, J. C., Kissling, G. E., Plauche, W. C., & Marier, R. L. (1988a). Evaluation of a teaching skills improvement programme for residents. *Medical Education, 22*, 514-517.

Edwards, J. C., Kissling, G. E., Brannan, J. R., Plauche, W. C., & Marier, R. L. (1988b). Study of teaching residents how to teach. *Journal of Medical Education, 63*, 603-610.

Edwards, J. C., Kissling, G. E., Plauche, W. C., & Marier, R. L. (1986). Long-term evaluation of training residents in clinical teaching skills. *Journal of Medical Education, 61*, 967-970.

Edwards, J. C., & Marier, R. L., (Eds.). (1988). *Clinical teaching for medical residents: Roles, techniques, and programs.* New York: Springer.

Greenberg, L. W., Goldberg, R. M., & Jewett, L. S. (1984). Teaching in the clinical setting: Factors influencing residents' perceptions, confidence, and behaviour. *Medical Education, 18*, 360-365.

Irby, D. M. (1979). Teaching and learning style preferences of family medicine preceptors and residents. *The Journal of Family Practice, 8*, 1065-1067.

Jewett, L. S., Greenberg, L. W., & Goldberg, R. M. (1982). Teaching residents how to teach: A one-year study. *Journal of Medical Education, 57*, 361-366.

Johnson, C. E., Bachur, R., Priebe, C., Barnes-Ruth, A., Lovejoy, F. H., & Hafler, J. P. (1996). Developing residents as teachers: Process and content. *Pediatrics, 97*, 907-916.

Kassebaum, D. G. (1988). Teaching residents how to teach. *Journal of Medical Education, 63*, 660.

Kates, N. S., & Lesser, A. L. (1985). The resident as a teacher: A neglected role. *Canadian Journal of Psychiatry, 30*, 418-421.

LaPalio, L. R. (1981). Time study of students and house staff on a university medical service. *Journal of Medical Education, 56*, 61-64.

Lawson, B. K., & Harvill, L. M. (1980). The evaluation of a training program for improving residents' teaching skills. *Journal of Medical Education, 55*, 1000-1005.

Lewis, J. M., & Cappelman, M. M. (1984). Teaching styles: An introductory program for residents. *Journal of Medical Education, 59*, 355.

Liaison Committee on Medical Education. (1993). *Functions and structure of a medical school.* Washington, DC: Association of American Medical Colleges.

Litzelman, D. K., Stratos, G. A., & Skeff, K. M. (1994). The effect of a clinical teaching retreat on residents' teaching skills. *Academic Medicine, 69*, 433-434.

Lowry, S. F. (1976). The role of house staff in undergraduate surgical education. *Surgery, 80*, 624-628.

Meleca, C. B., & Schimpfhauser, F. T. (1976). A house staff training program to improve the clinical instruction of medical students. *Proceedings of the 15th Annual Research in Medical Education Conference* (pp. 267-273). Washington, DC: Association of American Medical Colleges.

Meyers, A., Margolis, C. Z., Sheehan, J., Aita, S. J., & Risser, W. (1974). A time study of the pediatric resident's day. *Pediatrics, 53*, 712-715.

Orlander, J. D., Bor, D. H., & Strunin, L. (1994). A structured clinical feedback exercise as a learning-to-teach practicum for medical residents. *Academic Medicine, 69*, 18-20.

O'Sullivan, P. S., Weinberg, E., Boll, A.G., & Nelson, T. R. (1997). Students' educational activities during clerkship. *Academic Medicine, 72*, 308-313.

Pristach, C. A., Donoghue, G. D., Sarkin, R., Wargula, C., Doerr, R., Opila, D., Stern, M., & Single, G. (1991). A multidisciplinary program to improve the teaching skills of incoming housestaff. *Academic Medicine, 66*, 172-174.

Satran, L., & Harris, I. (1992). Medical student teaching by residents. *Resident and Staff Physician, 38*, 113-116.

Schwenk, T. L., & Whitman, N. A. (1984). *Residents as teachers: A guide to educational practice*. Salt Lake City, UT: University of Utah School of Medicine.

Sheets, K. J., Hankin, F. M., & Schwenk T. L. (1991). Preparing surgery house officers for their teaching role. *The American Journal of Surgery, 161*, 443-449.

Skeff, K. M., Stratos, G. A., Berman, J., & Bergen, M. R. (1992). Improving clinical teaching: Evaluation of a national dissemination program. *Archives in Internal Medicine, 152*, 1156-1161.

Snell, L. (1989). Improving medical residents' teaching skills. *Annals of Royal College of Physicians and Surgeons of Canada, 22*, 125-128.

Spickard, A., Corbett, E. C., & Schorling, J. B. (1996a). Improving residents' teaching skills and attitudes toward teaching. *Journal of General Internal Medicine, 11*, 475-480.

Spickard, A., Wenger, M., & Corbett, E. C. (1996b). Three essential features of a workshop to improve resident teaching skills. *Teaching and Learning in Medicine: An International Journal, 8*, 170-173.

Susman, J. L., & Gilbert, C. S. (1995). A brief faculty development program for family medicine chief residents. *Teaching and Learning in Medicine: An International Journal, 7*, 111-114.

Tonesk, X. (1979). The house officer as a teacher: What schools expect and measure. *Journal of Medical Education, 54*, 613-616.

Tremonti, L. P., & Biddle, W. B. (1982). Teaching behaviors of residents and faculty members. *Journal of Medical Education, 57*, 854-859.

Troupin, R. H. (1990). The mini-fellowship in teaching: A senior resident elective. *Investigative Radiology, 25*, 751-753.

Vu, T. R., Marriott, D. J., Skeff, K. M., Stratos, G. A., & Litzelman, D. K. (1997). Prioritizing areas for faculty development of clinical teachers by using student evaluations for evidence-based decisions. *Academic Medicine, 10*, (Suppl.): S7-S9.

Wargula, C. A. (1988). *Characteristics of effective resident teaching as perceived by third-year medical students and residents*. A study conducted at the State University of New York at Buffalo. [dissertation]

Weinholtz, D., & Edwards, J. C. (1992). *Teaching during rounds: A handbook for attending physicians and residents*. Baltimore: Johns Hopkins University Press.

White, C. B., Bassali, R. W., & Heery, L. B. (1997). Teaching residents to teach: An instructional program for training pediatric residents to precept third-year medical students in the ambulatory clinic. *Archives in Pediatric and Adolescent Medicine, 151*, 730-735.

Wilkerson, L., Lesky, L., & Medio, F. J. (1986). The resident as teacher during work rounds. *Journal of Medical Education, 61*, 823-829.

Wipf, J.. E. , Pinsky L. E., & Burke, W. (1995). Turning interns into senior residents: Preparing residents for their teaching and leadership roles. *Academic Medicine, 70*, 591-596.

Wray, N. P., Friedland, J. A., Ashton, C. M., Scheurich, J., & Zollo, A. J. (1986). Characteristics of house staff work rounds on two academic general medicine services. *Journal of Medical Education, 61*, 893-900.

Xu, G., Brigham, T. P., Veloski, J. J., & Rodgers, J. F. (1993). Attendings' and residents' teaching role and students' overall rating of clinical clerkships. *Medical Teacher, 15*, 217-222.

Xu, G., Veloski, J. J., & Brigham, T. P. (1995). A correlation study of students' perceptions of their active role as related to their clerkship experiences. *Medical Teacher, 17*, 199-203.

Yedidia, M. J., Schwartz, M. D., Hirschkorn, C., & Lipkin M. (1995). Learners as teachers: The conflicting roles of medical residents. *Journal of General Internal Medicine, 10*, 615-623.

CHAPTER SIXTEEN

Muddy Problems, Compassionate Care: Continuing Medical Education in the 21st Century

Nancy Bennett
Harvard Medical School

Continuing medical education (CME) will play a vital new role in health care during the 21st century. The evolving change results from a sharpening of its role based on a rapidly growing body of research and thoughtful interpretation of what we know about how to support physicians as they learn. Continuing medical education is the component of health care that will link all of the resources for physicians to learn effectively, beginning with the needs of each individual physician as practice settings shift, employers provide new options, and science grows.

Although CME is changing rapidly, some critical components of medicine are not. Patient problems will remain complicated with difficult solutions. Patients will not have "textbook" cases, and the problems will be difficult to manage with many ambiguous or "muddy" facets. A physician cannot predict with certainty which patients will respond to a drug or therapy, how several health problems will affect each other to diminish response to an effective protocol, or when an intervention will create new problems. A physician must make complicated choices about watchful waiting versus treatment, often without definitive data. Weighing choices to balance several problems for the overall health of the patient is difficult, and, physicians struggle with ways to be responsible for ethical and compassionate care in new environments. Although those in CME will not find simple answers to muddy problems, uniting disparate pieces of the health care system will support physicians as they struggle with these issues. This chapter describes components of a new CME system emerging for the 21st century that will address ways to look at learning for muddy problems and compassionate care.

Predicting the future of CME requires some understanding of the past. Through the 1970s and 1980s there was an enormous expansion of traditional CME, most often defined as a skillfully delivered lecture with instructional objectives, good attendance, helpful material, and a comfortable setting. This assumed that better practice came from more knowledge. Information was presented to a group of physicians, each of whom could pick out what he or she needed. Although significant effort went into describing the needs of learners, CME focused primarily on selecting good teachers. Evaluating whether the audience found the lecture helpful and enjoyable was far easier than defining what each person in the audience understood from that lecture. Traditional CME was comfortable for physicians, and often interesting, but it was not effective in changing physicians' behavior (Bennett & Casebeer, 1995; Davis, Thomson, Oxman, & Haynes, 1995; Fox, Mazmanian, & Putnam, 1989). The success of the system was measured in numbers, such, as how many people attended, how many hours of content were presented, and how many dollars were earned. Consequently, CME as a learning support system for physicians was tangled with CME as a business. It is clear that just as health care has been in turmoil, so has CME.

LEARNING FROM EXPERIENCE

Drafting the future system begins with understanding how physicians learn from their own experiences and how learning can improve health outcomes. Physicians must understand and use their own clinical experiences to assess what practices remain appropriate, what practices must be dropped, what must be added, and what problems remain troublesome. Patients present with problems that often are complex to define. Moreover, patients live complicated lives that prevent them from taking care of themselves in optimal ways. What is the role of a physician in working with a patient who does not want to stop smoking? When will surgery for prostate disease outweigh the benefits of medical management for an active 60-year-old or for a less active 80-year-old? When will an intensive regimen for control of blood sugars in diabetes be warranted when the patient does not seem to find diet changes consistent with family demands? To create a common baseline to see a new support system for learning, three forces that influence on learning shape a picture.

First, physicians who know how to provide optimal care do not always have improved outcomes for their patients. Nowlen (1988) used a double helix to describe factors that predict the patterns of practice for professionals. One of the interwoven strands of the helix is the culture in which medicine exists, which is made up of societal standards and community expectations. The other strand is each individual's personal history made up of experiences, relationships, and training, with their strengths and limitations. The two are interwoven to reflect the way individuals practice within the parameters of our culture.

Providing care includes technical skills as well as psychosocial skills and compassionate, ethical care. The picture of the double helix explains why a physician who increases his or her competence in an area may not see better results in patient care if society does not value that change. Alcoholism is one example. Some effective ways exist to help patients who have problems related to alcohol use, but the general public has conflicting feelings about the role of alcohol in socializing and their own experiences with drinking. As a result, reimbursement for such efforts as well as funding for innovative programs is uneven and inconsistent, and patients get mixed support from friends and family. Smoking cessation, preventative care, and weight loss are other examples of areas in which the available medical access and options conflict with societal ambivalence (Pincus, Esther, DeWalt, & Callaha, 1998).

LEARNING FROM REAL PROBLEMS

As a second force that influences learning, real patient problems are confusing and messy to diagnose and treat, and there may be more than one reasonable practice. Schön's model of reflective practice (Coles, 1996; Schön, 1987) describes the way physicians understand clinical problems as a result of their from education and experience. Whereas most education uses examples of problems that are overly simplistic or on the "high ground," most real-life problems are in the "swampy lowland" of confusing, messy, muddy problems that do not respond to simple answers. Many problems in medicine have no definitive answer, and some will not have a successful solution. Problems may have no single response, but may be treated in a variety ways according to how a physician sees the problem.

Schön (1987) referred to complicated problems as existing in the zone of indeterminacy. Solving a problem involves first defining what it is or framing the question. Framing the question means we must know how to think about it. If the problem resides in an area in which we have little experience, we can think about it only in simple terms. Schön supposed that we only ask questions for which we already have answers. A partial diagnosis, a somewhat ineffective treatment plan, or a less than optimal follow-up may be based on lack of experience so that the questions asked reflect a lack of appreciation for the complexity of the problem. In other words, a physician was not able to extract enough information from previous similar problems to shape a new response, or he or she had not been involved in a sufficient number of experiences to build a knowledge base sufficiently helpful for the new problem. Helping a patient with diabetes to change lifestyle and eating habits demands some sense of the family dynamics, access to and understanding of adaptations for diet and medication, and resources. Treating depression demands recognizing depression as a problem, differentiating it from other problems, and understanding the causes and options for treatment. Cultural differences, physical limitations, and "home" or alternative remedies are a few of the major contributors to how a patient complies with the kind of protocol the physician suggests.

LEARNING IN ORGANIZATIONS

Third, physicians understand the practice of medicine from their own experiences. Physicians do not practice in isolation, and their experiences are not in isolation. Physicians interact with other health professionals and administrators, consult with colleagues about difficult problems, and admit patients to hospitals. Each setting represents an organization, and each organization has a personality with a culture, rules, and functions that result from how its members learn, change, and work with each other. The potential power of adding together what each individual in a group knows makes organizational learning an important feature of CME. Sharing expertise among colleagues at the point of practice is part of learning. The business literature over the past decade has devoted much attention to whether organizations can learn and therefore make changes. Senge (1990) said that an organization learns by testing experiences, and transforming them into knowledge relevant to its core purpose, accessible to the whole organization. Other authors take the stance that only individuals create knowledge, and the organization provides a setting for that to happen (Confessore, 1991; Watkins & Marsick, 1993). All of these ideas suggest ways that CME will provide opportunities for physicians to "know" more ways to address patient problems as a result of working within different kinds of organizations.

CONTINUING MEDICAL EDUCATION IN THE 21ST CENTURY

Continuing medical education in the 21st century will focus on supporting individual physicians using a responsive learning system. We can draw from the models in this chapter to shape a picture. Specifically, CME educators will support a system so that each physician will have a self-directed curriculum of learning for which he or she will be accountable. Each physician will have opportunities to learn from a group of colleagues, formally and informally, and each physician will contribute to the way his or her organization learns. Skillful use of change strategies for both individual physicians and their organizations will be part of daily life. Learning will take place in more kinds of settings, especially at the point of service, making use of new formats. Electronically assisted learning and other new formats will continue to emerge as a critical element in accessing and managing information.

Educators in CME will support physicians in three overlapping and interconnected learning systems. The most basic and essential layer is the self-directed curriculum designed by each physician to reflect on personal experience about what works and what does not. An individual's learning system forms the basis for giving meaning to the huge amount of available material. Physicians sort, categorize, classify, and incorporate pieces of what they see in order to make changes. Without a self-directed curriculum, a physician cannot make decisions about what is necessary and appropriate to learn, and about which changes reduce the gap between current and desired practice. Physicians will choose from among a wide range of options for learning according to the nature of the problem and what would be an effective way to address it. Individual learning style, stage of professional development, goals for practice and many other factors will contribute to the decisions.

The second learning system includes informal and formal group learning. Ranging from hallway chats to formal, traditional programs by groups such as medical schools and professional organizations, group learning serves as a source of interaction and helps to shape the image of a change. Individuals do not make changes based on learning from one source (Anderson, Wheeler, Goldberg, Hosmer, Forcier, et al., 1994; Fox, Parboosingh, Rankin, Smith & Costie,1997; Rankin & Fox, 1995). Group learning provides a variety of resources to support the self-directed curriculum.

The third learning system is the societal definition of health care that provides the standards physicians use to create a rationale for care. It is Nowlen's (1988) second part of the double helix that reflects beliefs, norms, ethics, and standards. Accreditation bodies, social service agencies, and government units all are bodies that reflect societal demands in different ways. Societal systems create some of the rules that govern practice, and the rules that govern how learning is provided.

To be part of the new system, educators in CME must understand how, when, where, and why physicians learn as well as ways to integrate the components of the learning system. Learners must understand how they use each part of the learning system and ways to make that process more effective and efficient. In the next era, both physicians and educators will be held accountable for their use of the learning systems to reach agreed-on goals (Davis & Fox, 1994).

The CME learning system is centered on the self-directed curriculum. One option for use in a self directed curriculum, learning in groups, will remain an important part of CME, as it is now. Lectures, journal clubs, grand rounds, case management review sessions, and hallway consultations will continue to be some of the important ways physicians learn from each other. Formal learning has a role in shaping ideas and helping learners to reflect on ideas from new sources. It is one way to summarize and evaluate available information efficiently. Teachers can act as coaches who demonstrate the translation of experience into expertise by guiding physicians as they think about how to frame a problem in a new way, or how to recognize a "surprise." Both formal and informal group learning are ways of encouraging physicians to expand their ability to frame a broader array of questions.

Each approach to learning is useful in specific ways. We know that a lecture does not help support an individual in doing a new procedure, but it may be helpful in listing pros and cons of that procedure. Actual practice in a workshop or laboratory improves performance and allows a physician to imagine how a new procedure fits into his or her practice. Lectures do not "remind" or warn physicians about a drug interaction as they prescribe new medications, but computerized records with software "smart agents" do. Problem-based learning provides specific problems to solve, with guidance from a coach or group of peers to expand the way an individual looks at a specific problem, and may expand the repertoire of possible solutions for other problems. Solid links between institutional priorities and actual data will ensure that individuals have the expertise to perform at the highest level by making problems appropriate to a given setting. Educators will create a portfolio of formal learning options that respond to real needs identified by physicians. Educators also will support physicians in creating opportunities for informal learning by helping to foster organizational learning, supporting those things that contribute to reflection, and providing access to information in a timely manner. Electronically assisted learning will be a critical resource.

What are the details of CME in the 21st century? Each physician will use his or her own quantitative data such as patient panel data to compare personal results with more comprehensive data from the organization and from national sources. Qualitative data will come from personal experience, colleagues, and patients. Using data and reflection, physicians will become more skilled at defining the gaps between current practice and desired practice. A CME educator will help to identify sources for data and the kinds of available options that might address the identified gap. These might include such things as a formal program given by a medical school, reading as a result of a literature search, or information available on an Internet site. Educators will create and foster a climate that encourages organizational learning, and new kinds of communication with societal agencies will encourage expectations for physicians that are a blend of what science can do and what society wants.

Educators in CME will innovatively and capably support physicians as they change their performance by facilitating opportunities that are effective for learning. When we can list the kinds of changes we want, we can design learning to address those desired changes. The design cannot be overly simplistic or inexpensive in terms of time and money if effectiveness is the goal. However, we know how to be effective in planning learning that results in change. The new CME system will be able to list the desired changes, support physicians in making them, and foster organizations as they learn and adapt.

REFERENCES

Anderson, F. A., Wheeler, H. B., Goldberg, R. F., Hosmer, D. W., Forcier, A., & Patwardhan, N. A. (1994). Changing clinical practice: Prospective study of the impact of continuing medical education and quality assurance programs on use of prophylaxis for venous thromboembolism. *Archives of Internal Medicine, 154,* 669-677.

Bennett, N. L., & Casebeer, L. (1995). The evolution of planning. *Journal of Continuing Education in the Health Professions, 15*(2), 70-79.

Coles, C. (1996). Approaching professional development. *Journal of Continuing Education in the Health Professions, 16*(3), 152-158.

Confessore, S. (1991). Building a learning organization: Communities of practice, self-directed learning, and CME. *Journal of Continuing Education in the Health Professions, 17*(1), 5-11.

Davis, D. A., & Fox, R. D. (Eds.), (1994). *Physicians as learners*. Chicago: The American Medical Association Press.

Davis, D. A., Thomson, M. A., Oxman, A. D., & Haynes, B. (1995). Changing physician performance: A systematic review of the effect of continuing medical education strategies. *Journal of American Medical Association, 274,* 700-705.

Fox, R. D., Mazmanian, P. E., & Putnam, R. W. (Eds.), (1989). *Change and learning in the lives of physicians*. New York: Praeger.

Fox, R. D, Parboosingh, J., Rankin, R., Smith, E., & Costie, K. A. (1997, Summer). Learning and the adoption of innovations among Canadian Radiologists. *Journal of Continuing Education in the Health Professions, 17*(3), 173-186.

Nowlen, P. (1988). *A new approach to continuing education for business and the professions*. New York: Collier Macmillan.

Pincus, T., Esther, R., DeWalt, D. A, & Callaha, L. F. (1998). Social conditions and self-management are more powerful determinants of health than access to care. *Annals of Internal Medicine, 129,* 406-411.

Rankin, R., & Fox, R. D. (1995). Innovation adoption: Interview with Canadian radiologists. *Annals of the Royal College of Physicians and Surgeons of Canada, 28,* 100-103.

Schön, D. A. (1987). *Educating the reflective practitioner: Toward a new design for teaching and learning in the professions*. San Francisco: Jossey-Bass.

Senge, P. (1990). *The fifth discipline*. New York: Doubleday.

Watkins, K., & Marsick, V. (1993). *Sculpting the learning organization: Lessons in the art and science of systematic change*. San Francisco: Jossey-Bass.

PART III

MAJOR CURRICULUM
MOVEMENTS

CHAPTER SEVENTEEN

Major Curriculum Movements

Quinn Mast-Cheney

EDITORS NOTE

The idea of collecting the thoughts of a number of experts and putting them into a book that would pave the way for medical educators in the new millennium came from Terrill Mast, PhD. Terry organized the concept of the book and made numerous contacts with colleagues to set the stage for the various chapters. He had begun to organize his chapter when his health began to fail, and unfortunately the writing was never completed. He had intended to describe the major movements in medical education, a theme that reflected some of the major curricular movements at the Southern Illinois University School of Medicine during Terry's evolving career. His daughter Quinn, taking over from Terry's unfinished, rough notes, has provided her insights regarding some of these movements as they were played out at this school.

Theory and practice in the educational world outside of medical education often have stimulated instructional practice in the medical environment. In other cases, medical education has influenced the rest of the educational world. One of the educational practices discussed in this chapter has its roots in the general educational arena, and three have their roots in medical education.

A significant outside educational movement that had an impact on medical and surgical education was the emphasis on developing behavioral objectives, statements aimed at identifying what students would be able to do as a result of instruction. The Southern Illinois University School of Medicine was one school that adopted an objectives-based approach in the late 1970's (Silber, Williams, Pavia, Taylor, & Robinson, 1978). That curriculum centered around five central points: Learning objectives were shared with students before instruction began; the competencies tested corresponded to those specified in the objectives; criteria for measuring performance were developed in advance; multiple opportunities to achieve competency were afforded to students; and remedial assistance was offered to students to aid them in overcoming any difficulties. To ensure that students retained the learned material, a continuing cycle of practical applications and tests accompanied the stated goals.

Learning objectives became the basis on which all decisions regarding what and how to teach were made. Here, as in many places, objectives were usually part of a larger organizational unit--the organ system. With Case Western Reserve University School of Medicine leading (Hamm, 1962), the use of organ systems became a major organizational structure for the delivery of the basic sciences. Often, teaching teams were formed, composed of educators from each basic science discipline and one or more physicians, and when possible, topics were presented as problem units such as headache or diabetes. This approach assisted students in understanding relevance, and provided them with a framework to organize their knowledge. Whereas the early use of objectives focused on the content, skills, and behaviors that students should acquire, objectives currently tend to focus on performance outcomes in terms of how well students can orchestrate their knowledge, skills, and behaviors in the resolution of undifferentiated patient problems.

Most recently, the Medical School Objectives Project (MSOP), initiated by the Association of American Medical Colleges (AAMC: Medical School Objectives Writing Group, 1999), was designed to assist medical schools in developing objectives that reflected the changes in society's expectations of physicians. Specifically, MSOP was designed to determine the attributes that medical students should possess and be able to demonstrate at graduation. To be considered successful, physicians, in addition to being knowledgeable and scholarly, must be altruistic, skillful, and dutiful, treating patients and their families with compassion, patience, honesty, integrity, and respect.

Ensuring that students possessed specified skills such as these as a condition of graduation led to the development of performance-based assessment practices, including the Objective Structured Clinical Examination (OSCE; Harden & Gleeson, 1979) and, later, the Clinical Performance Examination (CPX); Barrows, Williams, & Moy, 1987; Williams & Barrows, 1987). A Josiah Macy Junior Foundation-supported curriculum reform conference concluded that the most effective way to change the medical education process was to change the way students are assessed, thus providing the impetus for changing medical schools' reliance on multiple-choice examinations to evaluate performance-assessment practices. Demonstrations for deans and medical educators of the Southern Illinois University School of Medicine's performance-based, senior examination used to assess students' readiness for postgraduate education led to a national interest in the technique and the development of multiple consortia funded by Macy. Currently, the use of performance assessments by 85% of the medical schools (AAMC, 1998), the Canadian licensure association, and the Educational Commission on Foreign Medical Graduates, as well as their planned use by the National Board of Medical Examiners on the United States Medical Licensing Examination, Step 2 demonstrates that it is becoming one of the most accepted methods for evaluating students' clinical acumen.

Performance-based testing would not have been possible had it not been for standardized patients (SPs). First developed by Dr. Howard Barrows (1964), standardized patients are persons trained to present a patient's illness in a standardized way, or actual patients trained to present their illness in a standardized way. Initially, standardized patients were used to provide a relevant context for students to learn and practice their clinical reasoning and problem-solving skills and for assessments during a neurology clerkship. Using standardized patients as a means for students to learn and demonstrate their patient care skills, having proven highly effective, has grown from a clerkship assessment tool to one that assesses students' history and physical examination skills, clinical reasoning skills, and knowledge.

The early work of Elstein, Shulman, and Sprafka (1978) as well as that of Barrows, Norman, Neufeld, and Feightner (1982) not only enhanced the ability of faculty to more easily assess components of the clinical reasoning process, but also stimulated the development of a provocative learning method that has captured the interests of educators across the educational spectrum. Introduced at McMaster University in 1968 (Spaulding, 1969), the use of (PBL) has increased significantly in medical schools around the world. Although few medical schools have adopted a total curriculum, many have incorporated components of the problem-based learning approach into the conventional curriculum.

In their book, *Medical Problem Solving: An Analysis of Clinical Reasoning*, Elstein, et al. (1978, p. vii) defined problem solving as "the process of making adequate decisions based on inadequate information." With the physician being the decision maker for more than 70% of our health care services, the need for medical and surgical education to focus on developing the problem-solving skills of students seems obvious.

These authors determined that diagnostic effectiveness varied from physician to physician, and related directly to the nature of the problem. A physician's previous experience with a related problem allowed him or her to determine which information was significant and how findings would be integrated into an appropriate hypothesis and conclusion. This assumption that effectiveness was related to experience suggested that a different approach to educating medical students was necessary, one that would give them repeated exposure to a variety of problems. These authors determined that "learning information is important but insufficient." What was needed instead was repetitive practice in applying information in a similar problem range.

Problem-based learning is centered around clinical problems as opposed to focusing on discrete subject-related concepts, the classic approach, which has left medical faculty concerned that what is learned during the preclinical years is not remembered or recalled during the clinical years of medical school and practice. When most of the preclinical material is taught out of the clinical context, students have difficulty in grasping the significance of what they are learning. Problem-based learning provides a link by actually demonstrating the significance of basic science information in the solution of patient problems, and also shifts the focus for learning from the faculty to the students because learning is a task for which they will be responsible their entire professional lives. In addition, students practice their clinical reasoning skills through repeated exposure to patient problems (Barrows, 1985).

These are the curriculum movements of which the author is most aware. They are special because they were developed and disseminated over a relatively short time, and they continue to have an impact on medical school curricula, as evidenced by the changing template of the AAMC Curriculum Directory (1998), and the accreditation standards of the Liaison Committee on Medical Education. They have provided the context for healthy debate among educators all over the world, have been the subject of innumerable articles published in the medical education literature, and chronicle very briefly the medical educational milieu in which the author's father participated.

REFERENCES

Association of American Medical Colleges. (1998, May). Emerging trends in the use of standardized patients. *Curriculum Issues in Medical Education, 1*(7). Washington, DC: AAMC.

Barrows, H. S. (1985). *How to design a problem--based curriculum for the preclinical years*. New York: Springer.

Barrows, H. S., & Abrahamson, S. (1964). The programmed patient: A technique for appraising student performance in clinical neurology. *Journal of Medical Education, 39*, 802-805.

Barrows, H. S. (1968). Simulated patients in medical education. *Canadian Medical Association Journal, 98*, 674-676.

Barrows, H. S., Norman, G. R., Neufeld, V. R., & Feightner, J. W. (1982). The clinical reasoning of randomly selected physicians in general medical practice. *Clinical and Investigative Medicine, 5*(1), 49-55.

Barrows, H. S., Williams, R. G., Moy, R. H. (1987). A comprehensive performance-based assessment of fourth-year students' clinical skills. *Journal of Medical Education, 62*(10), 805-809.

Elstein, A. S., Shulman, L., & Sprafka, S. (1978). Medical problem solving: *An analysis of clinical reasoning*. Cambridge, MA: Harvard University Press.

Hamm, T. H., (1962). Medical education at Case Reserve University. *New England Journal of Medicine, 267*(17), 868-874.

Harden, R. M., & Gleeson, F. A. (1979). Assessment of clinical competence using an objective structured clinical examination (OSCE). *Medical Education, 13*(1), 41-54.

Medical School Objectives Writing Group. (1999). Learning objectives for medical student education: Guidelines for medical schools: Report I of the Medical School Objectives Project. *Academic Medicine, 74*(1), 13-18.

Silber, D. L., Williams, R. G., Paiva, R. E. A., Taylor, D., & Robinson, R. (1978). The SIU medical curriculum: System objectives-based instruction. *Journal of Medical Education, 53*, 473-479.

Spaulding, W. B. (1969). The undergraduate medical curriculum (1969 Model): McMaster University. *Canadian Medical Association Journal, 100*(14), 659-664.

Williams, R. G., Barrows, H. S. (1987). Performance-based assessment of clinical competence using clinical encounter multiple stations. *International Conference Proceedings: Further developments in assessing clinical competence*, pp. 425-433. Ottawa, Canada: Can-Heal Publications.

CHAPTER EIGHTEEN

U. S. Medical Schools' Combined Degree Programs Leading to the MD and a Baccalaureate, Master's, or Other Doctoral Degree

Louise Arnold
Kenneth Roberts
University of Missouri-Kansas City School of Medicine

Physicians in the United States typically have two academic degrees, some three or more. Most earned their degrees after completing distinct curricula for each degree, often at different educational institutions, during discrete periods. However, some physicians followed a combined degree track that unified their studies toward dual degrees through a single admissions process, alternative curricula, or overlapping enrollment. Today U.S. medical schools offer combined-degree programs that lead to the MD degree along with a baccalaureate degree, a master's degree, a PhD, or another doctoral degree. This chapter focuses on baccalaureate-MD and PhD-MD programs because of their longevity, prevalence, student numbers, and availability of studies about them. These programs emerged in the 1960s. More than three decades later, in 1996-1997, one fourth of U.S. medical schools sponsored 53 baccalaureate-MD degree programs that admitted more than 900 students. In the same year there were slightly more than 100 PhD-MD degree programs that enrolled 300 students. This chapter also touches on combined JD-MD programs to illustrate the more recent development of curricula merging medicine with a host of other fields.

This chapter characterizes the programs' history, purposes, matriculants, defining features, innovations, and outcomes. It closes with speculation about the challenges they face and their future roles. The discussion rests on information from peer-reviewed publications, qualitative interviews with selected program directors, program documents, and private communications.

BACCALAUREATE-MD DEGREE PROGRAMS

History

The idea of a combined baccalaureate-MD degree first appeared in the Johns Hopkins Medical Bulletin in 1931 (Calkins & Jonas, 1981). World War II introduced accelerated medical education (Calkins & Jonas, 1981). In the early 1950s the medical school at Western Reserve University began to integrate basic and clinical science teaching (Olson, 1992). These were the forerunners of today's baccalaureate-MD programs.

By the late 1950s, several interrelated trends set the stage for the implementation of these programs. Federally funded biomedical research deepened the base of scientific knowledge relevant to medicine (Burdi, 1986). The space age dawned; governmental support for scientific research and development intensified (Arnold, Boex, Smith, & Veloski, 1988). Applicants to medical school declined to a ratio of less than two per place in the entering class (Wiggins, Leymaster, Ruhe, Taylor, & Tipner, 1961). The brightest of college students entered fields other than medicine where they would encounter exciting and challenging courses of study (Calkins & Jonas, 1981). The need to revise the scientific preparation of the physician and to interdigitate premedical and medical courses took hold (Alexander, 1964; Cooper & Prior, 1961).

The early 1960s saw four medical schools, in partnership with an undergraduate institution, offer a combined baccalaureate-MD degree (Alexander, 1964; Cooper & Prior, 1961; Keefer, 1964; Sodeman, 1963). Most of these programs selected a small number of gifted high school seniors, who usually spent two years in a baccalaureate curriculum, joined a class of college graduates in a regular four-year medical curriculum, and received their bachelor's degree after the first- or second-year of medical school. Another program introduced a six-year curriculum culminating in a Bachelor's and Master's of Medical Science degree, with a thesis, followed by two years of clinical training in medical school (Smith, 1989). All these ventures sought to prepare students better for patient care, teaching, or research. The particular solution each program crafted to improve physicians' education reflected not only national developments but also local traditions, needs, and the vision of charismatic leaders (Alexander, 1964; Cooper & Prior, 1961; Keefer, 1964; Smith, 1989; Sodeman, 1963).

The confluence of national trends, local circumstances, and institutional leaders continued to give birth to baccalaureate-MD degree programs in subsequent decades. In the late 1960s and early 1970s, the physician shortage, the need for primary care, the desire for better more humanistic health care in underserved communities, and a Carnegie Foundation call to reduce the high cost of medical education created a spurt of new combined-degree programs (Daubney, Wagner, & Rogers, 1981; Norman & Calkins, 1992). The thrust of the period was to graduate more physicians more quickly. However, some combined programs also sought to attract qualified students from underserved populations (Arnold et al., 1988; Gellhorn & Scheuer, 1978). Others seized the opportunity to create major innovations to graduate well-rounded humanistic physicians (Burdi, 1986; Dimond, 1988; Pritchard, 1976). Foundation grants to improve curricula encouraged some of these changes (Sandson, Blaustein, Stewart, Ravin, & Rock, 1979) that anticipated recommendations of Association of American Medical Colleges (AAMC's) General Professional Education of the Physician (GPEP) report of 1984 (Arnold et al. 1987; Muller et al. 1984).

New programs in the 1980s responded to the ongoing need for primary care physicians (Bloom, Vatavuk, & Kaliszewski, 1988; Interviews with selected directors, December, 1997) or to a recurring decline of medical school applicants (Interviews with selected directors, December, 1997). Some programs incorporated GPEP sentiments to reduce the "premed syndrome;" others joined technological and medical curricula (Norman & Calkins, 1992). In the 1990s combined programs designed to attract rural and underrepresented minority students to medicine emerged again (Interviews with selected directors, December, 1997). Several of these programs planned to increase the diversity of their students by networking with high schools. The greatest impetus for new combined-degree programs in the 1990s came from liberal arts institutions in the wake of competition for bright students (Guaranteed admission to medical school, 1997). These institutions believe combined programs can improve the quality of their student body.

Purposes

National and local needs of an era shaped the institutional purposes of the baccalaureate-MD degree programs. In summary, the initial purposes of the programs were to attract talented students into medicine, particularly gifted, rural, and minority high school students who might not otherwise become physicians; to assure them entry into medical school; to improve physician education by avoiding redundancy in high school and college curricula, creating vigorous yet flexible liberal arts and science courses, interdigitating college and medical school curricula and providing humane learning environments; to contain educational costs; to graduate physician scientists or clinicians, especially primary care providers; to produce well-trained, caring, socially conscious physicians in fewer calendar years; and to improve health care in surrounding communities by recruiting faculty to educate area students who hopefully would practice nearby. Not every program, it is important to note, subscribed to all the purposes.

Over time, program purposes have been generally stable. According to interviews with program directors, original purposes, such as graduating primary care physicians for practice in the surrounding region and educating minorities, have become even more relevant in the late 1990s. Other purposes such as improving the education of physicians express perennial intents of medical educators. More tightly integrating the phases of medical education that the early programs began has a contemporary ring. However, several initial purposes of baccalaureate-MD degree programs have lost their currency, for now. The need to graduate physicians faster has clearly faded (Norman & Calkins, 1992). Therefore, most baccalaureate-MD degree programs have lengthened their curricula, to enrich their students' preparation further. The need of liberal arts colleges to attract capable students has supplanted the need of medical schools to identify outstanding high school applicants (Interviews with selected directors, December, 1997). Emphasis on rigorous science preparation, especially for research careers, has moderated in some programs with that original intent (Smith, 1989; Interviews with selected directors, December, 1997).

Matriculants

Have combined programs found the high school students they sought--talented scholars who could become competent, caring physicians with career aspirations matching program goals? A partial answer lies in the nature of the matriculants themselves.

Baccalaureate-MD degree programs present opportunities for early bloomers (Olson, 1992). As multi-institutional research has determined, the combined-degree matriculants of 1990 chose medicine for a career at a far younger age than traditional medical students (Epstein, Hayes, Arnold, O'Sullivan, Ruffin, et al., 1994). Indeed, the shorter the program, the earlier the matriculants had identified medicine as their vocation. In the same study, combined-degree and traditional medical students found medicine attractive because of its service orientation and intellectual challenge. But unlike their peers, combined-degree students thought research opportunities and the extrinsic rewards of medicine also were important factors. Optimistic about medicine's future, the combined-degree matriculants expressed an openness to the type of medical career they would follow although they were drawn to clinical practice, a preference varying with program length. Earlier work showed that more combined-degree matriculants valued a culturally sophisticated, intellectual, and socially concerned academic orientation than did a national sample of college freshmen; whereas more combined-degree students were conventional and pragmatic than their college counterparts (Sloan & Brown, 1978).

Academic characteristics of matriculants have been impressive. In a multi-institutional study of entering students in 1990-1991 (Van Eyck & Arnold, 1993), entering students presented academic credentials that exceeded expected minimum levels for standardized test scores (1100-1300 SAT and 27-33 ACT), grade point averages (3.6-3.9), and class rank in high school (80th to 95th percentile). This work (Van Eyck & Arnold, 1993) and a later companion study in 1996 (Van Eyck,

Huggett, & Barnet, 1996) ascertained that, overall, the vast majority of matriculants met requirements for entry into the medical school phase of the programs.

From their inception (Kanter, 1969), baccalaureate-MD degree programs enrolled a larger percentage of women in their entering classes than did traditional medical schools (Grant, Arnold, Blaustein, Brown, Eder, 1986). These programs also attracted substantial proportions of students from Asian backgrounds (Grant, et al., 1986). After initial disappointments, several programs dedicated to the education of underrepresented minorities have successfully attracted target students (Roman & McGanney, 1994; Smith, 1993). For example, in one program the 1992-1993 underrepresented minority enrollment rate of 27% was more than double the national rate (Roman & McGanney, 1994).

In short, the students who have enrolled in baccalaureate-MD degree programs have typically matched program purposes on entry.

Defining Features

Baccalaureate-MD degree programs are not identical (Norman & Calkins, 1992). Dimensions along which they compare and contrast can identify the following regularities in defining features of the late 1990s (Interviews with selected directors, December, 1997; Medical School Admission Requirements 1998-1999, 1997):

- *Point of selection and matriculation: During the senior year of high school through the sophomore year of college.* Identifying students for the study of medicine during high school is a practice long typical of overseas programs in medical education. Of the 53 combined-degree programs in the United States, 85% select high school seniors through a single admissions process for entry into the program as college freshmen. Of the remaining 15% of the programs, most select students during the first-year of college for matriculation the following year. All but one guarantee students a spot in medical school if they meet performance standards. Only one fourth of these programs use the Medical College Admission Test (MCAT) as a factor in deciding if students will move into the medical school phase of the program.

- *Length of program: Six-, seven-, or eight- years with options for students to extend or shorten their course of study.* Slightly more than half of the 53 programs are *eight-years* long. Only four are currently six-years in length.

- *Field of study: Liberal arts or science.* Approximately two thirds of the programs say they encourage broad or liberal arts study for the baccalaureate degree. Their articulated emphasis coexists with permission for students to major in any discipline. About two thirds of the programs give students a choice of major, in which case most students major in science. The other one third of the programs require a science major. These programs tend to be in technologically oriented institutions. A few, however, have designed special science majors to encourage the study of humanities and social sciences, and the remainder are silent about a commitment to the liberal arts.

- *Integration between baccalaureate and medical school studies: Dual credit for coursework, and inclusion of medically relevant courses in the baccalaureate phase.* About half of the programs assign credit for a certain amount of coursework to both degrees. Programs that do are typically, but not exclusively, less than eight years in length. Of 27 programs reporting information, two thirds offered medically relevant courses in the baccalaureate phase. A richer index of integration was constructed for a study of curricular characteristics in 1983-1987 (Arnold, Xu, Epstein, & Jones, 1996). It included not only integration of medically relevant courses in the early curricular years, but also integration of liberal arts courses in the medical school phase. Of the eight programs studied, most achieved only low scores for curricular integration. The integration that occurs between baccalaureate and medical school studies is complex, and worthy of future study.
- *Track or freestanding programs.* The vast majority of baccalaureate MD degree programs are tracks during the undergraduate and medical school phases. Just four are stand-alone programs offering the combined-degree pathway as the major route to medicine.
- *Type of institutions: State or private.* Nearly half of the programs involve cooperation between public medical schools and public undergraduate institutions. An equal proportion consists of partnerships among private medical schools, colleges, and universities. A very few are liaisons between private and public institutions.

Innovations

To render the baccalaureate preparation of physicians more stimulating yet humanistic has been a leitmotiv of the combined-degree programs. Steps toward this goal have included a single admissions process; flexible requirements for an undergraduate major; elimination of unnecessary redundancy between high school, college, and medical school courses through advanced placement credits, double credits, and streamlined course content; and relatively generous performance requirements for advancing to the medical school phase, including elimination of the MCAT (Medical School Admission Requirements 1998-1999, 1997; Interviews with selected directors, December, 1997).

Other ways these programs energized the undergraduate curriculum and promoted problem-solving skills entailed opportunities for substantial research projects; strong health, society, and human values sequences; extensive service projects in medically related and other community agencies; early clinical clerkships, internships, and preceptorships; solid community medicine courses; and study abroad. (Medical School Admission Requirements 1998-1999, 1997; Interviews with selected directors, December, 1997).

Several programs have major support systems for students including proactive faculty and staff advisors (Hayes, Munro, Arnold, & Duckwall, 1993; Interviews with selected directors, December, 1997), appointment of psychologists and psychiatrists to work with students in the combined-degree programs (Hayes, Munro, et al., 1993; Interviews with selected directors, December, 1997), peer counselors (Interviews with selected directors, December, 1997), offices for professional development (Interviews with selected directors, December, 1997), formal partnerships between junior and senior students who teach and counsel each other as members of ongoing health care teams (Duckwall, Arnold, Willoughby, Calkins, & Hamburger, 1990), and student assignment to long-term learning communities with faculty mentors programs (Calkins, & Epstein, 1994; Hayes, et al., 1993).

Program innovations in medical education have been less frequent but significant. Some of the first programs revamped the basic science curriculum to reflect research advances of the era (Alexander, 1964; Campbell & De Muth, 1976; Cooper & Prior, 1961). Several planned for study of the humanities and social sciences during the medical phase of the program, only to find that practical considerations such as distances between cooperating institutions and conflicts in class schedules precluded implementation of the plans (Herbut, Sodeman, Conley, & Ascah, 1969; Interviews with selected directors, December, 1997). Such factors still constrain the intertwining of the humanities and social sciences with clinical medicine (Interviews with selected directors, December, 1997). However, several programs of the 1970s were and continue to be successful in this regard. Their humanities, social science, and community medicine sequences are remarkable (Interviews with selected directors, December, 1997). Service projects have been designed to promote medical student learning about community processes other than health care delivery (Interviews with selected directors, December, 1997). Flexible scheduling of medical school courses to meet students' own interests and needs is a contemporary reality in a few programs (Interviews with selected directors, December, 1997).

Longitudinal ambulatory care experiences have long been and still are hallmarks of three baccalaureate-MD degree programs (Arnold, Feighny, Hood, Stearns, Prislin, & et al., 1997b). Alternative teaching-learning formats--ongoing small groups called affinity or docent groups, formal mentoring, and student partnerships--have been central to medical education in several programs for decades (Calkins & Epstein, 1994; Duckwall et al., 1990). Nontraditional methods of student assessment such as progress testing and peer and self-evaluation also have been used (Arnold & Willoughby, 1990; Arnold, Willoughby, Calkins, Eberhart, & Gammon., 1981a; Arnold, Calkins, & Willoughby, 1985). Most, but not all, of these innovations in medical education have occurred in the free-standing combined-degree programs.

Outcomes: Students

Performances of baccalaureate-MD students and accomplishments of the programs themselves can document program success. Total attrition varies across programs and time. It is clear, however, that attrition of combined-degree students is much lower than that of premedical students, and in the medical school portion of the programs comparable to that of traditional medical students (Loftus & Willoughby, 1997). Attrition among women in combined-degree programs is higher than for men, but lower than the rate among premedical women (Loftus & Willoughby, 1997). Attrition among underrepresented minority students has been higher than for nonminority students (Loftus & Willoughby, 1997). However, more recent experience of a program targeted to the education of underrepresented minorities found convergence in attrition rates among minority and nonminority students (Roman & McGanney, 1994). Another program reported lower attrition among its minority combined-degree students than among minority students in a regular premedical curriculum (Smith, 1993). Attrition among rural and urban students is equivalent (Willoughby, Arnold, & Calkins, 1981).

In basic science and clinical medicine, the attainments of combined-degree students have on balance been comparable with those of traditional medical students (Loftus & Willoughby, 1997). This generalization applies to grade point averages (GPAs) (Golmon, 1981; Herbut et al., 1969; Kennedy & Austin, 1988; Lanzoni & Kayne, 1976), United States Medical Licensing Examination scores (Arnold, Willoughby, Calkins, & Jensen, 1981b; Blaustein, Meiselas, Brown, & Arnold, 1983; Gellhorn & Scheuer, 1978; Golmon, 1981; Herbut et al., 1969; Kanter, 1969; Lanzoni & Kayne, 1976), and clinical performance ratings in medical school (Blaustein et al., 1983; Golmon, 1981; Lanzoni & Kayne, 1976) and residency (Flair, 1969; Salzman, Arnold, & Willoughby, 1994). The most methodologically sound study of this topic concluded that a carefully chosen group of high school students can achieve high academic standards in a combined-degree program, graduate as younger physicians able to perform well in postgraduate training, and have highly productive careers in medicine (Callahan, Veloski, Xu, Hojat, Zeleznik, & et al., 1992).

Because selection of combined-degree students typically occurs in the senior year of high school, interest in predictors of their subsequent performance has practical and intellectual significance. Achievement of these students in high school can predict their academic performance in college and medical school (Arnold, Calkins & Willoughby, 1983). Furthermore, according to several studies, the clinical performance of these students can be predicted (Arnold et al., 1983; Arnold & Feighny, 1995; Arnold & Willoughby, 1993; Jones, 1991; Keck, Arnold, Willoughby, & Calkins, 1979; Willoughby, Gamon, & Jonas, 1979), an important result in as much as earlier work provided little evidence of a capacity to predict clinical performance (Loftus & Willoughby, 1997). Notably, other work on combined-degree students has determined that predictors of performance vary by gender (Calkins, Arnold, & Willoughby, 1987; Oggins, Inglebart, Brown, & Moore,

1988; Willoughby et al., 1979) and by ethnic and racial backgrounds of students (Calkins, Willoughby, & Arnold, 1982; Calkins & Willoughby, 1992).

Regarding career patterns, collaborative research involving eight baccalaureate-MD degree programs examined graduates' professional and personal characteristics that may be associated with curricular features of the programs (Arnold et al., 1996). The few differences obtained among the graduates concerned their practice patterns and accomplishments. They were accounted for primarily by program length. Graduates of six-year programs felt best prepared for careers focused on the physician's role as clinician and were most active in those careers. In contrast, graduates of seven- or eight-year programs said they were best prepared for and most accomplished in careers focused on the physician's role as scholar. A subsequent study showed that the work setting was the strongest correlate of the physician role that graduates played (Arnold, Willoughby, Xu, Epstein, & Jones, 1997c).

The same database also afforded a study of the career patterns followed men and women graduates of the baccalaureate-MD programs (Jones, Arnold, Epstein, & Xu, 2000). Differences were few and effect sizes small. Distinctions uncovered revealed that women were more likely to have traditional careers than men, an unexpected finding for women who had followed a nontraditional pathway to medicine.

Outcomes: Programs

Several indicators are available to judge the success of the programs themselves. First, early programs hoped to attract students who otherwise would not enroll. A contemporary study dramatically attested to the validity of that impetus (Albanese, Van Eyck, Huggett, Barnet, & Sugden, 1997b). Moreover, in that same program, the credentials of combined-degree students maintained the quality of the entire entering medical class during the nadir of national applications to medical school (Albanese, Van Eyck, Huggett, & Barnet, 1997a). In another program, the number of applicants never dipped during the nadir, and their outstanding qualifications remained constant (Calkin, Arnold & Huggett, 1997). The success of programs retaining racial and ethnic minorities, women, and rural students already has been reviewed.

Second, two studies of the courses that baccalaureate-MD students chose validated their programs' desire to encourage broad-based undergraduate work (Arnold et. al., 1988; Jacobs, Hinkley, & Pennell, 1988).

Third, the generally strong satisfaction of students with their programs has been reported consistently across institutions (Arnold et. al., 1996; Gottheil, Conley, & Menduke, 1972; Grossman, Conley, Menduke, & Graff, 1972; Jacobs et. al., 1988).

Fourth, concern for students' maturity to handle the pressures of their program has surfaced periodically. A body of work on this topic, however, found less perceived stress and greater ability to manage stress among combined-degree students than among traditional medical students (Arnold & Jensen, 1984; Calkins, Arnold, & Willoughby, 1994; Gottheil, et. al., 1972; Nathan, Nixon, Bairnsfather, Allen, & Hack, 1989).

Fifth, specialty choices of baccalaureate-MD graduates are of interest, particularly for programs that aspire to produce primary care physicians. Several studies suggest that programs with strong intent to graduate primary care providers were more likely to achieve this outcome than programs without such a commitment (Arnold et al., 1988; Bloom et al., 1988; Grant et al., 1986; Roman & McGanney, 1994), but not consistently (Callahan et. al., 1992). Predicting which students will enter primary care careers proved elusive when admissions data from one program were used systematically (Arnold et al., 1997a). A later study from the same school may provide an explanation (Munro, Feighny, & Arnold, 1997). It determined that students' career choices dramatically changed from the point of admissions to match day, as did their self-concepts and their images of specialties. These results also provide some evidence for the potential of combined-degree programs to guide students in their formative years.

Sixth, the number of programs has grown, increasing six-fold since the 1960s. Once begun, most combined-degree programs have continued. Only six have closed, and none were stand-alone programs.

Finally, these programs have been models for other combined-degrees in dentistry, engineering, business, and law. Some of their innovations such as integrated science courses, flexible scheduling, and early clinical experience have been adopted by traditional tracks in medical schools (Interviews with selected directors, December, 1997). Combined baccalaureate-MD programs, then, have been laboratories for exploring changes in professional education.

The Future

Can baccalaureate-MD degree programs demonstrate that their benefits outweigh the costs? The future of these programs hinges on the answer to that question (Interviews with selected directors, December, 1997). At least a few programs that closed seemingly did not consider their student outcomes distinctive enough to warrant the costs. In interviews, directors underscored their record of graduating substantially higher percentages of matriculants than those in the standard premedical curricula, with savings to students, institutions, and society. Although program costs have not been published, multiple positive outcomes have been documented. However, unless student outcomes remain positive, combined-degree programs will not be able to withstand imminent challenges. These include reduced student numbers that will make the programs too expensive to run, changes in medical education that will complicate current attempts of combined programs to integrate medical school and undergraduate studies, and attitudes toward education in managed care settings that may devalue liberal education and engender student concerns for their very livelihood (Interviews with selected directors, December, 1997).

Yet in these challenges may lie opportunities for baccalaureate-MD degree programs. After all, in the past these programs have responded to national and local needs effectively. Their record of attracting and graduating students who would not otherwise become physicians may give them a value-added edge. Their approach of networking with high schools, colleges, and medical schools to recruit area students from underserved populations, train them locally, encourage them to practice nearby, and improve the health of the region may create a powerful niche for these programs. Their scientific and humanistic curricula may enable graduates to grapple with medicine's growing technical and social complexities in changing health care settings.

Now that there is formal recognition of patient satisfaction as a key factor in health care outcomes, the humanistic thrust of the baccalaureate-MD programs may serve their graduates particularly well. Plans to deepen the abilities of combined-degree students by incorporating master's degree sequences into combined baccalaureate-MD curricula may prove sagacious. A useful step in this regard may be to offer baccalaureate-MD degree students a master's degree option in medical education inasmuch as some baccalaureate-MD programs are prone to graduate physicians who subsequently assume faculty positions in academic medicine (Arnold et al., 1996; Callahan et al., 1992).

MD-PHD PROGRAMS

History and Purpose

As organized academic entities, MD-PhD programs first appeared in the mid-1960s. The most visible of these were the medical science training programs (MSTPs) funded by the National Institutes of Health (NIH) (Shannon, 1976; Sutton & Killian, 1996). The impetus for these programs reflected a perceived need to correct fundamental science deficiencies of medical school graduates so they could become effective researchers. Because these deficits could not easily be addressed after awarding the MD degree (Shannon, 1976), the concept emerged of offering concurrent training in both medicine and research to interested medical students. That combined training, it was reasoned, would result in MD-PhD graduates who could best apply new basic science knowledge to the investigation of disease and its treatment (Sutton & Killian, 1996; Wyngaarden, 1979).

By the 1970s, the number of clinical investigators relative to research opportunities and open faculty positions declined (Bickel, Sherman, Ferguson, Baker, & Morgan, 1981; Davis & Kelley, 1982; Wyngaarden, 1979). Federal research funding continued to increase. New MD-PhD degree programs, therefore, opened, and their numbers rose steadily through the 1980s. A continuing decrease in clinical investigators, the potential of MD-PhD researchers to mine the rapid advances in biomedical science (Martin, 1991), and the emerging emphasis on population-oriented medicine (Watanabe, 1992) were factors in this growth. These same factors along with the need to replace clinical faculty account for the presence of MD-PhD programs in the 1990s (Interim Report of the NIH Director's Panel, December, 1996; Martin, 1991; McClellan & Talalay, 1992; Schrier, 1997; Sutton & Killian, 1996; Wartman, 1992, Fall). Recently, the clinical research role of MD-PhDs has been redefined to include patient-oriented research covering mechanisms of disease, therapeutic interventions, and clinical trials, epidemiologic and behavioral studies, outcomes research, and health services research (Interim Report of the NIH Director's Panel, December, 1996).

Despite the need for physician-scientists, less than 2% of all physicians are biomedical scientists (Cadman, 1990; Neilson, Ausiello, & Demer, 1995), and only 1.4% of senior medical students want to pursue a research career (Schrier, 1997).

Matriculants

What kinds of students decide to enter MD-PhD programs? Relatively little data are available to answer this question. In general, however, students have pursued this track from the outset of medical school because they have had prior research experience with an influential mentor or an already existing interest in research (Cadman, 1990; Wilkerson & Abelmann, 1993). Research experience and expressed interest are crucial factors in the preselection of students who matriculate into MSTP programs. The intellectual stimulation of research-oriented training and faculty role models are other reported motivators for MD-PhD matriculants (Wilkerson & Abelmann, 1993).

Why students do not choose these programs may be surmised from the more voluminous studies on why medical students are disinterested in research careers. Reasons for their disinterest include the prospect of longer research training (Schrier, 1997); the financial disadvantages of a research career relative to a medical practice (Silverman & McGugan, 1992); most importantly, the insecurities associated with a research career (Watanabe, 1992) such as limited job opportunities and limited job security, both perceived (Kennedy, 1994; Martin, 1991; Watanabe, 1992) and real (Kennedy, 1994); uncertain prospects for funding research in the short (Interim Report of the NIH Director's Panel, December, 1996; Martin, 1991; Schrier, 1997) and long term (Kennedy, 1994); and the amount of debt students face at the end of residency (Interim Report of the NIH Director's Panel, December, 1996; Kennedy, 1994).

Defining Features

Matriculation through MD-PhD programs takes approximately seven years (Kennedy, 1994). Biochemistry is the most common discipline that both MSTP and non-MSTP students pursue. Other top disciplines that MSTP students choose strongly reflect laboratory sciences such as neuroscience, molecular biology, and cell biology. In contrast, other top choices of non-MSTP students appear to be more clinical (e.g., pharmacology, physiology, and anatomy; Sutton & Killian, 1996). In general, research training of students tends to mirror the basic science problems of the disciplines within which they will receive the PhD (Sutton & Killian, 1996).

Possibly because graduate programs are flexible, discussions of other curricular characteristics in the literature are sketchy. Of interest would be future studies detailing the nature of required coursework, approaches used to reduce potential redundancies in basic science coursework for the two degrees, and the temporal sequencing of work toward each degree including course requirements, clinical clerkships laboratory or other research activities, and the onset of residency training.

Outcomes

Nearly 400 new MD-PhDs graduated from the 115 MD-PhD programs extant in 1995 (Sutton & Killian, 1996). Of these, nearly 60% came from non-MSTP programs (Sutton & Killian, 1996). The vast majority of MD-PhD graduates find research positions, primarily with academic appointments in clinical departments rather than basic science departments (Bradford, Pizzo, & Cristakos, 1986; Frieden & Fox, 1991; Martin, 1991; McClellan & Talalay, 1992; Wilkerson & Abelmann, 1993). These results suggest that MD-PhD programs are effective. Moreover, MD-PhD researchers are as successful as their PhD counterparts in obtaining NIH funding (Sutton & Killian, 1996). Finally, the rate at which they secure employment in clinical departments suggests a continuing demand for MD-PhD researchers in clinician-scientist roles (McClellan & Talalay, 1992).

However, as indexed by the topics of grant applications submitted to NIH, the vast majority of MD-PhDs are engaged in basic science research, not clinical research (Interim Report of the NIH Director's Panel, 1996; Sutton & Killian, 1996), just as their PhD colleagues are. Although these data clarify the research contributions of MD-PhD graduates, they raise some important issues. First, it is unclear if current MD-PhD training is fully addressing the continuing need for clinical researchers. Second, there is growing concern about the cost effectiveness of MD-PhD training (Kennedy, 1994; Perry, 1992) in terms of the indebtedness that students incur as well as the trainee costs that governmental agencies and educational institutions bear. Several issues underlie this concern. First, MD-PhD programs contribute a relatively small number of graduates to the biomedical investigator pool (Ammons & Kelly, 1997; Sutton & Killian, 1996). In particular, MSTP programs currently contribute less than half of the MD-PhD graduates. Second, the research topics and funding rates for MD-PhD compared with PhD graduates do not differ significantly, yet it may be that PhD students are cheaper to train. Third, there is an unresolved debate about whether the nation is overproducing basic biomedical researchers (Domer, Garry, Guth, Walters, & Fisher, 1996; Kennedy, 1994) which is the pool that current MD-PhD researchers appear to enter.

Future

The success of MD-PhD programs in producing biomedical scientists and clinical faculty is well documented. In light of the MD-PhD's redefined future role (Interim Report of the NIH Director's Panel, 1996) and the centrality of cost in health care delivery, MD-PhD programs have an opportunity to broaden their impact on medical research and patient care by expanding their training to include patient-oriented research. Research areas here include population health and prevention as well as demographic, epidemiologic, and behavioral studies. A reasonable result of this shift could be abatement of current cost-benefit controversies in medical and health care.

COMBINED MD-JD PROGRAMS

History and Purpose

Currently, only a few combined MD-JD degree programs exist in the United States (Medical School Admission Requirements 1998-1999, 1997), eight at most, (T. R. LeBlang, personal communication, March, 1998). The oldest of these programs opened in the early 1970s. The combined MD-JD programs endeavor to meet the needs of students committed to a career in medicine, but who simultaneously want to learn about the relationships among law, the practice of medicine, and health care delivery. The rise in medical malpractice litigation; legislation regulating the manner in which physicians relate to patients, hospitals, third-party payers, and clinical laboratories; issues surrounding medical care at the beginning and at the end of the life span; and other factors, have sparked an interest in these programs.

Defining Features

The extent to which the combined curricula integrate the study of law and medicine varies across programs. A rare tightly interdigitated program involves students who obtain degrees in law and medicine through required courses and extracurricular events throughout six years (LeBlang & Basanta, 1998). During the first two years of this program, students pursue standard law school courses while also participating in substantial curricular and extracurricular experiences in legal and clinical medicine. Then during the next three years, students follow a standard medical school curriculum including medical humanities work in law and medicine as they continue their extracurricular contact with legal medicine. In the final year, they are required to participate in a specially designed set of law, medicine, and health policy electives. The curricular design of this integrated program supports continuity in social relationships among the combined-degree students as well as their peers and faculty in law and medicine. On the other hand, students in less integrated programs must first complete all of their law courses before they undertake their medical studies, which are designed as a discrete curriculum without additional formal course work in the law, or they must rely on their own ad hoc arrangements to develop a law and medicine curriculum.

Outcomes

Because only a few students pursue the combined MD-JD programs each year (Matriculating Student Survey Results, 1996, 1997), only a few students graduate from these programs. Seven students responding to the AAMC graduating student questionnaire in 1996 and another four replying to the same survey in 1997 said that they were completing a combined MD-JD program (Medical School Graduation Questionnaire, 1996, 1997). So far, the aforementioned program has produced six graduates since it began in 1988. These physician attorneys are in residency programs in primary care, emergency medicine, radiology, and forensic pathology (LeBlang & Basanta, 1998). A more far-reaching description of the MD-JD programs and their outcomes awaits a national study.

SUMMARY

This review of combined-degree programs suggests that they are not isolated aberrations, but rather an integral part of the local and national fabric of educational, intellectual, economic, political, and social trends. They have introduced innovations in the education of physicians. Their outcomes point to student success, although how much of that success is because of the programs is unclear. Their future depends on the value they can add to medical education. One approach to adding value may be to emphasize population health in the baccalaureate-MD degree programs by regional recruitment, training, and retention of students to improve the health of an area; in the MD-PhD programs by educating researchers to study prevention, population health, and health outcomes; and in the MD-JD programs by emphasizing public policy studies. A more fundamental approach to adding value to combined-degree programs lies in their continuing commitment to educational innovation that fosters in-depth study of medicine, but in relation to rich exploration of allied fields. That has been and will be the contribution and promise of combined-degree programs. As they nurture study across fields, combined-degree programs can chart approaches to interdisciplinarity that may well characterize teaching, learning, and research in the academy in the 21st century.

ACKNOWLEDGMENTS

The authors thank the Group on Baccalaureate-MD Degree Programs for its contributions to the discussion, study, and advancement of these programs through the years. They are especially appreciative of the thoughtful comments and information they received from Theodore Brown, Alphonse R. Burdi, E. Virginia Calkins, Clara A. Callahan, Louis Cregler, Lynn C. Epstein, Robert E. Hinkley, Katie Huggett, Bonnie J. Jones, Sara Kremer, Lloyd Michael, Henry Pohl, David Seiden, Stephen R. Smith, Michael Stemerman, and Selma Van Eyck. The authors are responsible for the content and opinions that found their way into the final version of the chapter.

REFERENCES

Albanese, M., Van Eyck, S., Huggett, K., & Barnet, J. (1997a). Academic performances of early-admission students to a BA/MD program compared with regular-admission students in relation to applicant pool fluctuations. *Academic Medicine, 72*, S66-S68.

Albanese, M., Van Eyck, S., Huggett, K., Barnet, J., & Sugden, N. (1997b). *Alumnae perceptions of BA/MD program goal attainment*. Washington, DC: Annual Meeting, Group on Baccalaureate/MD Degree Programs.

Alexander, R. S. (1964). The Rensselaer-Albany medical biomedical program. *Federal Bulletin, 51*, 40-48.

Ammons, S. W., & Kelly, D. E. (1997). Profile of the graduate student population in U.S. medical schools. *Academic Medicine, 72*, 820-830.

Arnold, L., Boex, J. R., Smith, S. R., & Veloski, J. (1988). A symposium: A natural history of an innovation in medical education: The case of baccalaureate-MD degree programs. *Research in Medical Education Proceedings of the 27th Conference*. Chicago: 99th Annual Meeting of the Association of American Medical Colleges.

Arnold, L., Calkins, E. V., Meiselas, L., Roth, W., Allen, J., & Titus-Dillon, P. (1987). Baccalaureate-MD programs. *Journal of Medical Education, 62*, 952-953.

Arnold, L., Calkins E. V., & Willoughby, T. L. (1983). Can achievement in high school predict performance in college, medical school and beyond? *College and University, 59*, 95-101.

Arnold, L., Calkins, E. V., & Willoughby, T. L. (1985). Self evaluation in undergraduate medical education. *Journal of Medical Education, 60*, 21-28.

Arnold, L., Calkins, E. V., & Willoughby, T. L. (1997a). Antecedent and concurrent correlates of primary care practice. *Teaching and Learning in Medicine: An International Journal, 9*, 192-199.

Arnold, L., & Feighny, K. M. (1995). Students' general learning approaches and performance in medical school: A longitudinal study. *Academic Medicine, 70*, 715-722.

Arnold, L., Feighny, K. M., Hood, J., Stearns, J., Prislin, M., & Erney, S. (1997b). Educational correlates of students' perceptions of learning in longitudinal ambulatory primary care clerkships. *Academic Medicine, 72*, S136-S139.

Arnold, L. & Jensen, T. B. (1984). Students' perception of stress in a baccalaureate-MD degree program. *Perceptual Motor Skills, 58*, 651-662.

Arnold, L. & Willoughby, T. L. (1990). The quarterly profile examination. *Academic Medicine, 65*, 515-516.

Arnold, L. & Willoughby, T. L. (1993). The empirical association between student and resident physician performances. *Academic Medicine, 68*, S35-S40.

Arnold, L., Willoughby, T. L., Calkins, E. V., Eberhart, G., & Gammon, L. (1981a). Use of peer evaluation in the formal assessment of medical students. *Journal of Medical Education, 56*, 35-42.

Arnold, L., Willoughby, T. L., Calkins, E. V., & Jensen, T. (1981b). The achievement of men and women in medical school. *Journal of American Medical Women's Association, 36*, 213-221.

Arnold, L., Willoughby, T. L., Xu, G., Epstein, L. C., & Jones, B. (1997c). Models for predicting career patterns of graduates of combined baccalaureate-MD degree programs. In A. J. J. A. Scherpbier, C. P. M van der Vleuten, J. J Rethans,. & A. F. W. van der Steeg (Eds.), *Advances in medical education.* (pp. 538-541). Maastricht, The Netherlands: Kluwer Academic Publishers.

Arnold, L., Xu, G., Epstein, L. C., & Jones, B. (1996). Professional and personal characteristics of graduates as outcomes of combined baccalaureate-MD degree programs. *Academic Medicine, 71*, S64-S66.

Bickel, J. W., Sherman, C. R., Ferguson, J. F., Baker, L., & Morgan, T. E. (1981). The role of MD-PhD training in increasing the supply of physician-scientists. *New England Journal of Medicine, 304*, 1265-1268.

Blaustein, E. H., Meiselas, L., Brown, D. R., & Arnold, L. (1983). *Integrating and accelerating medical education: The combined baccalaureate-MD programs at Boston University, the City College of New York, the University of Michigan, and the University of Missouri-Kansas City.* New York: The Commonwealth Fund.

Bloom, F. J., Vatavuk, M. K., & Kaliszewski, S. E. (1988). Evaluation of the Gannon-Hahnemann program to provide family physicians for an undeserved area. *Journal of Medical Education, 633*, 7-10.

Bradford, W. D., Pizzo, S., & Cristakos, A. C. (1986). Careers and professional activities of graduates of a medical scientist training program. *Journal of Medical Education, 61*, 915-918.

Burdi, A. R. (1986). The challenges of a changing environment-INTEFLEX: Michigan's alternate pathway toward the MD degree In R. H. Bartlett, G. B. Zellenock, W. E. Strodel, M. L. Harper, & J. G. Turcotte, (Eds.), *Medical education: A surgical perspective* (pp. 209-222). Chelsea, MI: Lewis Publishers.

Cadman, E. C. (1990). The New Physician-Scientist: A guide for the 1990s. *Clinical Research, 38*, 191-198.

Calkins, E. V., & Epstein, L. C. (1994). Models for mentoring students in medicine: Implications for student well-being. *Medical Teacher, 16*, 253-260.

Calkins, E. V, Arnold, L, & Huggett, K. (1997) *The decline and rise in number of applicants to a combined degree program and their academic, demographic, and psychosocial characteristics.* University of Missouri-Kansas City School of Medicine, Kansas City, MO.

Calkins, E. V., Arnold, L., & Willoughby, T. L. (1994). Medical students' perceptions of stress: Gender and ethnic considerations. *Academic Medicine, 69*, S22-S24.

Calkins, E. V., Arnold, L. M., & Willoughby, T. L. (1987). Gender differences in predictors of performance in medical training. *Journal of Medical Education, 62*, 682-685.

Calkins, E. V., & Jonas, H. S. (Eds.), (1981). *Proceedings of a symposium. Issues and challenges: A decade of experience with cost-effective models for medical education.* Kansas City, MO: The W. K. Kellogg Foundation and the University of Missouri-Kansas City School of Medicine.

Calkins, E. V., & Willoughby, T. L. (1992). Predictors of black medical students' success. *Journal of the National Medical Association, 84*, 253-256.

Calkins, E. V., Willoughby, T. L., & Arnold, L. M. (1982). Predictors of performance of minority students in the first two years of a BA/MD program. *Journal of the National Medical Association, 74*, 625-632.

Callahan, C. A., Veloski, J. J., Xu, G., Hojat, M., Zeleznik, C., & Gonnella, J. S. (1992). The Jefferson-Penn State accelerated medical school program: A 26-year experience. *Academic Medicine, 67*, 792-797.

Campbell, C., & De Muth, G. R. (1976). The University of Michigan integrated premedical-medical program. *Journal of Medical Education, 51*, 290-295.

Cooper, J. A. D., & Prior, M. (1961). A new program of medical education at Northwestern. *Journal of Medical Education, 36*, 80-90.

Daubney, J. H, Wagner, E. E., & Rogers, W. A. (1981). Six-year BS/MD programs: A literature review. *Journal of Medical Education, 56*, 497-503.

Davis, W. K., & Kelley, W. N. (1982). Factors influencing decisions to enter careers in clinical investigation. *Journal of Medical Education, 57*, 275-281.

Dimond, E. G. (1988). The UMKC medical education experiment. *Journal of America Medical Association, 260*, 5-8.

Domer, J. E., Garry, R.F., Guth, P. S, Walters, M. R., & Fisher, J. W. (1996). On the crisis in biomedical education: Is there an overproduction of biomedical PhDs? *Academic Medicine, 71*, 876-885.

Duckwall, J. M., Arnold, L., Willoughby, T. L., Calkins, E. V., & Hamburger, S. C. (1990). An assessment of the student partnership program at the University of Missouri-Kansas City School of Medicine. *Academic Medicine, 65*, 697-701.

Epstein, L. C., Hayes, J., Arnold, L., O'Sullivan, P. S., Ruffin, A. L., Roger, L., Jones, B., Van Eyck, S., Brown, D., Hinkley, R., Linde, H., O'Bryan, P., & Roth, W. (1994). On becoming a physician: Perspectives of students in combined baccalaureate-MD degree programs. *Teaching and Learning in Medicine: An International Journal, 6*, 102-107.

Flair, M. D. (1969). Honors program in medical education at Northwestern University. *Journal of Medical Education, 44*, 1127-1131.

Frieden, C., & Fox, B. J. (1991). Career choices of graduates from Washington University's Medical Scientist Training Program. *Academic Medicine, 66*, 162-164.

Gellhorn, A., & Scheuer, R. (1978). The experiment in medical education at the City College of New York. *Journal of Medical Education, 53*, 574-582.

Golmon, M. E. (1981). The nontraditional medical student at Northwestern University. *Proceedings of a symposium. Issues and challenges: A decade of experience with cost-effective models for medical education* (pp. 97-112). Kansas City, MO: The W. K. Kellogg Foundation and the University of Missouri-Kansas City School of Medicine.

Gottheil, E., Conley, S. S., & Menduke, H. (1972). Adaptation to an accelerated medical school program. *Journal of Medical Education, 47*, 539-546.

Grant, L., Arnold, L., Blaustein, E. H., Brown, D. R., Eder, S., & Meiselas, L. (1986). Combined premedical-medical programmes: Programme structure and student outcomes at four universities. *Medical Education, 20*, 91-93.

Grossman, W. K., Conley, S. S., Menduke, H., & Graff, H. (1972). Medical students view their accelerated program. *Journal of Medical Education, 47*, 287-288.

Guaranteed admission to medical school becomes a tool for recruiting undergraduates. (1997, June 27). *Chronicle of Higher Education, 43*, A41-A42.

Hayes, J., Munro, S., Arnold, L., & Duckwall, J. (1993). A support program for freshman medical students. *Journal of Freshman Year Experience, 5*, 77-92.

Herbut, P. A., Sodeman, W. A., Conley, S. A, & Ascah, R. (1969). The Jefferson-Penn State accelerated medical student program. *Journal of Medical Education, 44*, 1132-1138.

Interim Report of the NIH Director's Panel on Clinical Research (CRP). (1996, December). Available: www.nih.gov

Jacobs, J. P., Hinkley, R. E., & Pennell, J. P. (1988). Student evaluation of the accelerated program at the University of Miami. *Journal of Medical Education, 63*, 11-18.

Jones, B. J. (1991). Can trait anxiety, grades, and test scores measured prior to medical school matriculation predict clerkship performance? *Academic Medicine, 66*, S22-S24.

Jones, B. J., Arnold, L., Epstein, L. C., & Xu, G. (2000). Gender differences in the preparation and practice of young physicians from baccalaureate-MD degree programs. *Journal of the American Medical Women's Association. 55*:1-3.

Kanter, G. S. (1969). The Rensselaer Polytechnic Institute-Albany Medical College six-year biomedical program. *Journal of Medical Education, 44*, 1139-1143.

Keck, J. W., Arnold, L., Willoughby, T. L., & Calkins, E. V. (1979). Efficacy of cognitive/noncognitive measures in predicting resident-physician performance. *Journal of Medical Education, 54*, 759-765.

Keefer, C. S. (1964). The training of the physician: Experiment with the medical school curriculum at Boston University. *New England Journal of Medicine, 271*, 401-403.

Kennedy, F. S., & Austin, J. C. (1988). Comparison of performance in programs at LSU Medical School in Shreveport. *Journal of Medical Education, 63*, 1-6.

Kennedy, T. J., Jr. (1994). Graduate education in the biomedical sciences; Critical observations on training for research careers. *Academic Medicine, 69*, 779-799.

Lanzoni, V., & Kayne, H. L. (1976). A report on graduates of the Boston University six-year combined liberal arts-medical program. *Journal of Medical Education, 51*, 283-289.

LeBlang, T. R., & Basanta, W. E. (1998). MD/JD dual degree program. In American College of Legal Medicine, *Legal Medicine*, (pp. 17-19). St. Louis:Mosby.

Loftus, L., & Willoughby, T. L. (1997). Evaluation of student performance in combined baccalaureate-MD degree programs. *Teaching and Learning in Medicine: An International Journal, 9*, 248-253.

Martin, J. B. (1991). Training physician-scientists for the 1990s. *Academic Medicine, 66*, 123-129.

Matriculating Student Survey Results: All Schools Summary, 1995, 1996. Washington, DC: Association of American Medical Colleges, 1996, 1997.

McClellan, D. A., & Talalay, P. (1992). MD-PhD training at the Johns Hopkins University School of Medicine, 1962-1991. *Academic Medicine, 67*, 36-41.

Medical School Admission Requirements 1998-1999: United States and Canada. 48th Edition. Washington, DC: Association of American Medical Colleges, 1997.

Medical School Graduation Questionnaire, 1996, 1997. Washington, DC: Association of American Medical Colleges, 1996-1997.

Muller, S., (Chairman), et al. (1984). Physicians for the twenty-first century: Report of the project panel on the general professional education of the physician and college preparation for medicine. *Journal of Medical Education, 59*, 1-208.

Munro, J. S., Feighny, K. M., & Arnold, L. (1997). Revisiting self-perception and specialty choice in primary and nonprimary care. *Annals of Behavioral Science and Medical Education, 4*, 21-36.

Nathan, R. G., Nixon, F. E., Bairnsfather, L., Allen, J. H., & Hack, M.A. (1989). Comparison of students in six-year and traditional eight-year medical school programs on measures of personality and stress early in medical school. *Academic Medicine, 64*, 690.

Neilson, E. G, Ausiello, D., & Demer, L. (1995). Physician-scientists as missing persons. *Journal of Investigative Medicine, 43*, 534-542.

Norman, A. W., & Calkins, E. V. (1992). Curricular variations in combined degree programs. *Academic Medicine, 67*:785-791.

Oggins, J., Inglebart, M., Brown, D. R., & Moore, W. (1988). Gender differences in the prediction of medical students' clinical performance. *Journal of American Medical Women's Association, 43*, 171-175.

Olson, S. W. (1992). Combined degree programs: A valuable educational alternative for motivated students with an early career choice. *Academic Medicine, 67*, 783-784.

Perry, D. R. (1992). Questioning public funding of MD-PhD programs. *Academic Medicine, 67*, 316.

Pritchard, H. N. (1976). The Lehigh-Medical College of Pennsylvania six-year B.A.-MD program. *Journal of Medical Education, 51*, 296-298.

Roman, S. A., & McGanney, M. L. (1994). The Sophie Davis School of Biomedical Education: The first 20-years of a unique B.S.-MD program. *Academic Medicine, 69*, 224-230.

Salzman, G., Arnold, L., & Willoughby, T. L. (1994). Clinical performance of graduates from an experience-based medical school curriculum. *Annals of Behavioral Science and Medical Education, 1*, 93-99.

Sandson, J. I., Blaustein, E., Stewart, P. A., Ravin, A. W., & Rock, M. B. (1979). New experiments to improve premedical and medical education. In *Proceedings of the Annual Conference on Research in Medical Education* (pp. 317-27). Washington, DC: Association of American Medical Colleges.

Schrier, R. W. (1997). Ensuring the survival of the clinician-scientist. *Academic Medicine, 72*, 589-594.

Shannon, J. A. (1976). Federal support of biomedical sciences: Development and academic impact. *Journal of Medical Education, 51*, S1-S98.

Silverman, M., & McGugan, S. (1992). Results of recent initiatives such as the MD/PhD program in the training of clinician-scientists. *Clinical Investigative Medicine, 15*, 224-228.

Sloan, T. S., & Brown, D. R. (1978). The Clark-Trow typology and applicants to a six-year A.B./MD program. *Journal of College Student Personnel, 19*, 6-9.

Smith, S. R. (1989). *Continuum medical education at Brown University: A retrospective.* Providence, RI: Brown University.

Smith, S. R. (1993). Retention of traditional premedical students in a medical career pathway compared with students in a combined baccalaureate-medical degree program. *Journal of the National Medical Association, 85*, 529-532.

Sodeman, W. A. (1963). A cooperative Jefferson Medical College-Pennsylvania State University program. *Federal Bulletin, 50*, 346-350.

Sutton, J., & Killian, C. D. (1996). The MD-PhD researcher: What species of investigator? *Academic Medicine, 71*, 454-459.

Van Eyck, S., & Arnold, L. (1993). Selecting high school students for combined baccalaureate-MD degree programs. *College and University, 68*, 32-37.

Van Eyck, S., Huggett, K., & Barnet, J. (1996). *How do we select our students?* Results of a survey of baccalaureate-MD degree program admissions/selection procedures. San Francisco: Annual Meeting, Group on Baccalaureate-MD Degree Programs.

Wartman. S. A. (1992, Fall). Multidisciplinary madness; The trials and tribulations of the MD-PhD *The Pharos*, 2-6.

Watanabe, M. (1992). How to attract candidates to academic medicine. *Clinical Investigative Medicine, 15*, 204-215.

Wiggins, W. S., Leymaster, G. R., Ruhe, C. H. W., Taylor, N., & Tipner, A. (1961). Medical education in the United States. *Journal of American Medical Association, 178*, 640.

Wilkerson, L., & Abelmann, W. H. (1993). Producing physician-scientists: A survey of graduates from the Harvard-MIT program in health sciences and technology. *Academic Medicine, 68*, 214-218.

Willoughby, L., Calkins, E. V., & Arnold, L. (1979). Different predictors of examination performance for male and female medical students. *Journal of American Medical Women's Association, 34*, 316-320.

Willoughby, T. L., Arnold, L., & Calkins, E. V. (1981). Personal characteristics and achievements of medical students from urban and nonurban areas. *Journal of Medical Education, 56*, 717-726.

Willoughby, T. L., Gamon, L. C., & Jonas, H. S. (1979). Correlates of clinical performance during medical school. *Journal of Medical Education, 54*, 453-460.

Wyngaarden, J. B. (1979). The clinical investigator as an endangered species. *New England Journal of Medicine, 301*, 1254-1255.

CHAPTER NINETEEN

Standardized Patients

Linda C. Perkowski
University of Texas - Houston Medical School

OVERVIEW AND TERMINOLOGY

Simulations have been used extensively in medical education for more than three decades. The instructional value implicit in simulation is its ability to provide an active, participatory, "real-life" situation to which the learner's knowledge can be applied (Spannaus, 1978). The advantages of simulations over actual clinical experiences and observation-based evaluations are their ready availability and portability, their standardization across learners, and their appropriateness for the level of the learner (Barrows, 1993). In medical education simulations provide opportunities to teach and assess both basic and complex clinical skills such as interviewing, physical examination techniques, clinical reasoning and problem solving (Norman, Muzzin, Williams, & Swanson, 1985).

The use of trained patients in simulations has increased dramatically in the past two decades. Originally referred to as "programmed patients" (Barrows & Abrahamson, 1964) and then "simulated patients" (Barrows, 1971), these are individuals with or without a disease who are coached to simulate an illness and portray a patient role in a realistic and consistent way. Initially, simulated patients were primarily used for teaching. Paula Stillman (1976) developed "patient instructors" who were individuals with and individuals without real physical findings who used their own bodies and findings to teach medical students to do physical examinations and to detect abnormalities. *Currently, simulated patients are used*

217

extensively in teaching students and residents history-taking, physical examination,
patient education and patient-physician interaction skills.

In addition to their value in teaching, simulated patients were perceived as useful
in the assessment of clinical   skills. In the late 1970s, simulated patient-based
examinations of clinical skills were introduced (Harden, Stevenson, Downie, &
Wilson, 1975). The commonly agreed-on term for a simulated patient today is
"standardized patient," often abbreviated as SP (Barrows, 1993). The use of the term
"standardized patient" reflects the main objective of SP encounters when they are
used for assessment purposes: to provide a realistic clinical challenge that does not
vary from student to student.

In recent years, the trend in medical education has been toward more
performance-based or authentic assessment" (Wiggins, 1989). The Liaison
Committee on Medical Education (LCME) is now requiring medical schools "to
develop a system of assessment which assures that students have acquired and can
demonstrate on direct observation the core clinical skills and behaviors needed in
subsequent medical training" (Functions and Structure of a Medical School, 1993,
p. 15). To address this need, SPs often are used in performance-based examinations.
These examinations consist of a series or circuit of different patient problems or
clinical encounters termed a "station." Stations vary in length from five- to 50-
minutes and make up the basic unit of the examination. Performance of the clinical
skills in these stations is assessed by means of a checklist or a rating scale completed
by either the SP or a clinician. These case-specific checklists focus on whether a
behavior was observed (i.e., asked if the pain radiated down my leg) or was
performed correctly (i.e., percussed the abdomen in all four quadrants). Total scores
are derived by summing across items on these checklists. A global skill such as
history-taking may be assessed by summing performance on similar items across all
cases in the examination.

Standardized patient-based examinations are designed by completing an
examination "blueprint." This process provides guidance for selection of an adequate
sample of cases that students should be capable of resolving (Newble, Dawson,
Daupinee, Macdonald, & Mulholland, et al., 1994). A blueprint is a matrix that helps
in conceptualizing the areas of clinical competence to be assessed. For example, a
blueprint may have clinical skills (e.g., history-taking, physical examination, patient
counseling, interpersonal skills) along one axis and body systems (e.g., respiratory,
neurologic, gastrointestinal) along the other axis. In addition, case selection may
address the nature of the clinical presentation (e.g., acute, chronic, behavioral) and/or
patient demographics (i.e., gender, age, ethnicity). Cases are then identified and
developed for sampling from these various categories. As an example, an acute
appendicitis case might be developed primarily to assess physical examination skills
(Fig 19.1).

SYSTEMS ➤	GI	NEURO	RESPIRATORY	GYN	CVS
CLINICAL SKILL ↓					
HISTORY		70-year old Female Vertigo			50-year old Male Chest pain
PHYSICAL EXAMINATION	25-year old Female Acute Appendicitis				
PATIENT COUNSELING			16-year old Male Non-compliant asthmatic		
PHYSICIAN AND PATIENT INTERACTION				45-year old Female Malignant breast mass	

FIG. 19.1. Standardized patient-based examination blueprint matrix.

Currently, there are two commonly adopted formats for SP-based assessments. The Objective Structured Clinical Examination (OSCE) was first introduced by Harden and his colleagues more than 20 years ago (Harden, Stevenson, Downie, & Wilson, 1975; Harden & Gleeson, 1979). Its purpose is to assess very specific clinical skills (e.g., percussing the abdomen, eliciting the history of chest pain). The examination typically consists of very short stations, five- to 10- minutes each. The OSCE is deemed most appropriate when used as an assessment tool during early clinical training (Barrows, 1993). Logistically efficient, the OSCE can be administered to a large number of students in relatively brief time.

The second format for SP-based assessments is the Simulated Clinical Encounter (SCE) (McGuire, 1993) or the Clinical Practice Examination (CPX) (Barrows, 1993). This examination format is best used at the end of the clerkships (Barrows, 1993). In the CPX, students are required to perform more complete workups. A station is designed to assess simultaneously several aspects of clinical competence (e.g., history-taking, physical examination, and patient counseling). The stations are longer than in the OSCE, usually 20- to 50-minutes each. The CPX "not only tests the student's ability to perform interview and physical examination techniques; it also tests the student's ability to apply those techniques when appropriate with a particular patient problem" (Barrows, 1987, p. 112).

In both assessment formats, the clinical encounter with the SP can be followed by non-SP based stations or postencounter exercises. The challenges for these stations include providing a differential diagnosis, ordering diagnostic tests, interpreting labs, presenting a patient's findings, and answering questions that explore the student's knowledge about the patient and the problem. The format of these stations may be paper-and-pencil or computer-based, or a faculty member may be present to ask questions.

DEVELOPMENT OF STANDARDIZED PATIENTS

Howard Barrows, a neurologist and medical educator, is credited with first conceptualizing and using the simulated (standardized) patient for teaching in a neurology clerkship. Numerous individuals have subsequently been instrumental in further developments. The development of this method is beautifully chronicled in a recent article by Peggy Wallace (1997).

The use of SPs for instruction has permeated all aspects of medical training. Lack of imagination and resources are the only limits to the instructional uses for SPs. In addition to basic interviewing and physical examination skills, standardized patients have been used effectively to teach a variety of more complex clinical skills such as interviewing difficult patients, counseling patients, delivering bad news, administering family therapy, dealing with death and dying, and taking a spiritual history.

In an environment wherein competition for faculty time is fierce and the length of patient hospital stays are decreasing, the use of SPs as teaching tools and even as trained instructors can be a real asset. Individuals with actual findings may be used as SPs to assist students in learning how to detect physical abnormalities. For faculty and resident teacher training, SPs have been used to portray "students" in ward teams on rounds, in classroom settings, and in one-on-one teaching/advising sessions. These simulations provide opportunities for instructors to practice and receive feedback on their abilities to teach, evaluate, and counsel learners.

Before the use of SP-based examinations, the assessment of clinical skills relied primarily on written tests and patient management problems (PMPs) to supplement faculty observations and ratings. There are limitations in these approaches. Written assessments are not able to evaluate hands-on skills such as the physical examination techniques or the interpersonal aspects of the physician-patient interaction. This is of concern because it has been documented that students often graduate without being observed by faculty completing a routine history and physical (Stillman, Regan, Swanson, Case, & McCahan, et al., 1990). Furthermore, when faculty did observe students, those observations were selective and few in number. Given there rarely are predetermined criteria for clinical competence, faculty ratings often are inconsistent assessments of students' performances. Furthermore, the patient challenge usually varies because different students are rated on encounters with different patients who have different problems (Mast, Schermerhorn, & Colliver, 1992; Schwartz, Donnelly, Young, Nash, White, et al., 1992). With the emphasis on standardization, well-designed SP-based assessments addressed these deficiencies.

Recent developments have encouraged the use of SP-based assessments. Both training and licensing bodies have expressed a need for valid performance-based assessment approaches. The Medical Council of Canada has implemented an SP-based clinical practice examination as part of the Canadian licensing examination (Reznick. Smee, Rothman, Chalmers, & Swanson, et al., 1993; Reznick, Blackmore, Dauphinee, Rothman, & Smee, et al., 1996). The National Board of Medical Examiners (NBME) is proposing implementation of an SP-based examination as part of the USMLE Step II licensure process at the beginning of the next century (Highlights of the 1995 Annual Meeting of the Board, 1995). In 1994 the Educational Council for Foreign Medical Graduates (ECFMG) authorized an SP-based assessment as part of their certification process (Educational Commission for Foreign Medical Graduates Annual Report, 1995). Simultaneously, practical experience and research expertise have been advancing continually in the area of training and use of SPs and in the psychometrics of performance-based examinations (Rothman, 1995).

The growing interest in and research on the use of SPs for teaching and assessment of clinical skills is well documented (Ferrell, 1995). The Association of American Medical Colleges (AAMC) demonstrated this by hosting a consensus conference on standardized patients in December, 1992. Subsequent to that conference, special issues of *Academic Medicine* (Proceedings of the AAMC's consensus conference, 1993) and *Teaching and Learning in Medicine* (Annex to the proceedings of the AAMC consensus conference, 1994) focused on topics related to the use of SPs for teaching and assessment. Within the AAMC, in addition to presentations and workshops related to the use of SPs, the Group on Educational Affairs (GEA) sponsors a special interest group (SIG) devoted to promoting advancements in the use of SPs. This SIG on SPs holds open sessions at both the annual AAMC meeting and the regional GEA meetings. Internationally, the use of SPs has been well received (Sutnick, Friedman, & Wilson, 1995). There have been eight international conferences directly related to teaching and assessment of clinical skills. In 1991 and 1992 the Josiah Macy Jr. Foundation awarded grants to support six U.S. consortia charged with developing interinstitutional strategies for designing and implementing SP-based examinations of clinical skills (Morrison & Barrows, 1994). Accompanying these activities and conferences, the research literature related to the use of SPs is burgeoning (Vleuten & Swanson, 1990; Vu & Barrows, 1994).

In a 1993 national survey on the use of SPs in medical education, 80% of the 138 schools responding indicated that SPs were used for either teaching or evaluation at their institutions (Anderson, Stillman & Wang, 1994). Of the 111 responding schools, 35% required their students to take an SP examination before graduation. These numbers have increased in the succeeding five years.

USE OF STANDARDIZED PATIENTS

Scope

Standardized patient-based assessments are used throughout the continuum of medical training with undergraduates (Dunnington, Wright, & Hoffman, 1994; Petrusa, Blackman, Rogers, Saydjari, Parcel, & et al., 1987; Scott, Irby, Guilliland, & Hunt, 1993), residency (Cohen, Reznick, & Taylor, 1990; Robb & Rothman, 1985; Schwartz, Donnelly, Sloan, Johnson, & Strodel, 1994; Sloan, Donnelly, Johnson, Schwartz & Strodel, 1993; Sloan, Donnelly, Schwartz, & Strodel, 1995), and practicing clinicians (Tamblyn, Berkson, Dauphinee, Gayton, & Grad, et al., 1997). The variety of clinical problems simulated is extensive (Barrows, 1993) and represents the breadth of clinical situations (Barrows, 1993; Pololi, 1995).

Practicality

The initial training of a lay person to produce a high-fidelity simulation can be time consuming. The SP does not merely learn facts but also must "understand what it is like to be the actual patient with the feelings and the problems the patient has" (Barrows, 1993, p. 445). When the SP also is required to record student behaviors, rate interpersonal skills, or give constructive feedback, the task becomes even more complex and the training more intensive. The SP must learn to complete a checklist or rating scale with multiple items accurately and reliably. This requires remembering the behaviors of a given student while the SP is portraying the role, and then accurately recording those behaviors during the brief time between a series of students. In some cases, the SP must also be able to provide constructive feedback to the learner, recalling specific nonverbal or verbal behaviors that occurred during the encounter. Research indicates that if adequately trained, SPs are accurate in both their portrayal of the patient role and their recordings of examinees' performances (Colliver & Williams, 1993).

Cost-benefits

Concerns have been voiced frequently regarding the high costs and labor-intensive nature of SP-based instruction and assessments as compared with more traditional paper-and-pencil formats (Proceedings of the AAMC consensus conference, 1993). Limited systematically collected information is available regarding the costs of using SPs in teaching. Typically SPs used in a teaching session would be paid between $10 and $30 an hour. If an invasive physical examination (i.e., genital, pelvic, or rectal) were involved, or if the SP took on an instructor role, the charges per hour would be higher. Published cost estimates for SP-based examinations range widely, from $21 to $1,200 per examinee (Carpenter, 1995; Cusimano, Cohen, Tucker, Murnaghan, & Kodama, et al., 1994; Frye, Richards, Philp, & Philp, 1989; Poenaru, Morales, Richards & O'Connor, 1997; Reznick, Smee, Rothman, Chalmers, & Swanson, et al., 1992; Stillman, Regan, & Swanson, 1987). These estimates vary depending on the model used for the examination (i.e., CPX vs. OSCE); the geographic location; and the expenses chosen for inclusion in the cost calculations.

Since the cost of conducting assessments with SPs has been reported, it is easier to define these expenses. Many of these same categories are directly applicable to the use of SPs in teaching. The costs of these examinations lie in three major areas: the SP (recruitment, training, and performance), administration (e.g., space, food, laundry, examination materials, audiovisual equipment, computers), and personnel (e.g., faculty time for case development, examination design, observation and rating; SP trainer; staff for examination; clerical support; data analyses). The costs reported typically represent an initial setup of the examination. As with any investment, some costs are amortized over time (e.g., purchase of equipment, recruitment and training of SPs, case development, procurement and duplication of examination materials, programming).

It is worthwhile to delineate ways in which costs can be reduced. A significant proportion of all the costs incurred are in personnel time, especially that of faculty. Sharing in the development of the cases or an examination, as is currently being done with regional consortia (Morrison & Barrows, 1994), can reduce faculty time and produce substantial cost savings. Using students and volunteers whenever possible may also be cost effective. In contrast to one-on-one instruction and practice with the SP and learner, a single SP can be used with a group of learners and a faculty facilitator to teach and practice clinical skills. This can be a very cost-efficient and effective use of simulation. Using computers to record and score the checklists and postencounter exercises will reduce data entry time (Blackwell, Ainsworth, Dorsey, Callaway, & Rogers, et al., 1991; Richards, Philp, & Philp, 1989). Shortening the length of the SP encounters and the examination time directly reduces all costs. A word of caution is needed. Although station length may be reduced without compromising the reliability of the examination (Shatzer, Darosa, Colliver, & Barkmeier, 1993; Shatzer, Wardrup, Williams, & Hatch, 1994; Vleuten & Swanson, 1990), as van der Vleuten and Swanson (1990) note, the criterion for determining station length should be the challenge presented to the student, not the costs.

The use of sequential testing has been suggested as a more effective and cost-efficient method of testing (Vleuten & Swanson, 1990). In this format, all examinees take a short screening test consisting of a few of the stations selected from a longer SP-based examination. Examinees who score above a specified cutpoint are then excused from taking the remainder of the examination. Only those examinees below the cutpoint are required to complete the entire examination. Such testing methods have been estimated to produce a 44% to 49% savings in number of encounters depending on the test cutpoint (Colliver, Mast, Vu, & Barrows, 1991).

Despite the cost of these SP-based examinations, researchers and educators conclude that they are financially feasible if the information they provide is valuable to the institution from both an educational and evaluative perspective (Cusimano et al., 1994). Some advantages inherent in SP-based examinations are that they can assess a broad range of competencies, provide comparisons of students/residents with an absolute standard of performance, make meaningful comparisons among students/residents identifying any deficits, and provide feedback on the curriculum, the training program, and faculty performance (Williams & Barrows, 1987).

IMPLICATIONS FOR THE 21ST CENTURY

The new century promises proliferation and refinement with respect to SPs. The use of SPs has expanded rapidly at both the institutional and national certifying and licensure levels. Given this increase in application and the related research, medical educators in this field have a responsibility to monitor and improve this method continually. Quantitative research addressing the measurement characteristics of SP-based assessments must and will continue, hopefully with an emphasis on validity and standard setting (Vleuten & Swanson, 1990). In addition, research is needed to address the impact of SP-based instruction and assessment on the curriculum and, more specifically, on student learning (Vleuten & Swanson, 1990). The large-scale administrations of national licensing organizations will be providing rich databases for such investigations. Qualitative research should be initiated on various unique parameters of this method: characteristics of individuals who serve as SPs and the impact of simulation on those individuals, SP training strategies and their efficacy, case development procedures, cost-benefit analyses, SP program development and management, quality assurance, and ethical issues involved with using SPs in various types of simulations.

With the existence and development of various national groups, networks, and internet-based information sources devoted to SPs, sharing of resources and technical expertise will become easier and more timely. This experiential base will continue to support improvements in the method and increase the sophistication of simulations. Standardized patient encounters will be adapted from clinical scenarios representative of the emerging health care system: interdisciplinary health care teams, diversity challenges, continuity of care, and alternative and evidence-based medicine. As the work of Robyn Tamblyn (1997) exemplifies, SP-based assessments are being used already to investigate physician practice and patient outcomes. The use of SP-based instruction and assessment will become more extensive with practicing physicians who are "at risk," or who choose to improve their clinical skills to adapt to the changing medical care delivery system.

Unlike other more short-lived educational "fads," SPs are likely to survive and flourish well into the new millennium. Standardized patients are real, sentient human beings and, as such, form the basis for the doctor-patient relationship. As noted by George Miller (1993), "Standardized patients can serve a unique education purpose, one that cannot be adequately exploited using other education and evaluation techniques" (p. 472-473).

REFERENCES

American Association of Medical Colleges (AAMC). (1993). Proceedings of the AAMC's consensus conference on the use of standardized patients in the teaching and evaluation of clinical skills (special issue). *Academic Medicine, 68,* 437-483.

American Association of Medical Colleges (AAMC). (1994). Annex to the proceedings of the AAMC consensus conference on the use of standardized patients in the teaching and evaluation of clinical skills (special section). *Teaching and Learning in Medicine: An International Journal, 6,* 2-35.

Anderson, M. B., Stillman, P. L., & Wang, Y. (1994). Growing use of standardized patients in teaching and evaluation in medical education. *Teaching and Learning in Medicine: An International Journal, 6,* 15-22.

Barrows, H. S. (1971). *Simulated patients.* Springfield, IL: Charles C Thomas.

Barrows, H. S. (Ed.), (1987). Multiple station. In I. R. Hart & R. M. Harden (Eds.), *Further developments in assessing clinical competence* (pp. 111-113). Ottawa, Canada: Can-Heal Publications.

Barrows, H. S. (1993). An overview of the uses of standardized patients for teaching and evaluating clinical skills. *Academic Medicine, 68*(6), 443-453.

Barrows, H. S., & Abrahamson S. (1964). The programmed patient: A technique for appraising student performance in clinical neurology. *Journal of Medical Education, 39,* 802-805.

Blackwell, T. A., Ainsworth, M. S., Dorsey, N. K., Callaway, M. R., Rogers, L. P., & Collins, K. E. (1991). Extending the skills measured with standardized patient examinations. *Academic Medicine, 66,* S40-S42.

Carpenter, J. L. (1995). Cost analysis of objective structured clinical examinations. *Academic Medicine, 70*(9), 828-833.

Cohen, R., Reznick, R. K., & Taylor, B. R. (1990). Reliability and validity of the objective structured clinical examination in assessing surgical residents. *American Journal of Surgery, 160,* 302-305.

Colliver J. A., Mast, T. A., Vu, N. V., & Barrows, H. S. (1991). Sequential testing with a performance-based examination using standardized patients. Academic Medicine, 66, S64-S66.

Colliver, J. A., & Williams, R. G. (1993). Technical issues: test application. *Academic Medicine, 68*(6), 454-460.

Cusimano, M. D., Cohen, R., Tucker, W., Murnaghan, J., Kodama, R., & Reznick, R. K. (1994). A comparative analysis of the costs of administration of an OSCE. *Academic Medicine, 69*(7), 571-576.

Dunnington, G. L., Wright, K., & Hoffman, K. (1994). A pilot experience with competency-based clinical skills assessment in a surgical clerkship. *Association for Surgical Education, 167,* 604-607.

Educational Commission for Foreign Medical Graduates Annual Report, 1995. (1996). *Educational Commission for Foreign Medical Graduates,* Philadelphia.

Ferrell, B. G. (1995). Clinical performance assessment using standardized patients: A primer. *Family Medicine, 27*(1), 14-19.

Frye, A. W., Richards, R. F., Philp, E. B., & Philp, J. R. (1989). Is it worth it? A look at the costs and benefits of an OSCE for second-year medical students. *Medical Teacher, 11,* 291-293.

Harden, R. M., Stevenson, M., Downie, W. W., & Wilson, G. M. (1975). Assessment of clinical competence using objective structured examinations. *British Medical Journal, 1,* 447-451.

Harden, R. M., & Gleeson, F. A. (1979). Assessment of clinical competence using an objective structured clinical examination (OSCE). *Medical Education, 13,* 41-54.

Highlights of the 1995 Annual Meeting of the National Board of Medical Examiners. (1995). *The National Board Examiners, 42,* 1-3.

Liaison Committee on Medical Education. (1993). *Functions and structure of a medical school.* Association of American Colleges and the American Medical Association.

Mast, T. A., Schermerhorn, G. S., & Colliver, J. A. (1992). Medical education. In M.C. Alkin, (Ed.), *Encyclopedia of Educational Research,* (pp. 814-825). New York: Macmillan.

McGuire, C. (1993). Perspectives in assessment. *Academic Medicine, 68*(Suppl 2), S3-S8.

Miller, G. E. (1993). Conference summary. *Academic Medicine, 68*(6), 471-474.

Morrison, L. J., & Barrows, H. S. (1994). Developing consortia for clinical practice examinations: The Macy Project. *Teaching and Learning in Medicine: An International Journal, 6*, 23-27.

Newble, D., Dawson, B., Daupinee, D., Macdonald, M., Mulholland, H., Page, G., Swanson, D., Thomson, A., & van der Vleuten, C. (1994). Guidelines for assessing clinical competence. *Teaching and Learning in Medicine: An International Journal, 6*(3), 213-220.

Norman, G. F., Muzzin, L. J., Williams, R. G., & Swanson, D. B. (1985). Simulation in the health sciences education. *Journal of Instructional Development, 8*(1), 11-17.

Petrusa, E. R., Blackwell, T. A., Rogers, L. P., Saydjari, C., Parcel, S., & Guckian, J. C. (1987). An objective measure of clinical performance. *American Journal of Medicine, 83*, 34-42.

Poenaru, D., Morales, D., Richards, A., & O'Connor, H. M. (1997). Running an objective structured clinical examination on a shoestring budget. *The American Journal of Surgery, 173*, 538-541.

Pololi, L. H. (1995). Standardized patients: As we evaluate, so shall we reap. *Lancet, 345*, 966-968.

Reznick, R. K., Smee, S., Rothman, A., Chalmers, A., Swanson, D., Dufresnel, L., Lacombe, G., Baumber, J., Poldre, P., & Levesseur, L. (1992). An objective structured clinical examination for the licentiate: Report of the pilot project of the Medical Council of Canada. *Academic Medicine, 67*, 487-494.

Reznick, R. K., Smee, S. Baumber, J. S., Cohen, R., & Rothman, A. T. (1993). Guidelines for estimating the real cost of an objective structured clinical examination. *Academic Medicine, 68*(7), 513-517.

Reznick, R. K., Blackmore, D., Dauphinee, W. D., Rothman, A. T, & Smee, S. (1996). Large-scale high-stakes testing with an OSCE: Report from the Medical Council of Canada. *Academic Medicine, 71*, S19-S21.

Richards, B. F., Philp, E. B., & Philp, J. R. (1989). Scoring the objective structured clinical examination using a microcomputer. *Medical Education, 23*, 376-380.

Robb, K., & Rothman, A. I. (1985). Assessment of clinical skills in general internal medicine residents: Comparison of the objective structured clinical examination to a conventional oral examination. *Annals of the Royal College of Physicians and Surgeons of Canada, 18*, 235-238.

Rothman, A. I. (1995). Understanding the objective structured clinical examination. *Australian New Zealand Journal of Surgery, 65*, 302-303.

Schwartz, R. W., Donnelly, M. B., Sloan, D. A., Johnson, S. B., & Strodel, W. E. (1994). Assessing senior residents' knowledge and performance: An integrated evaluation program. *Surgery, 116*(4), 634-637.

Schwartz, R. W., Donnelly, M. B., Young, B., Nash, P. P., White, F. M., & Griffen, Jr., W. O. (1992). Undergraduate surgical education for the twenty-first century. *Annals of Surgery, 216*(6), 639-647.

Scott, C. S., Irby, D. M., Guilliland, B. C., & Hunt, D. D. (1993). Evaluating clinical skills in an undergraduate medical education curriculum. *Teaching and Learning in Medicine: An International Journal, 5*(1), 49-53.

Shatzer, J. H., Darosa, D., Colliver, J. A., Barkmeier, L. (1993). Station-length requirements for reliable performance-based examination scores. *Academic Medicine, 68*, 224-229.

Shatzer, J. H., Wardrup, J. L., Williams, R. G., & Hatch, J. F. (1994). The generalizability of performance on different station length standardized patient cases. *Teaching and Learning in Medicine: An International Journal, 6*, 54-58.

Sloan, D. A., Donnelly, M. B., Schwartz, R. W., & Strodel, W. E. (1995). The objective structured clinical examination: The new gold standard for evaluating postgraduate clinical performance. *Annals of Surgery, 222*(6), 735-742.

Sloan, D. A., Donnelly, M. B., Johnson, S. B., Schwartz, R. W., & Strodel, W. E. (1993). Use of an objective structured clinical examination (OSCE) to measure improvement in clinical competence during the surgical internship. *Surgery, 114*(2), 343-351.

Spannaus, T. W. (1978, May). What is simulation? *Audiovisual Instruction, 23*(5) 16-17.

Stillman, P. L. (1976). The use of paraprofessionals to teach interviewing skills. *Pediatrics, 57*, 769-774.

Stillman, P. L., Regan, M. B., & Swanson, D. B. (1987). Fourth year performance assessment task force group: A diagnostic fourth-year performance assessment. *Archives of Internal Medicine, 65*, 320-326.

Stillman, P. L., Regan, M. B., Swanson, D. B., Case, S., McCahan, J., Feinblatt, J., Smith, S. R., Willms, J., & Nelson, D. V. (1990). An assessment of clinical skills of fourth-year medical students at four New England medical schools. *Academic Medicine*, *65*(5), 320-326.

Sutnick, A. I., Friedman, M., & Wilson, M. P. (1995). ECFMG international ventures in clinical competence assessment. *Proceedings of the Sixth Ottawa Conference on Medical Education*. Ontario, Canada: University of Toronto Bookstore Custom Publishing.

Tamblyn, R., Berkson, L., Dauphinee, W. D., Gayton, D., Grad, R. P., Huang, A., Issac, L., McLeod, P., & Snell, L. (1997). Unnecessary prescribing of NSAIDs and the management of NSAID-related gastropathy in medical practice. *Annals of Internal Medicine*, *127*(6), 429-438.

Vleuten, C. V. D., & Swanson, D. (1990). Assessment of clinical skills with standardized patients: State of the art. *Teaching and Learning in Medicine: An International Journal*, *2*, 58-76.

Vu, N. V., & Barrows, H. S. (1994). Use of standardized patients in clinical assessments: Recent developments and measurement findings. *Educational Researcher*, *23*(3), 23-30.

Wallace, P. (1997). Following the threads of an innovation: The history of standardized patients in medical education. *Caduceus*, *13*(2), 5-28.

Wiggins, G. (1989). A true test: Toward more authentic and equitable assessment. *Phi Delta Kappa*, *70*, 703-713.

Williams, R. G., & Barrows, H. S. (Eds.), (1987). Performance-based assessment of clinical competence using clinical encounter multiple stations. In I. R. Hart & R. M. Harden (Ed.), Further developments in assessing clinical competencies (pp. 425-433). Ottawa, Canada: Can-Heal Publications.

CHAPTER TWENTY

Reliability and Validity Issues in Standardized Patient Assessment

Jerry A. Colliver
Southern Illinois University School of Medicine

Mark H. Swartz
Mount Sinai School of Medicine

Clinical performance is the major concern of medical education, and many approaches to its assessment have been used, ranging from the traditional bedside oral examination to written simulations of patient management problems (Mast, Schermerhorn, & Colliver, 1992). However, the bedside orals were thought to be unreliable, because different examinees were assessed by different examiners in encounters with different patients with different problems. Furthermore, the written simulations elicited more actions (e.g., history-taking questions, physical examination maneuvers, tests ordered) than performed with real patients, which cast doubt on the validity of the measurements.

STANDARDIZED PATIENTS

Standardized patients (SPs) introduced by Barrows and Abrahamson in 1963 to overcome these difficulties, are the major approach currently considered for the assessment of clinical performance (Barrows & Abrahamson, 1964; Colliver & Williams, 1993; van der Vleuten & Swanson, 1990). An SP is a nonphysician who has been trained to portray a specific patient case in a consistent standardized fashion. In the interaction with the examinee, the SP presents the case history in response to questioning by the examinee and undergoes physical examination at the examinee's direction.

Examinees interact with SPs the same way they would interact with a real patient. In addition, SPs also complete checklists after the student-SP encounter on which they document actions performed by students on history-taking, physical examination, and behaviors related to interpersonal and communication skills. Scoring typically is based on the number (or percentage) of actions recorded on the SP checklist.

Standardized patients are being used increasingly worldwide in local medical school testing programs, and plans are underway for the use of SPs in licensure and certification testing. A survey of the 142 curriculum deans of U.S. and Canadian medical schools conducted in 1993 showed that 111 (80%) of the 138 schools responding indicated that SPs were being used in teaching and assessment at their schools (Anderson, Stillman, & Wang, 1994). For example, more than 1,000 students in the eight member schools of the New York City Consortium are tested each year on the seven-case SP assessment administered at The Morchand Center of Mount Sinai School of Medicine (Swartz & Colliver, 1996). At Southern Illinois University School of Medicine, starting with the class of 1986, all fourth-year students have taken the required 15-case SP assessment, for a total of 13 classes and more than 900 students tested at one school (Vu, Barrows, Marcy, Verhulst, & Colliver, et al., 1992). With respect to licensure and certification, the Medical Council of Canada (MCC) has used SPs in the Canadian licensure examination since 1993; the Educational Commission for Foreign Medical Graduates (ECFMG) initiated an SP component as a part of their testing program in 1998; and the National Board of Medical Examiners (NBME) is developing SP cases for use as a part of the United States Medical Licensing Examination (USMLE) Step 2 in the near future.

Because of this widespread interest in SPs, a considerable amount of research has been conducted to evaluate the adequacy of SP assessment. A consensus conference on the use of SPs was convened by the Association of American Medical Colleges (AAMC) in December 1992 to review the findings (Annex to the proceedings of the AAMC consensus conference, 1994; Proceedings of the AAMC consensus conference, 1993). One major area of research has been concerned with whether SPs can do the job. That is, are they realistic, are they accurate at portraying their roles, and are they accurate at checklist completion? With respect to SP realism, for example, research has shown that experienced physicians cannot differentiate SPs from real patients when SPs are sent unannounced into the physician's office. This finding is particularly impressive given that the physicians had agreed in advance to participate in the studies and knew that SPs would be coming to their offices. Studies also have shown that the clinical performance of house officers was quite similar to that of real patients and SP clones of the real patients. Other studies have demonstrated acceptable levels of accuracy of SPs at portraying their roles and completing checklists. The authors' conclusion is that SPs can do the job, and that the serious questions for SP assessment concern the measurements themselves, in particular, their reliability and validity.

RELIABILITY

Reliability is a major area in research in SP assessment (Colliver, Verhulst, Williams, & Norcini, 1989). *Reliability* refers to whether measurements obtained with a given measurement process are reproducible (i.e., consistent or stable) with repeated application of the process. The authors' sense of the many reported reliabilities of SP examinations is that they tend to fall short of the recommended reliability of 0.80 for educational and psychological tests, almost regardless of examination length. For example, the reliabilities of the New York City Consortium examination for the classes of 1995, 1996, and 1997 were 0.68, 0.64, and 0.65 respectively. For the Southern Illinois University School of Medicine examinations, the reliabilities for the 13 classes (1986 to 1998) were 0.72, 0.62, 0.56, 0.56, 0.62, 0.61, 0.59, 0.63, 0.70, 0.58, 0.50, 0.65, and 0.68, respectively.

Reliability is related to test length, which with SP assessment refers to the number of cases in the total examination. Therefore, the number of cases needed to achieve the recommended 0.80 level can be determined. For example, by increasing the length of the 1995 Consortium examination from seven to 13 cases, the reliability would reach the recommended 0.80 level. In actual practice, the reliability of pass-fail decisions is of more concern than the reliability of the examination scores. Fortunately, the reliability of pass-fail decisions is typically better than that of examination scores. For example, for the 1995 Consortium examination, the pass-fail reliability was 0.96. Therefore, although score reliabilities generally seem to fall short of the recommended 0.80 level, pass-fail reliabilities may reach an acceptable level.

One commonly expressed concern is that reliability might be seriously affected by the common practice of using two or more (multiple) SPs to simulate the same case (Colliver, Swartz, Robbs, Lofquist, & Cohen, et al., 1998). Because of the time required to administer all cases in an SP examination, especially with a large-scale testing program, multiple SPs are required to simulate the same case, which raises questions about the consistency of the simulation and the consistency of checklist completion by two or more simulators/raters.

Fortunately, studies have shown, at most, only a small effect of using multiple SPs on examination reliability. For example, the largest effect reported in a recent study of a large-scale testing program was for history-taking and physical examination checklist scores, for which the generalizability coefficient free of measurement error due to multiple SPs was 0.71, and the coefficient reflecting measurement error due to multiple SPs was 0.65. Other differences reported between these two types of generalizability coefficients have been smaller. In other words, multiple SPs are a source of unreliability, but the extent of that unreliability is not sufficient to raise concerns about the use of multiple SPs. Moreover, the usual reliabilities reported in the literature already reflect multiple-SP error and would be even higher if that source of unreliability were removed.

VALIDITY

Validity is the most important concern for any measurement process, including SP assessment, although research in this area has been limited (Colliver, 1995). *Validity* refers to whether an examination measures the dimension or construct it purports to measure, and the construct measured with SP assessment is called *clinical competence*. The validity of an SP examination, then, would be demonstrated by evidence showing that variation in SP test scores is indicative of actual variation in clinical competence. Thus, a generally accepted indicator of clinical competence is needed for use as a gold-standard criterion to validate SP examinations and to guide scoring and standard setting. One recurring suggestion for the gold-standard criterion has been global ratings by faculty-physician observers (Colliver, 1995).

In a recent study, a panel of five faculty physicians observed and rated videotaped performances of 44 medical students on the seven-case New York City Consortium SP examination (Swartz, Colliver, Badres, Charon, & Fried, et al., 1997). Correlations between the scores on the examination and the faculty ratings of clinical competence ranged from 0.60 to 0.70, which is high enough to suggest that they can be increased to the 0.80 level (also recommended for validity) on the basis of further studies to identify those measurable performance characteristics that reflect the gold-standard ratings. This research is underway, and these ratings are being used as a basis for the development and refinement of SP cases, checklists, scoring rubrics, and passing standards.

Other validity research has been less direct and thus less convincing, looking simply at relationships between SP examination scores and other variables to see what is and what is not reflected by the scores. Validity is demonstrated by showing that examination scores are consistent with our thinking about clinical competence and by testing whether the scores are related to what they should be related and not related to what they should not be. For example, a number of studies have shown that examinees' scores on an SP examination improve with additional training through medical school, residency, and practice, which of course is consistent with expectations (Barnhart, Marcy, Colliver, & Verhulst, 1995). However, the finding itself is indirect and provides only weak evidence for validity, although failure to find these results would raise serious doubts about the measurements, so the finding is important. Nevertheless, the evidence is weak, because scores on almost any dimension of medical performance should improve with more training, including scores on conventional multiple-choice examinations such as the USMLE Step examinations which are thought to measure cognitive knowledge of medical science rather than clinical performance. In other words, the improvement in SP examination scores with additional training does not show directly or convincingly that SP examinations are valid measures of clinical performance--that they are measuring something different from the less expensive, less time-consuming multiple-choice measures of knowledge.

However, findings from the aforementioned validity study showed that the gold-standard faculty ratings of clinical performance correlated only 0.16 and 0.30 with

USMLE Step 1 and Step 2, respectively, which suggests that the ratings of clinical performance are measuring something different from the traditional cognitive measures of medical knowledge (Swartz, et al. 1997). This finding lends credence to the thinking that motivates the continuing search for a measure of clinical performance such as SP assessment, namely, that conventional paper-and-pencil measures of cognitive knowledge may not be good indicators/predictors of clinical performance. Recently, the NBME has initiated work to develop written questions that require clinical problem solving, but research will need to be conducted to show that this paper-and-pencil format truly assesses clinical performance, such as it might be judged by expert observers.

Performance assessment by its very nature would seem to require (a) the observation of performance and (b) its holistic evaluation by expert observers. Otherwise, conventional paper-and-pencil measures would seem to suffice. At least, this seems to be the thinking of those who advocate performance assessment with SPs. For example, the Liaison Committee on Medical Education (LCME) calls for medical schools "to develop a system of assessment which assures that students have acquired and can demonstrate on direct observation the core clinical skills and behaviors needed in subsequent medical training" (LCME, 1991, p. 242). Clearly, this direct observation would have to be done by experts, and these experts should be given free reign to make their evaluations on the basis of their clinical experience and expertise (and of course the purpose of the examination, the level of students tested, etc.). Checklists, whether completed by SPs or faculty physicians, prestructure the task, so there is no guarantee that the checklist scores reflect the experts' holistic evaluations. Furthermore, checklist ratings would necessarily be subject to the same prestructuring. But if checklist scores do reflect the experts' global ratings of observed performance, checklist scores can be used as a proxy for the more expensive and time-consuming ratings, and SPs can complete the checklists as a part of their routine. Of course, global ratings by physicians must be obtained at some point to construct and test (i.e., validate) the checklist scores for subsequent use in actual testing (in place of the faculty global ratings). Global ratings by SPs are only of academic interest, because SPs lack the needed experience and expertise in clinical performance to give the ratings credibility, despite their potentially higher reliability compared with checklist scores.

SUMMARY AND CONCLUSION

Standardized patients offer a promising approach to the assessment of clinical performance: They present a high-fidelity simulation of the real clinical situation. They provide a standardized presentation of the same patient problem from examinee to examinee. They record the actions performed by examinees for use in deriving examination scores. For SP examinations at this writing, however, more SP cases are needed to achieve an acceptable level of score reliability, but the reliability of a pass-fail decision seems to be adequate. Validity research that informs scoring and standard setting is getting underway, but much work in this area is needed to provide meaningful feedback about clinical performance.

The immediate future of SP assessment seems bright, as the calls for clinical education and assessment of clinical performance continue. In the long run, however, concerns about the length and expense of SP examinations will need to be resolved. Currently, the cost of SP assessment for various testing programs at The Morchand Center of Mount Sinai has been estimated at approximately $200 to $400 per student tested, and about 10- to 20-hours of testing time per student are projected to achieve acceptable levels of reliability. However, sequential testing has been shown effective as a way to minimize the length and expense of SP assessment, whereby students who pass a short screening test with stringent standards would immediately receive a passing score on the full examination and thus would not be required to take the majority of the SP cases in the examination (Colliver, Mast, Vu, & Barrows, 1991). In addition, testing time and expense have been called "red herrings," in light of the years of training and overall costs of medical education, given that clinical performance is its primary goal. Therefore, more studies are needed to establish firmly that SP assessment measures something other than cognitive knowledge and that the something measured is clinical performance. Also, studies need to show that this cannot be measured adequately with the more efficient and less expensive paper-and-pencil format. Findings such as these are needed to ensure the long-term future of SP assessment.

REFERENCES

Anderson, M. B., Stillman, P. L., & Wang, Y. (1994). Growing use of standardized patients in teaching and evaluation in medical education. *Teaching and Learning in Medicine: An International Journal, 6,* 15-22.

Association of American Medical Colleges (AAMC). (1993). Proceedings of the AAMC consensus conference on the use of standardized patients in the teaching and evaluation of clinical skills (special issue). *Academic Medicine, 68,* 437-483.

Association of American Medical Colleges (AAMC). (1994). Annex to the proceedings of the AAMC consensus conference on the use of standardized patients in the teaching and evaluation of clinical skills (special issue). *Teaching and Learning in Medicine: An International Journal, 6,* 2-35.

Barnhart, A. J., Marcy, M. L., Colliver, J. A., & Verhulst, S. J. (1995). A comparison of second-year and fourth-year medical students on a standardized-patient examination of clinical competence: A construct validity study. *Teaching and Learning in Medicine: An International Journal, 7*(3), 168-171.

Barrows, H. S., & Abrahamson, S. (1964). The programmed patient: A technique for appraising student performance in clinical neurology. *Journal of Medical Education, 39,* 802-805.

Colliver, J. A. (1995). Validation of standardized-patient assessment: A meaning for clinical competence (commentary). *Academic Medicine, 70,* 1062-1064.

Colliver, J. A., Mast, T. A., Vu, N. V., & Barrows, H. S. (1991). Sequential testing with a performance-based examination using standardized patients. *Academic Medicine, 66,* 64-66.

Colliver, J. A., Swartz, M. H., Robbs, R. S., Lofquist, M., Cohen, D. S., & Verhulst, S. J. (1998). The effect of using multiple standardized patients on the intercase reliability of a large-scale standardized-patient examination administered over an extended testing period. *Academic Medicine, 73,* 81-83.

Colliver, J. A., Verhulst, S. J., Williams, R. G., & Norcini, J. J. (1989). Reliability of performance on standardized-patient cases: A comparison of consistency measures based on generalizability theory. *Teaching and Learning in Medicine: An International Journal, 1,* 31-37.

Colliver, J. A., & Williams, R. W. (1993). Technical issues: Test application. *Academic Medicine, 68,* 454-460.

Liaison Committee on Medical Education. (1991). Functions and structure of a medical school. *Teaching and Learning in Medicine: An International Journal, 14.*

Mast, T. A., Schermerhorn, G. S., & Colliver, J. A. (1992). Medical education. In M. C. Alkin (Ed.), *Encyclopedia of educational research,* (6th ed. pp. 814-825). New York: Macmillan.

Swartz, M. H., & Colliver, J. A. (1996). Using standardized patients for assessing clinical performance: An overview. *The Mount Sinai Journal of Medicine, 63*(34), 241-249.

Swartz, M. H., Colliver, J. A., Badres, C. L., Charon, R., Fried, E. D., & Moroffi, S. (1997). Validating the standardized-patient assessment administered to medical students in the New York City Consortium. *Academic Medicine; 72*(7), 619-626.

van der Vleuten, C. P. M., & Swanson, D. B. (1990). Assessment of clinical skills with standardized patients: State of the art. *Teaching and Learning in Medicine: An International Journal, 2,* 58-76.

Vu, N. V., Barrows, H. S., Marcy, M. L., Verhulst, S. J., Colliver, J. A., & Travis, T. A. (1992). Six-years of comprehensive clinical performance-based assessment using standardized patients at the Southern Illinois University School of Medicine. *Academic Medicine, 67,* 42-50.

CHAPTER TWENTY-ONE

Performance-Based Assessment

Richard K. Reznick
Krishan Rajaratanam
University of Toronto

The formal assessment of students across the continuum of medical education was a challenge to medical educators for the better part of the 20th century. The quest has been to develop a set of assessment tools that are both reliable and valid, adaptable to the specific purpose of the assessment task. Often competence in a particular area is inferred from the results of examinations that test only some aspects of the domain or a group of competencies perceived as a precondition for performance in a particular domain. The best example of this has been the reliance on multiple-choice examinations to test the knowledge base of medical students and residents. From the results of these tests, decisions about constructs other than cognitive knowledge often have been made. In large part, the birth of performance-based testing in medical education grew out of a dissatisfaction from the lack of tests that would fundamentally allow the observation of performance, with it inferred instead from the results of assessment methods that were not designed for such inference. To paraphrase George Miller (1990), educators need to focus on assessment techniques wherein students "show how" they do things instead of relying on tests that examine whether students "know how" to do things.

This chapter focuses on performance-based testing. In doing so, the authors speculate on what might lie ahead in performance-based testing over the next several decades, specifically exploring how new technologies might be deployed. They comment on the use of performance-based testing at the individual institutional level as well as at the national licensure and certification levels. Finally, they review some of the current concepts about adaptive testing and its role in the future.

The most obvious place to start in performance-based assessment is with ongoing monitoring of a student or resident's capacities during his or her day to day work. For quite some time, in-training evaluation reports or rating assessments have been commonplace in medical education. They, however, have received fairly bad press because of their purported lack of reliability. In fact, reliability is perhaps not the main issue. Rather, the more likely issue is that of getting preceptors to fill out in-training reports accurately and having them use the full range of any measurement scale. All too often preceptors evaluating either medical students or residents have rated virtually every trainee as very good or excellent. Trainees found to be problematic are rarely identified as such, and evaluators have found it difficult to fail individuals when in-training reports or global rating scales are the sole measure of assessment. Consequently in-training reports have been branded as subjective evaluation tools that have added little to the objective measure of an individual's competence.

This, however, need not be the case. The ongoing monitoring of students' progress during the course of their training provides a wonderful opportunity for accurate assessment. The great need is to bring structure to what now is basically a chaotic, haphazard evaluation tool. One such attempt that seems to be showing promise is the critical incident technique. With this procedure, the evaluators identify performances that are either exceptionally good or exceptionally bad on an ongoing basis (Grey, 1996). This technique may be of value because it has the potential to create a portfolio of performance-based activities for every student or resident, which would then have the potential to paint a more accurate portrait of an individual than the random biopsies to which we are accustomed.

Performance-based assessment generally refers to those tests in which actual performance of a skill is observed and measured. The prototype for this form of assessment in medicine has become the "objective structured clinical examination "(OSCE) first developed by Harden and colleagues from Dundee (Harden, Stevenson, Downie, & Wilson, 1975). This examination framed the emerging technology of standardized patient portrayals into a structured examination format, wherein each examinee performed the same tasks and were marked from standardized scoring schemes. The OSCE had enjoyed an almost unprecedented popularity as an examination tool in undergraduate medical education. Most North American schools now employ some form of OSCE in their curriculum. Several testing agencies have used or are poised to use the OSCE for licensure and certification (Harden, 1975; Reznick, Blackmore, Dauphinee, Rothman, & Smee, 1996; Grand'Maison, Lescop, Rainsberry, & Brailovsky, 1992; Sutnick, Stillman, Norcini, Friedman, & Williams, et al., 1994).

In Canada, the Medical Council of Canada and La Corporation Professionelle des Médecins du Québec in conjunction with the four medical schools in Québec have implemented OSCEs for licensure in their jurisdictions. Both of these examinations have been running for more than five years, and the psychometric properties have proved to be very acceptable for high-stakes testing. Both of these certifying bodies have invested heavily in smoothing the logistics of mounting multisite OSCEs. In the United States, the Educational Commission on Foreign Medical Graduates (ECFMG) is set to launch a standardized patient-based examination as a part of their testing process for foreign medical graduates gaining entry to the United States. The National Board of Medical Examiners has been conducting research for several years in the development of a reliable and valid standardized patient-based examination with a view to incorporating it into the United States Medical Licensing Examination (USMLE) in the future.

Many lessons have been learned from the large-scale experiences with the OSCE to date. The most important message is that large-scale application of the OSCE is possible, albeit costly. It requires a substantial degree of buy-in from all the stakeholders in the examination, and a fair degree of time must be invested in paying attention to the political details surrounding the examination if the examination is to be successful. A minimum of four-hours of testing time is required for an examination such as this to be reliable. High-stakes OSCEs can be successfully given at multiple sites with parallel forms. More work needs to be done in the realm of predictive validity to ensure that the results from this type of examination correlate well with future performance.

The OSCE and standardized patient techniques also have been the subject of an enormous body of research, most of which focuses on the reliability and validity of these techniques. To summarize this large body of research in this short overview would be impossible. However, several generalizations can be drawn from the research into OSCEs over the past few decades. First, the OSCE is a labor-intensive and costly form of assessment. The rigor in conducting the OSCE usually is proportional to the level of the stakes in the examination. It has been perceived that the OSCE, as it currently exists, requires a level of financial and personnel commitment that not every program can afford.

Nonetheless, a second principle that emerges is that examiners usually get what they pay for. In this regard, the OSCE is viewed as a more valid form of assessment than many evaluations used to infer clinical competence, such as the essay examination, the oral examination, and global rating assessments of ward performance. The major strength of the OSCE lies in its ability to assess fundamental clinical skills such as taking a history, conducting a physical examination, solving a problem in light of the clinical reality, and communicating with a patient or his or her family. Despite the fact that many validity concerns have been addressed through studies on the OSCE, there is the general perception that much work on the validity of the OSCE is still to be done. This is particularly true concerning the measurement of predictive validity: Is the level of performance seen on a licensure OSCE, for example, predictive of future practice?

The third element that emerges from the body of studies on the OSCE is that it generally is a reliable form of assessment, with excellent results achievable in terms of interrater agreement, interstation reliability, standardization of patient portrayals, and standardization of delivery across multiple sites. Effecting these good results, however, requires a lengthy examination of usually at least four-hours, a fair degree of patient and examiner preparation, and meticulous attention to detail around creation of the scoring checklists.

There have been cries that the OSCE trivializes the medical task, and that its use should be limited to formative rather than summative assessment. The OSCE has its limitations. It is not an efficient method of assessing cognitive knowledge and probably should not be used to do so. Similarly, there may be existing or emerging ways of assessing problem-solving skills that may be more efficient than the OSCE, for example, paper-and-pencil or computer-based formats assessing clinical reasoning skills (Pangaro, Worth-Dickstein, MacMillan, Klass, & Shatzer, 1997; Page, Bordage, & Allen, 1995). The OSCE does a good job of assessing the clinical skills of medical students and likely junior residents, but it may not be the ideal format for measuring the clinical competence of senior level trainees. The OSCE awards thoroughness, but may disadvantage an expert who has learned, through experience, to be efficient in his or her clinical skills. This may be particularly true when a checklist approach is the exclusive scoring rubric used.

Recently, MacRae, Cohen, Regehr, Reznick, and Burnstein (1997) have introduced a new form of performance-based testing known as the "patient assessment and management examination" (PAME). This examination is a form of OSCE in which the candidate meets the standardized patient more than once during a station and the focus of the encounter is patient management. The PAME also incorporates a structured oral evaluation into the examination. This evaluation has been shown to be appropriate for senior level trainees, with an ability to separate final year residents from penultimate year residents.

The PAME is a relatively labor-intensive form of the OSCE that requires fairly sophisticated training for standardized patients as well as examiners. Similar to the OSCE, the PAME requires approximately four-hours of testing for a reliable examination. This translates to a minimum of six- to eight-long patient encounters to obtain adequate reliability. At this point, however, the PAME has not been used extensively, and further information will be needed before it can be promoted as a tool for high-stakes testing.

These points and counterpoints regarding the OSCE and similar examinations notwithstanding, the OSCE likely is here to stay, and so it should be. At this writing, it has been a very successful addition to the testing tool chest. There will be a growing familiarity with the OSCE by medical school faculties and licensing bodies. This will ultimately lead to more efficient delivery of the examination with the expectation of cost reduction. Ultimately, rationalization will be the key. Medical schools will need to develop centralized testing organizations that can deliver performance-based tests to many departments in the faculty, and schools will need to get together to share testing resources in consortia type models.

The expense and logistic complexities of mounting OSCEs, particularly those for licensure and certification, have prompted many individuals to consider how the computer may play a role in performance-based assessment. It certainly seems possible in the foreseeable future that some form of interactive test using a computer-based platform may either replace or supplement the OSCE. However, for the time being, the computer is serving an increasing role in the assessment of clinical reasoning skills and patient management skills (Clyman, Julian, Orr, Dillon, & Cotton, 1991). At this writing, computer-based testing has had a limited effect in this, largely because of the logistics in mounting large-scale operations using a computer platform, and because the technology has been advancing and changing rapidly over the past decade. Clearly, programs written for computer-based testing only a few years ago have become obsolete with the advent of newer technologies. However, it does seem likely that the computer will play an increasingly vital testing role in all domains in the very near future. It is clearly conceivable as audio and video capabilities become increasingly prominent on the Internet that a digitally based examination will become logistically easier to mount and be richer in its contextual capabilities. In this regard, the future appears to be extremely exciting and may well parallel the staggering growth witnessed in computer-based technology over the past decade.

An issue quickly emerging in performance-based assessment is evaluation of the technical competence of physicians engaged in procedural skills. A development in this regard has been the reporting of a new examination called "objective structured assessment of technical skills" (OSATS) by Martin, Regehr, Reznick, MacRae, Murnaghan, et al. (1997). This examination is an OSCE-like test wherein candidates rotate from station to station performing discrete elements of technical tasks. The test is now given using bench model simulations of the operative reality (Reznick, Regehr, McRae, Martin, & McCulloch, 1997). At this writing, the psychometric properties of this examination have been promising, but as yet its use has not become widespread. There are, however, compelling reasons why tests such as the OSATS will need to be developed and matured. Not only is there an increasing demand for certification of technical competence at the graduating specialist level, but there also is a definite need for the assessment of competence in emerging new surgical technologies. On entering an era of medicine that is becoming increasingly high-tech, the public will be appropriately demanding concrete evidence of competence in the use of these new technologies.

Currently, experience with OSATS is growing. This technique, pioneered at The University of Toronto, now has been used for the assessment residents across Ontario and has been exported to two major urban centers in the United States. It would appear that this technique, although labor intensive and expensive like any performance-based assessment, has the possibility of finding a regular niche in the assessment of technical competence for surgical residents.

Performance-based testing has been applied largely to undergraduate education and, to a lesser extent, graduate education. It has not, however, entered the field of continuing education in any substantial way. The authors predict that this will change in the future. Increasing demands will be made by the public and certifying bodies that practitioners' competence to practice medicine be monitored in an ongoing fashion. At this writing, most recertification efforts have used paper-and-pencil-based tests to infer ongoing competence. However, as is the case concerning dissatisfaction with these tests in the undergraduate medical education arena, so too, dissatisfaction in the continuing education domain is likely. Just as airline pilots are expected to demonstrate ongoing maintenance of competence, so too will physicians be required to do so in some rigorous way. It is extremely likely that in this area the kind of performance testing described in this chapter will be used in the future.

As mentioned, one of the difficulties in performance-based testing has been the complexity and expense of these assessments. As such, many testing bodies have been experimenting with the concept of adaptive testing. Adaptive testing, simply stated, implies that not all test takers need to take every last item to demonstrate competence. Rather, a portion of a test can be given to a group of test takers who might then be given further elements of the test with either increasing or decreasing difficulty depending on how they faired in the initial aspects of the test. As it relates to performance-based testing in general, and OSCEs in particular, this might manifest as sequential testing. The basic notion is to give an initial screening test by which it can be predicted with a large degree of certainty which candidates would ultimately succeed on the total test. The remainder of the test could then be focused on the candidate pool that falls in the marginal group or the group at risk for failure. This approach to testing, which might be particularly applicable to computer-based strategies, would potentially serve to streamline the approach to testing and be particularly applicable at a certification or licensure level.

A final aspect of performance-based assessment that has been the focus to a great degree in previous research is the issue of standard setting. Despite much work in this area, however, not many good models have emerged showing how to set the standard for these kinds of examinations. Both norm-referenced and criterion-referenced approaches have been used with varying degrees of success. Norm-referenced testing is the simplest, but it is considered by most authorities to be inappropriate because of the arbitrariness in the way the standard is set. However, groups that have attempted to use criterion-referenced approaches to setting standards for performance-based assessment have been disappointed by the results. Generally speaking, some form of normative or politically acceptable standard must be applied to any system being used.

Perhaps the most important challenge in the move to performance-based assessment, even more challenging than the issue of logistic feasibility, is the process of ensuring that these processes are valid. It may be that traditional concepts of validity are not entirely appropriate for performance-based assessment (Moss, 1992). Indeed, there are many challenges in ensuring that performance-based assessment actually tests the construct that it purports to test. Moreover, and perhaps as important, it will be incumbent on researchers evaluating performance-based assessment to focus on the extent to which tests taken in this domain translate to the realities of future performance. The authors believe it is clear that performance-based assessment in medicine is feasible, and if the tests given are performed with care and sufficiently extensive, they can be reliable assessment formats. What remains to be proved is that these tests live up to the real reasons for their birth and increasing popularity, namely the claim that they are more valid forms of assessment than previously used tests in medicine.

REFERENCES

Clyman, S. G., Julian, E. R., Orr, N. A., Dillon, G. F., & Cotton, K. E. (1991). Continued research on computer-based testing. *Proceedings of the Annual Symposium on Computer Applications in Medical Care*, 742-746.

Grand'Maison, P., Lescop, J., Rainsberry, P., & Brailovsky, C. A. (1992). Large-scale use of an objective, structured clinical examination for licensing family physicians. *Canadian Medical Association Journal, 146*, 1735-1740.

Grey, J. (1996). Primer on resident evaluation. *Annals of Royal College of Physicians and Surgeons of Canada, 29*, 91-94.

Harden, R., Stevenson, M., Downie, W. W. W., & Wilson, G. M. (1975). Assessment of clinical competence using objective structured examination. *British Medical Journal, 1*, 447-451.

MacRae, H. M., Cohen, R., Regehr, G., Reznick, R., & Burnstein, M. (1997). A new assessment tool: The patient assessment and management examination. *Surgery, 122*(2), 335-343.

Martin, J. A., Regehr, G., Reznick, R., MacRae, H., Murnaghan, J., Hutchison, C., & Brown, M. (1997). Objective structured assessment of technical skill (OSATS) for surgical residents. *British Journal of Surgery, 84*, 273-278.

Miller, G. (1990). *Service to medicine: A special review* (pp. 48-49). Philadelphia: National Board of Medical Examiners.

Moss, P. A. (1992). Shifting concepts of validity in educational measurement: Implications for performance assessment. *Review of Educational Research, 62*(3), 229-258.

Page, G., Bordage, G., & Allen, T. (1995). Developing key-feature problems and examinations to assess clinical decision-making skills. *Academic Medicine, 70*(3), 194-201.

Pangaro, L. N., Worth-Dickstein, H., MacMillan, M. K., Klass, D. J., & Shatzer, J. H. (1997). Performance of "standardized examinees" in a standardized-patient examination of clinical skills. *Academic Medicine, 72*(11), 1008-1011.

Reznick, R., Regehr, G., MacRae, H., Martin, J., & McCulloch, W. (1997). Testing technical skill via an innovative bench station examination. *American Journal of Surgery, 173*, 226-230.

Reznick, R. K., Blackmore, D. E., Dauphinee, W. D., Rothman, A. I., & Smee, S. (1996). Large-scale high-stakes testing with an OSCE: Report from the Medical Council of Canada. *Academic Medicine, 71*(1), S19-S21.

Sutnick, A. I., Stillman, P. L., Norcini, J. J., Friedman, M., Williams, R. G., Trace, D. A., Schwartz, M. A., Wang, Y., & Wilson, M. P. (1994). Pilot study of the use of the ECFMG clinical competence assessment to provide profiles of clinical competencies of graduates of foreign medical schools for residency directors. Educational Commission for Foreign Medical Graduates. *Academic Medicine, 69*(1), 65-67.

CHAPTER TWENTY-TWO

Clinical Practice Examinations

Linda J. Morrison
Southern Illinois University School of Medicine

The roots of the clinical practice examination initiative stem from early 1984 when the Josiah H. Macy, Jr. Foundation sponsored an invitational conference on How to Begin Reforming the Medical Curriculum, at the Southern Illinois University (SIU) School of Medicine at Springfield. The report of the Association of American Medical Colleges (AAMC) Project on the General Professional Education of the Physician (GPEP) had recently focused national attention on inadequacies in the medical curriculum (Panel on the General Professional Education of the Physician, 1984), providing the stimulus for the conference. Medical school deans and educators from around the country were the invited participants. Recognizing that changing student evaluation methods would provide one of the most effective means of stimulating curricular reform, conference participants encouraged movement toward evaluating the competencies needed by the practicing physician and away from the rote memorization and recall of isolated facts. Included in the consensus statements emerging from the conference was the following recommendation: The evaluation of medical students for promotion and progress must include examinations that assess more than cognitive skills such as memorization, recognition, and recall of facts and concepts (Barrows & Peters, 1984, p. v).

Dr. Howard S. Barrows at the SIU School of Medicine suggested that this recommendation could be met through the use of a new type of performance assessment, the "clinical practice examination" (CPX), and he offered to demonstrate the CPX station at a follow-up conference later in the year. The performance assessment most familiar in medical education at this time was the "objective structured clinical examination" (OSCE, which had been introduced by Dr. Ronald Harden in the mid-1970s.

An OSCE consists of short patient stations, each typically five- to 10-minutes in length, that focus on individual or component skills of the patient workup. In contrast, the CPX is designed to reproduce the full patient visit in one station. In a CPX station, students or examinees complete a full clinical encounter with a patient, from the opening introductions, through focused history-taking and physical examination, to the provision of treatment options and patient education appropriate to the problem. Examinees are tested not only on their individual clinical skills, but also on their ability to recognize which of those skills or components are applicable in any given situation and to orchestrate them into a coherent whole. Usually 15- to 20-minutes are allocated for a CPX station.

Newer Approaches to the Assessment of Clinical Performance, a follow-up conference for the purpose of demonstrating the CPX, was held at SIU School of Medicine in late 1984. It effectively exhibited the realism, face validity, and potential power of this type of clinical performance and provided a prototype for the use of the assessment in a multiple-station format (Barrows, 1985).

Given the anticipated development, implementation, and research costs, some conference participants were interested in creating a consortium of medical schools to explore the use of the multiple-station CPX. Funding for consortium development could not be found at the time, but the SIU School of Medicine began the independent development of a multiple-station CPX for its senior medical students. This 15- to 20-patient CPX was established in the fall of 1985 and has been administered to senior medical students annually since that time (Barrows, Colliver, Vu, Travis, & Distlehorst, 1992). The examination, regarded by the school as a final clinical assessment, evaluates a student's ability to interview, examine, diagnose, and manage a series of standardized patients (SPs) in realistic clinical presentations. Unlike departmental clerkship examinations in which students know the clinical orientation of the cases and the faculty examiners, the CPX presents patients in clinical settings that are uncued to specialty orientation. Students have the freedom to workup and diagnose their patients without the interference and possible bias that could be introduced by knowledge of case author specialty.

In 1988, one of the six major recommendations emerging from the international medical education conference on Adapting Clinical Medical Education to the Needs of Today and Tomorrow was to require medical students to pass comprehensive, clinical examinations. This recommendation was directed not only to medical school faculties and administrators, but also to state licensing agencies and the Liaison Committee on Medical Education (LCME). Acknowledging that further research would be needed to establish the normative value of performance examinations, the method was accepted as an important educational advance (Gastel & Rogers, 1989).

To increase the understanding and use of the CPX and to encourage its implementation through the establishment of regional medical school consortia, the Josiah Macy Jr. Foundation supported a series of CPX demonstration workshops held by the SIU School of Medicine for all North American medical schools. The endeavor was endorsed by the Association of American Medical Colleges (AAMC), the Educational Commission on Foreign Medical Graduates (ECFMG), and the National Board of Medical Examiners (NBME).

Deans and senior faculty from 90 medical schools participated in the workshops over the three-year course of the project. Feedback from the 130 participants was very positive. More than 80% of the schools reported either beginning or contemplating beginning CPX efforts within the next year (Barrows & Morrison, 1992). The major concern noted at this time, as in 1984, was the cost, both in dollars and human resources, of establishing and conducting CPX assessments. The Macy Foundation responded to that concern by offering to fund a small number of medical school consortia for the purpose of establishing regional CPX assessments. Sixteen proposals representing more than 60 schools were submitted, with funding ultimately awarded to six: the North Carolina Medical Schools Consortium, the Gulf Coast Regional Consortium for the Assessment of Performance, the Northwest Consortium for the Assessment of Clinical Performance, the Southern California Consortium for Assessment of Clinical Competency, the New York City Consortium, and the Upstate New York Clinical Competency Center (Morrison & Barrows, 1998).

Although all six consortia were similar in some respects, each had its own vision, purpose, and operational style that resulted from the particular needs, goals, and resource configurations of its member schools. This resulted in a rich seedbed for CPX research and development. The Northwest Consortium was particularly interested in the curriculum feedback provided by the CPX. The Gulf Coast Consortium focused on developing a preclinical CPX to be linked later to a senior CPX. The Southern California Consortium was interested in developing strong interschool consensus relationships and establishing common graduation objectives. The Upstate New York Consortium worked on creating an interdisciplinary health professional approach for its examination, involving faculty from nursing and physician assistant programs. The North Carolina Consortium sought to develop a statewide CPX with a strong emphasis on appropriate communication and patient interaction skills. The New York City Consortium developed a comprehensive citywide clinical assessment for senior medical students that culminated daily in a faculty-led debriefing emphasizing the important teaching aspects of the patient cases.

All schools entered their consortia with the belief that cooperative pooling of resources would improve the quality and scope of the resulting clinical assessment. At the end of the grant period, most of the 28 schools involved in the six consortia planned to continue their CPX and remain in their respective consortium. Many had identified funds and space in which to construct clinical assessment centers that would allow easier administration of their examinations as well as program expansion, an oft-cited goal. Because of what the schools had learned about their students and their curricula through this experience, the CPX had become an educational priority.

CPX DEVELOPMENT AND STRUCTURE

Development of a multiple-station CPX begins with the adoption of an examination matrix or blueprint. The examination matrix maps out the cases that make up the CPX, providing a guide for the subsequent development of those cases. Based on the goals of the curriculum and reflecting what faculty feel is important to assess, the examination matrix generally includes some or all of the following parameters: clinical settings, acuity of need, organ systems, specialties, common problems, patient demographics, and competencies to be tested, including specific communication skills such as giving bad news or providing patient education. Having a formal examination matrix in place makes the process of case review and revision more effective.

A CPX provides rich opportunities for assessing a variety of clinical skills, particularly history-taking, physical examination, interpersonal skills, communication, and patient education, but also clinical problem-solving, test interpretation, diagnosis, management, and case presentation, all within the context of a particular patient problem or set of problems. The choice of skill components to be assessed in each case depends on the critical skills involved in that case and on the curriculum objectives specified by the examination matrix.

Most CPX stations include an assessment of appropriate history and physical examination (H&P) skills. As used here, H&P skills refer to the ability to ask appropriate questions and perform basic physical examination maneuvers to gather the information needed to diagnose and manage patients. Because H&P skills often are learned by students as full menus that stress the complete workup, one of the first challenges a student in a CPX faces is deciding how to focus each investigation on the needs of the particular patient in the time allotted. Helping students to shift from doing a complete H&P to performing a more focused one was a definite change in educational strategy stimulated by the CPX.

The CPX also provides an excellent and unique opportunity to assess a student's communication and interpersonal skills. In some stations (e.g., where a patient presents with a suspicious mammogram), these skills will play a major role in the expectations for student performance.

Communication, H&P, and interpersonal skills all lend themselves to direct observation, so data can be easily and reliably collected by means of checklists. Checklists generally are completed by nonphysician raters, often by the SP himself or by another SP trained in the case and working in tandem with the presenting SP. In addition to completing checklists or scales rating what happened during the encounter and their satisfaction with it, SPs also may be asked to provide subjective comments as feedback for the students.

The SPs must be able to complete their checklists with a high degree of accuracy over the course of the examination. Research has demonstrated the ability of the SP to satisfy this criteria (Tamblyn, Klass, Schnabl, & Kopelow, 1991; Vu, Steward, &

Marcy, 1987), but a system of reliability checks is recommended if the CPX is being used for student promotion.

The remaining clinical skills (test selection and interpretation, diagnosis, patient management, and case presentation) must be assessed using other methods. Student follow-up exercises and faculty observation and participation are additional methods that can be used to provide performance data in a CPX.

Student follow-up or interstation exercises are typically short series of clinically relevant questions following each patient that ask the student some or all of the following: What was found on history or physical examination? What diagnostic ideas are being considered? What tests or procedures should be ordered, and what do the results mean? What is the diagnosis? What treatment or management plans should be recommended? Additional information (e.g., laboratory results) can be provided during the follow-up exercise for students to interpret. Questions can be multiple-choice or short answer, or instead of questions, students may be asked to write chart notes, orders, or a short H&P writeup.

Follow-up exercises provide students with the opportunity to exhibit their clinical understanding of the patient and his or her illness or condition. They reveal the knowledge the student can recall and apply clinically during his or her work with patient problems, all situated in a realistic practice setting. Computer applications being developed for use with the CPX are designed to match student-constructed responses with instructor expectations for both the clinical reasoning question approach and the chart note approach.

Faculty observation and participation can provide another valuable dimension to the assessment of performance on a CPX. Depending on the features and equipment available in the assessment facility, faculty can observe directly at the time of the examination or via videotape at a later, more convenient time. Real-time observation allows the provision of immediate feedback to students, maximizing the learning potential of the experience. Faculty typically rate student performance globally as satisfactory or unsatisfactory (and points in between), but also may use checklists developed by the case author that are designed to focus on particular components important to the case. Faculty also may participate by listening to case presentation skills and rating them, or by conducting oral examinations that probe student understanding of the cases and content involved.

It has been suggested that clinical faculty observation and rating of students can be used as a gold standard in measuring the clinical competence of medical students. Studies published in this area demonstrate mixed but encouraging findings (Herbers, Noel, Cooper, Harvey, & Pangaro, 1989; MacRae, Vu, Graham, Word-Sims, & Colliver, 1995; Swartz, Colliver, Bardes, Charon, Fried, et al., 1997). However, more work is needed to determine how and on what criteria faculty make judgments about student performance.

Among the reasons underlying adoption of the CPX by medical school faculty is the rationale that students are not routinely observed during the regular course of their medical education, particularly in the clinical years. The CPX is seen as an alternative method for this that also can objectively assess the student's clinical reasoning and mastery of the principles of medical practice. Because of the availability of checklists and student questionnaires for collecting performance data, a CPX reduces dependence on faculty raters, thus reducing or removing the error introduced by interrater variability. Obviously, direct faculty observation and participation are very time intensive, and these resource costs must be considered during examination planning.

SCORING AND STANDARD SETTING

Scoring and setting standards for student performance may be the issues of greatest current effort regarding the CPX. Although there seems to be wide agreement that the CPX is a valid and valuable experience for students, there is less confidence that scores derived from it are a reliable measure of student performance. The clinical performance of a physician, whether a novice (learner) or an expert, is a complex combination of knowledge, technical skills, interpersonal interaction, communication, and clinical reasoning all operating simultaneously. Therefore, these different components cannot be separated and evaluated independently. Depending on the particulars of a given case, one or more of these components may be more important or critical to the determination of clinical competency assessment than the others. Also, there is an element of art involved in the practice of medicine that complicates the assessment of competence. Faculty do not necessarily agree readily, particularly across departments, on what is important in any given clinical situation, or how it should be handled. Different clinical approaches to any examination case must be carefully discussed, with parallel credit awarded to appropriate alternatives.

As noted earlier, three ways have been identified and used to collect data for use in scoring student performance on the CPX: SP checklists, student follow-up exercises, and faculty ratings. All of these methods have their uses, but none of them are by themselves universally satisfactory. That is, none can capture all elements of the clinical encounter independently. With any data collection measure, scores can be attributed to each item or component and decisions made about how or if they are to be combined to create an overall score. Scores may be collected as either dichotomous (pass-fail) or continuous (percentage or total correct) data, or a combination of the two methods may be used. Criteria for passing each case as well as the examination as a whole must be established.

Different measures will elicit information about different types of competencies (Neufeld & Norman, 1985). Checklists are effective for collecting information about clinical skills, whereas student follow-up stations provide a method for collecting information about clinical reasoning and knowledge application. Faculty ratings can provide an independent global assessment of the overall competency or clinical adequacy displayed by the student in the patient encounter. To compare performance among students over a number of cases or across measures, numerical scores often are awarded to items or ratings. Unfortunately, the scores derived from the different measures do not necessarily correlate as highly as would be desired (Travis, Colliver, Robbs, Barnhart, & Barrows, et al., 1996). Perhaps the critical indicators of clinical competence, consistent from case to case, have not yet been clearly identified. Whether they can be determined is yet to be seen, but distilling the essence of a student's clinical skills and reasoning in and about a patient encounter down to meaningful numerical scores is a very complex issue.

Standard-setting procedures for performance-based examinations such as the CPX have been adapted from those used for other types of examinations, such as extensions of the Angoff and Ebel methods (Livingston & Zieky, 1982). For example, faculty raters, within the context of a small group, may review all checklist items individually, stating whether a hypothetical borderline medical student or examinee would have completed each one successfully. Results are then shared with the group and discrepancies between raters discussed. Faculty are asked to rate the items again, and the review process is repeated. The average of a third and final independent rating, often after performance data are shared, becomes the performance standard for that item (Norcini, Stillman, Sutnick, Regan, & Haley, 1993). The contrasting-groups approach, which has been used with some success, is an alternative method for standard setting that requires faculty raters to make judgments regarding individual performances instead of individual items (Ross, Clauser, Margolis, Orr, & Klass, 1996). The development of automated algorithms for scoring and standard setting are being investigated with promising results (Clauser, Ross, Fan, & Clyman, 1998).

Setting performance standards for cases and examinations at single schools, however, may be as simple in practice as a series of faculty review sessions during which faculty collectively relate performance expectations to curricular priorities. The issues of scoring and standard setting continue to be studied carefully as performance assessments are increasingly used for national certifying examinations.

USES OF THE CPX

The CPX has the dual goal of providing a valid and reliable measure of both student competence and curriculum effectiveness. Although originally envisioned as a summative examination, the CPX also has value as a formative examination. It can provide useful and pertinent feedback to students about their clinical strengths and weaknesses in a meaningful context. Until faculty are convinced of the ability of the CPX to provide meaningful numerical scores that can contrast and rank order students by their performance, reservations will remain about using the examination as a true summative measure of performance.

For some schools, curriculum feedback to the faculty is the most important product of the CPX. When cases are carefully selected and developed, the performance of students on a CPX can provide a clear picture of how they understand and apply the knowledge and skills gained through participation in the curriculum. Reported to the curriculum planning faculty, this performance can identify gaps or problems in student learning. As a result, curriculum revisions can be targeted to improve or clarify basic biomedical and clinical concepts.

STRENGTHS OF THE CPX

Faculty have noted that the CPX provides students with the opportunity to demonstrate their knowledge, skills, and behavior on a consistent standardized set of patient problems in a realistic and objective context. Important patient experiences not available to students in the "real world," such as giving bad news or making decisions in an emergency situation, also can be included in a CPX. Student understanding of the clinical practice of medicine can be assessed as well as the underlying concepts on which that practice is based.

A CPX can emphasize the specific skills, competencies, and clinical knowledge that faculty want students to develop. It shifts the emphasis in student performance from rote recall to applied knowledge. It has long been known that student study is directed by the type of examinations they are given, and it is generally believed that these examinations should reflect what the faculty believe is important in a particular area of study. For multiple-choice knowledge tests, students will study textbooks and other sources of factual material intensively, but for a CPX, the best way to study is to see patients. The CPX then encourages students to engage in the very behavior that will make them better doctors: increased clinical practice.

The CPX provides an opportunity for faculty to observe students working with patients, allowing them to provide feedback to the students about their demonstrated skills. This is beneficial from curriculum and faculty development standpoints, not just from a student progress standpoint. For students, the CPX provides an opportunity to practice and receive feedback in an environment safe from the actual repercussions of clinical mistakes. For the faculty, it shows how effectively students can manage a selected set of patients without disrupting clinic schedules or compromising the care of patients. Students with problems can be identified, and timely assistance can be provided. This is particularly beneficial when used early in the clinical curriculum as a formative assessment.

Students have been generally supportive of the CPX. Although there are some complaints that it is an unnecessary addition to an already full schedule, most students report that the CPX helps them identify their strengths and weaknesses, pointing them to areas in which they need further study. Some students are nervous, and some have difficulty with the "suspension of disbelief" that is needed for simulation, but most appear to feel that the examination is a valid, useful, and necessary component of their medical education. Two elements that particularly contribute to student support for a CPX are feedback (to maximize the learning potential of the examination) and clinical faculty participation during the examination itself (to allay student anxiety and acknowledge the importance or significance of the activity) (Morrison & Barrows, 1998).

CONCERNS ABOUT THE CPX

The thorny issue of attributing meaningful scores to the activities involved in the practice of being a physician has already been addressed. Although the reliability of the scores themselves tends to be below the level expected for examinations, the reliability of pass-fail decisions based on student scores has been shown as quite high (Colliver, Verhulst, Williams, & Norcini, 1989). The psychometric properties of performance assessments continue to need and receive study and research.

One early concern was whether examination security would be compromised with the small number of cases generally used in a CPX (fewer than 20). Studies have shown, however, that the sharing of examination information among students has no effect on the performance of subsequent students (Furman, Colliver, Galofre, Reaka, Robbs, & King, 1997; Swartz, Colliver, Cohen, & Barrows, 1995). It appears that having advance information in a performance examination does not necessarily result in a student being able to use that information directly to improve performance. Understanding the clinical context of the problems and using learned information and process skills to solve the clinical problems presented appear to be less susceptible to interference or improvement by security breaches.

One of the most critical elements in a CPX or any other examination that uses SPs is the quality and realism of the SPs. The integrity of the examination rests on their ability to relate as real patients with prescribed sets of physical signs and symptoms and to be both accurate and consistent in each portrayal. The ability of the SP to record the actions of the students accurately, particularly over time and on examinations that depend heavily on checklist scores, is a critical issue. As noted earlier, research has shown that SPs are acceptably reliable for both portrayal and checklist accuracy (Colliver & Williams, 1993).

A final set of concerns has to do with administrative issues, particularly curricular time, resource allocation, and resource use. Putting on a CPX is resource intensive for both faculty and staff and requires that a school develop or contract with an SP program to work with faculty to develop cases and to manage the patient training and administrative aspects of a performance assessment. This requires program development funds and a continuing budget for an SP trainer, staff, and simulators. Although it is possible to administer a CPX in active clinic space when it is not scheduled for patient use, for scheduling effectiveness, it is helpful to have a dedicated clinical examination center. The audiovisual modifications that allow faculty unobtrusively to observe student performance usually are not otherwise easily available.

FUTURE OF PERFORMANCE ASSESSMENT USING SPS

There has been unparalleled growth in the use of SPs in medical education during the past decade, in both OSCEs and CPXs. In 1993, acceptance of performance-based clinical assessments using SPs was firmly established with the AAMC's Consensus Conference on the Use of Standardized Patients in the Teaching and Evaluation of Clinical Skills (Proceedings of the AAMC Consensus Conference, 1993). In that year, the AAMC Curriculum Directory reported that 81% of North American medical schools used standardized patients, and that 49% used some type of performance assessment. In 1997, the directory reported that 95% of schools were using SPs, and that 69% were using performance assessment. This represents a 14% increase in the use of SPs and a 20% increase in the use of performance assessment. Data show that just with the Macy CPX Consortia Project, the number of schools administering a comprehensive CPX to senior medical students grew from only a handful of schools at the beginning of the decade to, at a minimum, approximately 30 by the end of 1995. Also, more schools have joined the number administering CPXs since that time. As preparations continue for the inclusion of an SP assessment in the United States Medical Licensing Examination (USMLE) in the near future, more and more medical schools are becoming involved in preparing their own examinations or in cooperating with the National Board of Medical Examiners (NBME) in the pilot trials of its examination. The impact of this expected event has been significant in the proliferation of performance assessments.

Medical education journals and meetings are now peppered with papers, studies, and reports on performance assessment using SPs. These range from studies on student skills (interpersonal expertise, communication, history-taking, physical examination) to gender and cultural diversity effects (involving both students and SPs) to examination properties (particularly related to scoring and standard setting to psychometric properties (generalizability, reliability, validity, predictability) and to multiple-site issues (reproducibility, length, screening examinations).

What have we learned in the past several decades of focused effort on the development and use of clinical practice examinations?

- A CPX is most effective when faculty involved in the direct teaching effort also are involved in the determination of the examination blueprint and the establishment of performance standards (expectations) for students, in an effort to match assessment to curriculum. In a CPX that crosses department boundaries, a transdisciplinary committee of faculty should be convened for this purpose.

- Students need to understand clearly who they are (i.e., what role they are to play), where they are, and what is expected of them. A CPX works best if students are just themselves (medical students), with variations in clinical settings, if necessary. Just as when they are working with a particular attending physician in a clinical setting, they need to understand what they are expected (and not expected) to do with the patient and also in any follow-up exercise. Setting the environment is a key factor in the ability of students to demonstrate a full range of competence.

- The more closely a clinical assessment parallels what actually happens in the practice of medicine, the more value students and faculty attribute to the assessment outcomes.

- The response of students to a CPX is most positive when they are allowed to work up and discuss the patients freely and in their own words. The clinical relevance of the activity and the pertinence of the feedback derived from it are then undeniable.

- Performance standards for tasks included in a senior CPX may be more rigorous than in prior clinical experiences or assessments, and students may be expected to demonstrate competency in more areas (e.g., diagnosis and management, in addition to H&P skills).

- Although certain logistical restrictions (e.g., time limits) are inherent in any testing situation with multiple takers, care should be taken to maintain clinical realism as much as possible. Anything that detracts from the impression of clinical realism (e.g., patient findings cards, bells, loudspeakers) should be kept to a minimum.

- Data collection measures should be matched to the purpose and goals of the examination. Multiple measures allow the multiple components of clinical expertise to be sampled and therefore may be more useful than a single measure.

- Finally, faculty use performance assessment not because the psychometric reliability has been established, but because it is an effective teaching tool. It provides a clinically consistent way to demonstrate and assess educational achievement and clinical ability, along with an opportunity to provide relevant feedback to the learner.

The performance assessment research effort certainly will continue as the national focus on performance assessment continues to be strong. Whether the focus is on the short structured stations of the OSCE or the longer less-structured stations of the CPX, it appears that performance assessment finally has achieved a place of acknowledged value in the medical education evaluation lexicon.

REFERENCES

Association of American Medical Colleges (AAMC). (1993). Proceedings of the AAMC Consensus Conference on the Use of Standardized Patients in the Teaching and Evaluation of Clinical Skills. *Academic Medicine, 68,* 437-511.

Barrows, H. S. (1985). *Newer approaches to the assessment of clinical performance.* Springfield, IL: Southern Illinois University School of Medicine.

Barrows, H. S., Colliver, J. A., Vu, N. V., Travis, T. A., & Distlehorst, L. H. (1992). *The clinical practice examination: A six-year summary.* Springfield, IL: Southern Illinois University School of Medicine.

Barrows, H. S., & Morrison, L. J. (1992). *Evaluation report of the CPX demonstration project*. Springfield, IL: Southern Illinois University School of Medicine.

Barrows, H. S., & Peters, M. J. (Eds.), (1984). *How to begin reforming the medical curriculum*. Springfield, IL: Southern Illinois University School of Medicine.

Clauser, B. E., Ross, L. P., Fan, V. Y., & Clyman, S. G. (1998). A comparison of two approaches for modeling expert judgment in scoring a performance assessment of physicians' patient-management skills. *Academic Medicine, 73*, S117-S119

Colliver, J. A., Verhulst, S. J., Williams, R. G., & Norcini, J. J. (1989). Reliability of performance on standardized patient cases: A comparison of consistency measures based on generalizability theory. *Teaching and Learning in Medicine: An International Journal, 1*, 31-37.

Colliver, J. A., & Williams, R. G. (1993). Technical issues: Test application. *Academic Medicine, 68*, 454-460.

Furman, G. E., Colliver, J. A., Galofre, A., Reaka, M. A., Robbs, R. S., & King, A. (1997). The effect of formal feedback sessions on test security for a clinical practice examination using standardized patients. *Advances in Health Sciences Education, 2*, 3-7.

Gastel, B., & Rogers, D. E., (Eds.), (1989). *Clinical education and the doctor of tomorrow*. New York: New York Academy of Medicine.

Herbers, J. E., Noel, G. L., Cooper, G. S., Harvey, J., Pangaro, L. N., & Weaver, M. J. (1989). How accurate are faculty evaluations of clinical competence? *Journal of General Internal Medicine, 4*, 202-208.

Livingston, S. A., & Zieky, M. J. (1982). *Passing scores: A manual for setting standards of performance on educational and occupational tests*. Princeton, NJ: Educational Testing Service.

MacRae, H.., Vu, N. V., Graham, B., Word-Sims, M., Colliver, J. A., & Robbs, R. S. (1995). Comparing checklists and databases with physicians' ratings as measures of students' history and physical-examination skills. *Academic Medicine, 70*, 313-317.

Morrison, L. J., & Barrows, H. S. (1998). *Educational impact of the Macy consortia: Regional development of clinical practice examinations*. Final report of the EMPAC Project. Springfield, IL: Southern Illinois University School of Medicine.

Neufeld, V. R., & Norman, G. R. (Eds.), (1985). *Assessing clinical competence*. New York: Springer.

Norcini, J. J., Stillman, P. L., Sutnick, A. I., Regan, M. B., Haley, H. L., Williams, R. G., & Friedman, M. (1993). Scoring and standard setting with standardized patients. *Evaluation and the Health Professions, 16*, 322-332.

Panel on the General Professional Education of the Physician. (1984). Physicians for the twenty-first century: The GPEP report. *Journal of Medical Education, 59*(11, pt2), 1-208.

Ross, L. P., Clauser, B. E., Margolis, M. J., Orr, N. A., & Klass, D. J. (1996). An expert-judgment approach to setting standards for a standardized-patient examination. *Academic Medicine, 71*, S4-S6.

Swartz, M. H., Colliver, J. A., Cohen, D. S., & Barrows, H. S. (1995). The effect of deliberate, excessive violations of test security on a standardized examination: An extended analysis. In A. Rothman & R. Cohen, (Eds.), *Proceedings of the Sixth Ottawa Conference on Medical Education*, (pp. 280-284). Toronto, Canada: University of Toronto Bookstore Custom Publishing.

Swartz, M. H., Colliver, J. A., Bardes, G. L., Charon, R., Fried, E. D., & Moroff, S. (1997). Validating the standardized-patient assessment administered to medical students in the New York City Consortium. *Academic Medicine, 72*, 619-626.

Tamblyn, R. M., Klass, D. J., Schnabl, G. K., & Kopelow, M. L. (1991). The accuracy of standardized-patient presentations. *Medical Education, 25*, 100-109.

Travis, T. A., Colliver, J. A., Robbs, R. S., Barnhart, A. J., Barrows, H. S., Giannone, L., Henkle, J. Q., Kelly, D. P., Nichols-Johnson, V., Rabinovich, S., Ramsey, D. E., Riseman, J., Rockey, P. H., Ross, D. S., Schrage, J. P., & Steward, D. E. (1996). Validity of a simple approach to scoring and standard setting for standardized-patient cases in an examination of clinical competence. *Academic Medicine, 71*, S84-S86.

Vu, N. V., Steward, D. E., & Marcy, M. L. (1987). An assessment of the consistency and accuracy of standardized patients' simulations. *Journal of Medical Education, 62*, 65-67.

CHAPTER TWENTY-THREE

Authentic Problem-Based Learning

Howard S. Barrows, MD
Southern Illinois University School of Medicine

Problem-based learning first emerged as an educational method in the early 1970s at McMaster University in Hamilton, Ontario, Canada. The founding fathers of that new medical school wanted to avoid the general disenchantment medical students had with medical education. They decided that medical school would be more exciting and rewarding if patient problems were used as the focus of learning (Spaulding, 1991). The creator of problem-based learning (PBL) as a defined teaching-learning method, was James Anderson, a physician, anatomist, and anthropologist who by his diffident nature was the perfect tutor (he would seemingly never directly answer any questions put to him). He also established a very successful high school program based on PBL.

Because the medical school at McMaster was a new school without old teaching traditions to change this revolutionary approach to education, PBL flowered there. Following McMaster's lead with many workshops and exchanges with McMaster's faculty came two other new medical schools: Newcastle in Australia and Maastricht in The Netherlands. Soon thereafter, the University of New Mexico's School of Medicine pioneered an alternative PBL curriculum in primary care, which paralleled its traditional curriculum. They also had workshops and exchanges with the McMaster faculty. Those brave faculty members had the difficult task of getting PBL underway within a traditional, already established curriculum.

Soon, a small number of other schools undertook curricular changes to PBL, both in the United States and globally. However, most of the older, well-established medical schools showed little interest in this curricular innovation, and its dissemination as a teaching-learning method in medical education was slow. This changed after Harvard's medical school moved to PBL (first as an alternative curriculum and later across the whole curriculum integrated with more traditional approaches) and after the Association of American Medical Colleges (AAMC) published *Physicians for the Twenty-First Century-The Report of the Panel on the General Professional Education of the Physician and College Preparation for Medicine*. This report encouraged medical schools to adopt a number of curricular reforms, many that were supported by PBL.

Now, at the turn of the century, PBL has become popular in medical education, and countless medical schools throughout North America and around the world have used or are in the process of using what they each refer to as PBL. However, the methods they use are so diverse, and some so poorly designed (far from the original concept of PBL), that it would be impossible now to generalize about PBL as a teaching method. With many of the approaches, it would be hard to be enthusiastic about PBL. Unfortunately, many medical school teachers are unaware that PBL is not a monolithic method, the same wherever used. If they witness a poorly designed endeavor called PBL, they may generalize that experience to all PBL. Understanding PBL is further complicated by a rash of other terms used for what many assume are similar approaches such as case-based learning, project-based learning, theme-based learning, contextual learning, action learning, practice-based learning, and so forth.

The purpose of this chapter is to describe the characteristics that should be present in PBL if it is to be considered "authentic" and capable of taking advantage of the many educational objectives possible with PBL as an active, student-centered learning method.

AUTHENTIC PROBLEM BASED LEARNING

The term "authentic" is used in education to describe any learning method that requires the learner to carry out the same activities in learning that will be required of the learner in the real world--and does not require the learner to carry out activities during learning that are not valued in the real world. The "real world" in this context is that of clinical practice.

Problem-Based Learning should be authentic from three perspectives. First, the problems used in PBL should be those that the student will most likely encounter in subsequent practice. Second, the problem simulation formats used should be designed to challenge the same reasoning skills required in clinical work. Third, the sequence of activities the students go through working with a problem in the small group learning process, should be the same activities that will be carried out in their subsequent practice. Many PBL methods do not meet one or more of these perspectives concerning authenticity. In authentic PBL, students are practicing and perfecting the skills required in their professional work. However, students are not just playing doctor prematurely, but are acquiring a deep understanding of the sciences basic to medicine as well. This is accomplished through the crucial role of the "tutor' who, in this context, is the facilitator of the learning process in the small group. The role and preparation of the tutor also is a major variable in many PBL methods. These three perspectives for authenticity (problem selection, problem simulation format, PBL process) are examined in more detail.

PROBLEM SELECTION

In PBL, a problem, usually a patient problem, is presented to the students to challenge their problem-solving skills and to stimulate their need to know and desire to learn. To be authentic, the PBL problems must be actual patient problems, and not problems created by the faculty to stimulate learning in specific content areas. Students tend to become more motivated and involved with problems they know are real. Problems in community health, practice management, patient advocacy, and community health education must also be included because they represent an important part of a physician's responsibility in the community.

The problems used in authentic PBL curricula should be those that occur frequently and are likely to be encountered by students despite the particular career or specialty they choose. The problems also should be those that have a high impact in terms of mortality, morbidity, and health care costs even if not frequent. Whatever students must learn to understand, the basic mechanisms responsible for these patient problems and the understanding needed to diagnose, treat, educate and care for those patients determine the curriculum. Whatever basic science and clinical content is needed to understand the problems down to the appropriate level and detail of learning is the curriculum. In this way the PBL curriculum is authentic and will always be contemporary and relevant to practice because new problems and issues that appear in medicine and health care can be added and those becoming outdated or replaced can be eliminated. The problems also should present an appropriate balance of age groups, ethnic backgrounds, and socioeconomic status.

PROBLEM SIMULATION FORMAT

The only way a patient problem can be presented to a small working group of students is through simulation. The lowest order of simulation with the least authenticity is the writeup of a patient case printed on paper. The audiovisual-tactile reality of the patient is reduced to verbal descriptions. Clinicians with patient experience can recreate what the reality of a patient must be like when reading a paper case, but not medical neophytes. An even more important problem with the printed case is that it already presents most of the important information needed to analyze the patient problem. The author of the case writeup did the problem-solving work writing up the case, so there is little challenge for the student to use problem-solving skills.

Sequentially presented written cases are also prevalent in PBL curricula. In this format, a paragraph of information is given about the patient (usually more than was available when the patient appeared in the real clinical situation), and students are asked to analyze this information, decide what they think might be going on, and determine what questions or examinations they might like to perform and why. After that, the students read another paragraph, and the process continues. Although the students generate hypotheses as to what they think might be going on with the patient and think of information from the patient they would need to establish their hypotheses, their inquiry is never directly answered. As a result, their problem-solving strategies can never be carried out. Patients never present clinically in that manner. These formats are not authentic, so they are unable to realize the learning potential offered by patient problem simulation in PBL.

The Problem-Based Learning Module (PBLM) (Distlehorst & Barrows, 1982) also is a printed simulation of the patient problem, but it provides greater authenticity by presenting the patient problem exactly as it presented clinically and allowing the students to ask any questions of the patient, perform any item of a physical examination, and order any laboratory or diagnostic test in any sequence and learn the results of these actions as in actual practice.

A number of computerized patient simulations are available. Many present all of the patient information in words only, even though the computer has the ability to present audio and visual patient data. Most computer patient simulations do not offer a natural language interface that allows the students to interact with the patient through typed or verbal questions. Often, the complete history is presented to the student, as are the results of the physical examination if requested. This is the same as a printed case writeup. Other computer simulations offer screens with various menus presenting different actions for the student to consider (e.g., present illness, past history, review of systems) that are cumbersome and not authentic to the clinical setting. The computer has great potential if a natural language interface is used and the patient is presented with audiovisual representation, possibly a virtual patient.

The use of standardized patients (SPs) to present patient problems to the group offers far greater authenticity because a patient surrogate is present in audiovisual-tactile reality, and the student can interview and examine the patient. The use of the SP also challenges the students to develop skills in patient communication, interpersonal doctor-patient relationship, and patient feedback and education. There is a limitation to the SP because invasive diagnostic and treatment interventions are not possible, so the students must return to printed simulations to carry out these tasks.

Of the aforementioned formats, the PBLM and the SP allow the students to interview and examine the patient, using free inquiry to develop clinical problem-solving skills as they learn about the patient problem, thus enhancing later recall and application in the clinical setting. Until better computer programs are available with natural language interfaces and audiovisual presentation of the patient, these formats are more authentic.

The problems of community health, practice management, patient advocacy, and the like should be included in a PBL curriculum. These problems also should be presented to students in the way they appear in practice, designed so that students can deal with them using the cognitive, reasoning, or problem-solving skills required in practice.

THE PROBLEM-BASED LEARNING PROCESS

The PBL process is the sequence of events carried out by students and tutor in the small group as students learn. The model for the process in authentic PBL is the sequence of activities undertaken by physicians with a patient. As in an apprenticeship, which the PBL process resembles, the students are practicing and perfecting the important complex skills required for their profession as they acquire an integrated knowledge base in medicine and the sciences basic to medicine.

The following description shows the parallelism that should occur between the physician's activities with a patient and the student group's learning activities in authentic PBL. This description does not cover all of the steps in the PBL process itself. That information can be found elsewhere (Barrows, 1994). The physician's activities in the patient encounter are described in the indented paragraphs.

> By whatever route the patient is encountered by the physician (walk-in, referral, or ambulance) the physician assumes responsibility for the patient. The patient is his or her problem.

This scenario must also occur in PBL. The design of the simulation and the actions of the tutor can cause it to happen.

A printed or sequentially revealed case engenders little feeling of responsibility because it is a long way from the visual-auditory-tactile reality of a patient. It is a passive format requiring no interaction with the patient by the student. These formats present the patient problem as an intellectual exercise, and there is nothing to engender feelings of responsibility and the need to learn in order to help the patient. This is where the reality of the problem in the simulation format and the ability of that format to support free inquiry, through history-taking and physical and laboratory tests, are important.

Although the PBLM is principally a verbal format (including pictures of the patient, x-rays, scans, funduscopic photos, etc.), it does support free inquiry. Anything the students can do with an actual patient in terms of history-taking, physical examination, and laboratory and diagnostic tests can be done to the PBLM, and the students can obtain the patient's answers to their questions, findings on items of the physical examination they choose to do, and results of the laboratory test they ordered. The students are engaged and assume responsibility. The standardized patient is so close to clinical reality that it is the most engaging simulation next to the actual patient. Responsibility for the patient in the PBLM and standardized patient formats can be encouraged further by the tutor: "Here is your patient. What are you going to do?" Experience has shown that students will take on responsibility for the problem with engaging formats and initial encouragement by the tutor. In the future, medical education might look to more realistic, computationally supported, multimedia simulations of the patient problem.

> On first encountering the patient, the physician almost automatically generates multiple hypotheses concerning possible diagnoses and approaches to treatment and carries out a patient-focused deductive inquiry to understand the problem well enough to decide on the most likely diagnosis/differential diagnosis and an appropriate treatment plan (Barrows & Feltovich, 1987).

This activity also occurs in authentic PBL. Using problem simulation formats that permit free inquiry, the students can practice and develop these same reasoning skills. Tutors can model this activity initially by asking the students the questions they would be asking themselves concerning the patient problem such as, "What could be going on here?" "What might be wrong with this patient?" and later, "What information do we need to decide which of these ideas are the right ones?" Later, as students develop their reasoning skills, intervention by the tutor becomes less frequent.

A number of PBL approaches do not incorporate this activity aimed at the development of clinical reasoning skills, and instead use complete cases or sequentially presented cases in which clinical inquiry cannot be successfully undertaken. Some use structured approaches to reasoning with the problem such as the "seven-step" procedure that does not parallel clinical reasoning. These are not authentic, and an important opportunity to develop problem-solving skills is missed.

A major difference in this parallel between the authentic PBL process and the clinical process of the physician is the responsibility the students have for learning about the patient problem down to the cellular and molecular level in the sciences basic to medical practice as well as behavioral science, sociology, epidemiology, and ethics. The tutor helps them focus their discussions concerning symptoms and signs, possible diagnoses, treatment, questions and examinations of the patient, and their ideas about basic mechanisms to this level. The tutor asks, "Why?" "How does that work?" "Can you describe that in more detail?" until the students ask these questions of each other and of themselves in their ongoing problem-solving discussions and deliberations. Their discussions and deliberations bring out what they already know and reveal to them what they do not know and obviously will need to learn. The patient problem provides both the stimulus for learning and the opportunity for developing clinical reasoning skills. The physician aims to provide appropriate care for the patient, but in this process often finds that he or she needs to learn new information and skills to do this. The clinical context of learning and the excitement generated makes what is learned not only memorable for the students, but also likely to be recalled through rich association and applied to future patient problems.

To keep track of the group's activities with the problem, a blackboard, white board, or flip charts are used. The hypotheses generated, then modified during the groups ongoing discussions, are recorded. A growing summary of the information acquired from the patient in history and physical (and later laboratory and diagnostic) studies, and a list of the areas in which self-directed learning will need to occur also are recorded. Not only does this serve to focus discussions and organize student thinking, but this information also serves as a record of the group's thinking for later evaluation and critique. This is the group's parallel to the physician's patient notes.

The physician employs interpersonal, communication, and patient education skills to ensure as much as possible the patient's understanding, cooperation, and satisfaction. These should be practiced and developed when SPs are used in the small group. At some point the physician makes a commitment as to the likely diagnosis and management.

Each member of the group should make a similar commitment when the group is finished working with the patient problem. Just like the physician, they have done this with the knowledge already in their heads before going off for self-directed learning. Even if they feel there is too much they have to learn before making any commitment, it is good practice for them to try to make decisions at that time, carefully reasoning with the knowledge they already have even though data are missing or ambiguous. Physicians must do this frequently, and it makes the students' motivation for self-directed study even more compelling and focused.

As mentioned previously, the physician often needing to learn more to provide care to the patient will seek information from books, journals, online resources (MEDLINE, Internet), consultants, and colleagues.

The students have a lot to learn, and in authentic PBL should learn to use those same resources effectively that will be available to them in practice. There are rich information resources for them in the school's library, and there is a rich array of consultants available to them--the entire clinical and basic science faculty of the school--in addition to others they could call or contact online. Usually, PBL curricula provide students with a list of resource faculty willing to provide them with information and references for their study. These faculty are, in effect, consultants, and learning to work with them effectively will pay off for the students in their clinical work.

Self-directed study encompasses another set of skills that must be practiced, developed, and perfected. To help develop their self-study skills, the tutor asks the students to describe the learning resources they are going to use in their study. When they return, each student is asked to comment on his or her success in using those resources and estimate the accuracy and usefulness of the information obtained. Effective and efficient self-directed study skills best ensure that in the future whenever students realize they need to learn something, they can get it "just in time."

When physicians acquire new information from any of the aforementioned resources, they apply it to their thinking about the patient and may realize that more is needed from the patient on history or physical, and that other laboratory or diagnostic tests are needed to confirm their diagnostic ideas and to rule out others they had considered. On the basis of the new information from these resources, physicians may change some diagnostic ideas and thus again need more information from the patient and other laboratory and diagnostic tests.

This is exactly what the group needs to do in authentic PBL: apply the information they have acquired back to the patient problem by reviewing their hypotheses listed on the board, and discussing how these should be changed now that they have returned from self-directed study with new knowledge about the patient's problem and the underlying mechanisms involved. As changes are suggested by members of the group, they are asked to describe what in their self-directed study led them to want to make the change. The tutor encourages a general discussion about the changes and encourages contributions by every member in the group. Later, as more information is obtained from the patient and tests are ordered by the students, these discussions continue. What they have learned is applied in the context of the group's ongoing thinking and reasoning about the patients' problem. This is an essential step in authentic PBL. It enlarges the students' learning and understanding about medicine in relation to patients' problems, ensuring recall and application in their future clinical work. This also gives the students the opportunity to critique their prior thinking and reasoning with the problem before self-directed study to sharpen their reasoning skills.

This essential step often is not used in other PBL approaches. After returning from self-directed learning, students frequently recite and discuss what they have learned without actively applying it to their thinking about the problem. Not only is this boring, but it also poses the risk that much of the new information will be forgotten by the students and not recalled in their future work with patients.

OTHER STEPS NECESSARY IN THE AUTHENTIC PROBLEM-BASED LEARNING PROCESS

Once work with a problem is finished, it is important for the problem solver to reflect and verbalize on what has been learned. What new concepts, principles, or generalizations have been learned? How does learning with this problem relate to similar problems encountered in the past, and how can it be applied to other problems in the future. Such verbalizing encourages transfer of new knowledge to other problems in the future. The use of concept maps in the small group facilitates and organizes reflection and generalization about what has been learned. This should go on in the mind of the practitioner. Some of it does go on in clinical seminars and case discussions.

The student group should carry out self-assessment and peer assessment activities. Effective lifelong learning depends on physicians accurately assessing their own strengths and weaknesses. Physicians must realize when their own performance is not as it should be, what knowledge or training is needed, and how to get it. Effective self-directed learning in PBL depends on students being able to assess their thinking and knowledge, identify, weaknesses, and determine how to correct them. Peer assessment permits students to be seen in the light of their colleagues, and it often provides valuable new information about their performance. Physicians must work on many teams in health care. Effective team performance depends on skills in providing others with accurate and constructive feedback. Each student should assess her-himself with comments from others in the group. The tutor facilitates the practice and development of these skills.

THE TUTOR

The tutor's skill in facilitating student reasoning, self-directed learning, and self- and peer assessment without taking control and dispensing information or opinions is the backbone for authentic PBL (Barrows, 1988). The tutor's role is initially very active with a new group in the authentic PBL process. As students gain skills in the process and in their own skills, the tutor becomes less and less active, commenting only when it seems needed. Tutors need training for this difficult role, and they need support while they are tutoring.

ASSESSMENT

Assessment is a strong determinant of the way students will learn. Despite what the faculty may say are the objectives of a curriculum, students will learn in the way they think will result in their best performance on any assessment. They have learned this since primary school. If the assessment consists of multiple-choice questions chosen by the faculty, students will cram to memorize the information they think will be on the test, even if problem-solving and self-directed study skills are faculty objectives. Students in authentic PBL must be involved in assessing the same behaviors required in their learning: reasoning through a problem, engaging in self-directed study, and applying what is learned to the care of the patient.

EVALUATION OF AUTHENTIC PROBLEM-BASED LEARNING

Two meta-evaluations have been carried out on PBL, but their conclusions are limited by the great variability of the PBL methods evaluated in the studies they include (Albanese & Mitchell, 1993; Vernon & Blake, 1993). They show that students are very enthusiastic about PBL as a method, as are faculty involved in the method. Although the students did not do as well on standardized tests (not the kind that should be used in PBL), they were found to perform more effectively clinically. Two recent studies of authentic PBL at different schools indicate that PBL students do about the same as students in standard curricula on the United States Medical Licensing Examination (USMLE) Step I (they have learned as many facts), and perform significantly better in their clinical clerkships (Distlehorst & Robbs, 1998; Richards, Ober, Cariaga-Lo, Camp, Philip, et al., 1996). Another study suggests that graduates from a PBL school are more contemporary in their practice than graduates from a traditional medical school (Shin, Haynes, & Johnson, 1993). More evaluations that, like these latter ones, assess PBL student performance relevant to the objectives of PBL are needed.

CONCLUSION

Authentic PBL is modeled on the skills and activities that will be expected of students when they are practicing their profession. It avoids requiring any learning behaviors that are not of value to the students' future role as physicians (e.g., rote memorization and answering multiple-choice questions). The direct descendant of the method that began more than 30 years ago, PBL has improved over time with experience and modifications to enhance its authenticity.

Methods called PBL that do not address its authenticity to medical problems, physician reasoning, and practice pose the risk of trivializing it as an educational method, which could destine it to pass as a fad instead of growing in sophistication and value for medical students.

More needs to be done to further develop authentic PBL. Patient simulations must be devised to present richer, audiovisual-tactile patient data. Transitions of PBL to and through the clinical years maintaining its dedication to the development of the skills expected of the physician need to be developed. In the clinical years, the problems students face are real patient problems, and the students should continue to develop learning issues, carrying out self-directed study, reflection, and self-assessment both individually and in groups. The patient who is the responsibility of a student in a clinical PBL group can be used as the focus for PBL.

Computer enhancements of simulations should, in addition to creating a natural language interface, better track and record individual and group thinking. Computer support of information retrieval with the Internet and the World Wide Web is in its infancy and eventually should be able to support self-directed study in newer and more powerful ways. There is no reason why tutor and students need always to be face to face in their work. With appropriate computer enhancements, PBL group work can be carried out with students in their homes, in clinics, and at remote placements. In fact, groups could consist of members from around the world, each enriching the group's knowledge from their unique points of view and their access to information and expertise. It could be an exciting time for authentic PBL.

REFERENCES

Albanese M. A., & Mitchell S. (1993). Problem-based learning: A review of literature on its outcomes and implementation issues. *Academic Medicine, 68*(1), 52-81.
Barrows, H. S. (1988). *The tutorial process.* Springfield, IL: SIU School of Medicine.

Barrows, H. S. (1994). *Practice-based learning: Problem-based learning applied to medical education.* Springfield, IL: SIU School of Medicine.

Barrows, H. S., & Feltovich, P. J. (1987). The clinical reasoning process. *Medical Education, 21*(2), 86-91.

Distlehorst, L. H., & Barrows, H. S. (1982). A new tool for problem-based self-directed learning. *Journal of Medical Education, 57*(6), 486-488.

Distlehorst, L. H., & Robbs, R. S. (1998). A comparison of problem-based learning and standard curriculum students: Three-years of retrospective data. *Teaching and Learning in Medicine: An International Journal, 10*(3), 131-137.

Richards B. F., Ober, P., Cariaga-Lo, L., Camp, M. G., Philip, J., McFarland, M., Rupp, R., & Zaccara, D. J. (1996). Ratings of students' performance in a third-year internal medicine clerkship: A comparison between problem-based and lecture-based curricula. *Academic Medicine, 71,* 187-189.

Shin, H., Haynes, R., & Johnson, M. E. (1993). Effect of problem-based, self-directed undergraduate education on lifelong learning. *Canadian Medical Association Journal, 148*(6), 969-976.

Spaulding, W. B. (1991). *Revitalizing medical education: McMaster Medical School, the early years 1965-1974.* Philadelphia: B. C. Decker, Inc.

Vernon, D., & Blake, R. (1993). Does problem-based learning work? A meta-analysis of evaluative research. *Academic Medicine, 7,* 550-563.

CHAPTER TWENTY-FOUR

Implementing Problem-Based Learning In Medical Education

Earl L. Loschen
Southern Illinois University School of Medicine

What medical educators have come to identify as a problem-based learning (PBL) curriculum model had its origins in medical education at the McMaster Faculty of Health Sciences in Canada approximately 30 years ago. Although numerous aspects of PBL preceded this effort, it was at McMaster that the full model for medical education was first developed. Since that time, in North American medical schools there have been numerous developments of PBL in a variety of formats. These have included the use of PBL as a complete curriculum for basic sciences, in alternative or parallel tracks for part of a student class, or in some partial manner such as in a streamer or course for teaching clinical reasoning skills. Recently, there have been efforts to adapt PBL for clinical clerkship education in surgery, obstetrics/gynecology, and psychiatry. This chapter reviews these various developments and presents the status of PBL in North America.

Many medical schools are actively addressing the many problems facing them in a rapidly changing world including revising their educational programs. Not only are the sciences underlying medicine advancing rapidly, but there also is a revolution in how health care is delivered including an ever-increasing stress on such issues as quality of life, ethics of health care decisions, and the increasing role of alternative providers of health care.

As if this were not enough, the very technology making progress in medical care so possible is also complicating the very educational process meant to carry this information forward. The advent of computers has made progress in many areas of science possible, but these same machines provide new challenges to the delivery of the educational enterprise. The traditional lecture and laboratory experience just does not fit the bill very well anymore. Today's medical students need to be on the cutting edge of the information revolution because if they are not, they will be ill-prepared to work with patients who progressively have available to them the same information sources as their treating physicians. In addition, medical students must learn to work together in teams if they are to learn the survival techniques needed to work in a corporate medical setting with other physicians and a myriad of alternative health care providers.

The goals of PBL include more than the simple acquisition of knowledge (or "factlets"). Although there have been many critiques of PBL in its efforts to improve clinical reasoning skills (Berkson, 1993), most authors have not paid as close attention to other goals of PBL. In addition to the acquisition of knowledge and problem-solving skills, a well-designed curriculum will include objectives related to self-directed learning and to working in a group context. These objectives are particularly important to keep in mind given the brave new world of medicine we are entering.

A multitude of efforts were made to introduce PBL into medical schools during the last third of the 20th century. These efforts can be divided into several distinct patterns. Some schools, reflecting the first pattern, have developed a PBL curriculum that covers the whole of the medical school enterprise. As a second pattern, other schools have developed a separate track of PBL, either as a permanent option for students or as a developmental step in curricular reform that has not always resulted in a problem-based curriculum. A third pattern includes schools that have implemented PBL in a course or some other curricular unit in contrast to the rest of the curriculum. A fourth recently emerging pattern has been the modification of clinical clerkships to use PBL as the educational method for the didactic experiences of students on the clerkship. Finally, there is emerging a group of schools that implemented PBL as a track or similar curricular unit and now are attempting to combine PBL with more traditional lecture and laboratory formats. In the next several sections, these options are reviewed. This is not an exhaustive review of the literature nor are all schools that have undertaken curriculum reform to incorporate PBL included. This chapter tries to provide an overview of some innovations that have been attempted and some outcomes that have been reported in the literature.

THE COMPLETE PROBLEM-BASED LEARNING PROBLEM-BASED LEARNING CURRICULUM

The first effort to develop a different style of curricular delivery, one based on adult learning theory, occurred in Hamilton, Ontario with the establishment of McMaster University in 1966. The goals for this curriculum, as reported by Neufeld and Barrows (1974), included many of the goals now broadly recognized as essential to the preparation of the medical school graduate. These included such items as being able to locate information to solve patient problems and being able to solve clinical problems effectively, function as an effective self-directed learner, possess effective clinical skills, and operate as a member of a team.

The McMaster program was designed to use small tutorial groups as the primary educational activity, in which students would confront patient problems and attempt to resolve them under the guidance of a faculty tutor. In this process, the students would identify their learning needs, and at appropriate times recess the group to undertake self-directed study to meet these needs. The curriculum was divided into a variety of units, which allowed for allocation of resources and scheduling efficiencies as well as an opportunity to mix student groups. The major revolution introduced by this program was the change in emphasis from students gaining "content" to students learning "process." The emphasis was clearly on the students learning the process of clinical reasoning, self-directed learning, and clinical skills in addition to the accumulation of knowledge about the basic and clinical sciences.

The McMaster innovation provoked an era of change in medical school curricula, at first more widely noted internationally than on the North American continent. The University of Limburg in the Netherlands (more recently renamed Maastricht University) established a medical school in 1974 concentrating on training primary care physicians for the region but relying on the use of PBL as its instructional format (Bouhuijs, Schmidt, Snow, & Wijnen, 1978). Students enter medical school in the Netherlands immediately after secondary school, so the program there combines elements of both a college and a professional school education. The commitment has been to problem-based education throughout, however, and now other professional schools at the University also use this method. A similar effort occurred at the University of Newcastle in New South Wales, Australia, where a new medical school using PBL was established at the end of the 1970s (Engel & Clarke, 1978; Neame, 1982).

Although this pattern of newly established medical schools using PBL techniques has been common elsewhere in the world, only one new medical school in North America besides McMaster University was established using PBL as its curricular model, and that was Mercer University (Heestand, Templeton, & Adams, 1989).

CHANGING A TRADITIONAL CURRICULUM

Most medical schools have established problem-based curricula by switching from traditional methods to PBL. This change has used two patterns. Some schools have chosen to develop and implement an entirely new PBL curriculum serving all students. Other schools have chosen a more cautious approach, choosing instead to develop an alternative PBL curriculum for only a portion of each class of students. Each of these strategies has met with variable success.

Although there are many informal reports of schools changing to PBL, there are only a few reports that describe that process in any detail. The University of

Sherbrooke in Canada has described this process in some detail (Des Marchais & Dumais, 1990), beginning with the class of medical students entering in 1987. Careful planning of the curriculum and attention to detail including faculty development marks this program shift as one of the most thoughtful program changes reported in the literature. The Sherbrooke curriculum emphasizes PBL throughout all years of the program. The University of Hawaii also implemented a total curriculum change with the entering class of 1989 (McDermott & Anderson, 1991), as did Dalhousie University Faculty of Medicine with its entering class of 1992 (Kaufman & Mann, 1996). In each of these instances, the curricular change was for the entire curriculum.

Many schools have chosen to develop an alternative curriculum using PBL either as a strategy ultimately to convert the entire curriculum to PBL or to provide an alternative style for selected students. This approach was most notably chosen by the University of New Mexico School of Medicine with the development of the Primary Care Curriculum (Kaufman, Klepper, Obenshain, Voorhees, Galey, et al., 1982; Kaufman, Mennin, Waterman, Duban, Hansbarger, et al., 1989). This program began in 1979 as an alternative curriculum, but was much more than simply a PBL curriculum. Most notably, the curriculum's major goal was to train primary care physicians for rural areas of New Mexico. In keeping with that goal, the curriculum also included substantial early clinical experiences for medical students in various rural settings in the state.

In 1973 Michigan State University developed an alternative track curriculum called Track II, which used a series of "focal problems" around which patient case scenarios were developed. As opposed to problem-solving tutor groups, this program emphasized more of a small group discussion in which several faculty preceptors (including both clinicians and basic scientists) met with students to discuss not only the cases, but also related concepts and materials. This curriculum ceased to exist as a separate curriculum in 1992, but major aspects of the program were incorporated into the new general curriculum (Suwanwela, Xue-Min, McKeag, Ramos, Paul, et. al., 1993).

In 1984, Rush Medical College established the "Alternative Curriculum" for the basic science years of the school for a portion of its students. This curriculum uses a more Socratic approach to teaching in which the faculty tutors make greater use of an active questioning role than is commonly associated with the role of the tutor as facilitator in most PBL curricula.

Harvard University exemplifies a school that used the alternative curriculum approach to phase in PBL more broadly. In 1985 Harvard established the New Pathway as a pilot alternative track curriculum for 24 students and then expanded it to 40 students the next year. The underlying principles used PBL as a foundation for students receiving a general medical education emphasizing problem-solving skills and self-directed learning (Tosteson, 1990). After successfully piloting the program, the University extended the approach to much of the remaining curriculum.

Both Bowman Gray School of Medicine (Adams, 1989; Skipper, Pratto, Philip, Camp, & Hoban, 1989) and Southern Illinois University School of Medicine

(Loschen & Merideth, 1997) established alternative curricula using PBL as the major curricular method in the late 1980s. In both instances, the curriculum was designed around units of varying length during the first two years of basic science education and used small group tutorial sessions as the major focus of learning in the curriculum. The major differentiating feature between the two curricula was the use of short case scenarios in the Bowman Gray curriculum and the use of Problem-Based Learning Modules (PBLMs) in the Southern Illinois curriculum. This latter format, described by Distlehorst and Barrows (1982), allows the students to inquire freely and request examinations of a paper case, which more closely mimics the use of the clinical reasoning process usually seen in medical practice. Although the PBL curriculum is still an alternative track curriculum, Southern Illinois has recently made the commitment to change its undergraduate curriculum throughout into a single curriculum that focuses on the objectives used to establish the PBL curriculum.

CLERKSHIPS

Some efforts have been made to introduce PBL as the major focus of learning into a variety of medical school clerkships. The most well known and widely quoted effort has been in the surgery clerkship at the University of Kentucky (Nash, Schwartz, Middleton, White, & Young, 1991). In addition to the required clinical experiences common to all clerkships, this program has used small group tutorial sessions to confront surgical problems requiring self-directed learning on the part of the students. Similar programs have been developed for community medicine (Silver, Schechter, Walther, & Deuschle, 1991), primary care (Cooksey, Davnizer, Ervin, Groves, Tyska, et. al., 1995), internal medicine (Lawrence, Grosenick, Simpson, & van Susteren, 1992; McLeod & Whittemore, 1989), pediatrics (Wendelberger, Simpson, & Biernat, 1996), and obstetrics and gynecology (Cleave-Hogg & Gare, 1995). In addition, both the surgery and psychiatry departments at the Southern Illinois University School of Medicine use PBL as the major didactic component of their respective clerkships. In most of these programs, students spend most of their time working with real patients in an attending faculty model, but the lecture course work common to most clerkships is replaced in whole or in part by the use of small group tutorial sessions focusing on typical or prototypic problem cases for the specialty.

PARTIAL EFFORTS TO USE PROBLEM BASED LEARNING

Innumerable reports in the medical education literature describe the efforts of medical school faculty to use PBL methods in single courses, either as the major educational organizing principle or as an effort to demonstrate to the faculty at large the effectiveness of PBL in medical education, with the hope that the innovation will spread beyond the unit or course. Unfortunately, these reports often describe short-term programs, with few describing the long-term effects of such strategies. Anecdotally, one usually hears that the course or unit is offered for a limited number of times and then with a change in course directors or faculty, the curriculum reverts to a more "traditional" approach. It is, however, useful to learn something about some of these efforts, especially the extent and breadth of course work that has been tried with some success.

Faculty have used a variety of approaches in introducing PBL into basic science course work. For example, Farnsworth, Medio, Nelson, Mann, Norwell, et al., (1988) described a biochemistry course that used a combination of lectures and clinical problem-solving workshops in an effort to integrate biochemistry into a clinical context in a freshman course. The workshops used groups of 12 or 13 students each to discuss cases that reflected the content of the lecture series. Puett and Braunstein (1991) described a two-week endocrine course for freshman medical students at the University of Miami that likewise used a combination of lecture and problem-solving conferences. These conferences focused on cases illustrating issues covered in lectures and use student groups of 12 to 17 each with two or three faculty facilitators. This report is noteworthy in that it reports on a program of seven years duration and details results of student feedback (highly favorable) and student performance (predominantly A's and B's based on classroom grades).

Some schools have used problem-based methods in individual courses to present concepts often overlooked in the regular curriculum. An example of this is the use of a problem-based module on nutrition at the Medical College of Wisconsin presented as a pilot project to 13 volunteer students in 1991 (Bayard, Nitzke, & Nuhlicek, 1994). Another example exists at Dartmouth Medical School in the first-year Clinical Symposia course. There a prevention module was developed using both introductory lectures and small group exercises, in which students are given preventive medicine scenarios that they must then research and report to the class (Dietrich, Moore-West, Palmateer, Radebaugh, Reed, et al. 1990).

Also at Dartmouth, Almy, Colby, Zubkoff, Gephart, Moore-West, et al., (1992) described a senior medical student required course in which students in small groups are asked to apply behavioral and social science concepts to the care of patients outlined in various case scenarios. The groups are facilitated by faculty, but the students are expected to identify their own learning needs and to use widely varying learning resources. Although no evaluative data is presented on the effectiveness of this course, it is noteworthy because it has been presented on an ongoing basis since 1983 (Colby, Almy, & Zubkoff, 1986).

Sometimes courses are developed and delivered as a transition from a "traditional" curriculum to a PBL method. Vincelette, Lalande, Delorne, Goudreau, Lalonde, et al. (1997) reported on such an effort at the Université de Montréal, where a five-week course on the respiratory system was developed and delivered as a pilot experience for a more sweeping change to be implemented in the following year. The course involved a mixture of small group tutorial sessions, limited lectures, a variety of learning resources, and clinical skill sessions in a hospital setting.

Outcomes included revision of faculty development efforts and a reassurance of the faculty regarding the upcoming curricular reform.

Another example of this strategy was reported by Al-Jomard (1997) at the Jordan University of Science and Technology. Although the report states that one of the purposes of a new problem-based course in anatomy was to encourage development of PBL in the school, there are no outcomes described in the report that would suggest that this strategy is likely to be successful in this school.

COMBINING EDUCATIONAL METHODS

Some medical schools have now began to combine both "traditional" lecture-based curriculum activities with small group, "problem-based" activities. This is best exemplified by the University of New Mexico which has taken a combination of its traditional curriculum and integrated that into the more problem-based learning format of the Primary Care Curriculum (Sheline, Gorby, Small, Schuster, McCollum, et al., 1990). These newest efforts have not yet generated any substantial evaluative reports so it is still too early to tell if these diverse methodologics can be brought together and made to be compatible.

LESSONS LEARNED

Since the initiation of the first PBL medical school program at McMaster University, there have been many efforts to incorporate some aspects of the method into a variety of medical education programs. Interestingly, many of these efforts initiate a partial program but fail to fully use the approach over the long term. Either in the design or in the evolution of the program, the core approach of student-directedness is relinquished for increasing teacher-directedness. This may take the form of "optional" lectures, structured educational activities, or the use of objectives in an effort to "improve" the program. In fact, there are very few examples of "pure" PBL curricula that can serve as a prototype for educators to study and emulate. This is even more interesting given the outcome studies that generally show that students in PBL programs do as well as students from more traditional curricula but are clearly happier and more motivated by their curriculum (Vernon & Blake, 1993). This phenomenon of partial and incomplete program initiation is likely a transitional occurrence as medical education undergoes a substantial revolution.

On entering the 21st century, we will dramatically change the way we learn and work. Developments such as computers, the Internet, and distance education potentially will change our educational institutions and ultimately the workplace. The physician of the future will increasingly be required to seek out information to problem solve patient dilemmas that present in the clinical arena in new ways. In the past, much of this information was sought in various continuing education programs using passive, lecture-based activities. Now the physician can consult a variety of resources on the Internet or elsewhere specifically tailored to the physician's needs. Traditional curricula are not designed to teach this type of activity as effectively as PBL curricula. Teaching medical students the skill of self-directed learning is a strength of PBL, and because of this, such approaches will undoubtedly influence the development of the medical school curricula of the future.

REFERENCES

Adams, R. S. (1989). Making doctors: A new approach. *Teaching and Learning in Medicine: An International Journal, 1*(2), 62-66.

Al-Jomard, R. M. (1997). Problem-based learning trial in the Department of Anatomy, Jordan University of Science and Technology. *Medical Teacher, 19*(1), 58-59.

Almy, T. P., Colby, K. K., Zubkoff, M., Gephart, D. S., Moore-West, M., & Lundquist, L. L. (1992). Health, society, and the physician: Problem-based learning of the social sciences and humanities. *Annals of Internal Medicine, 116*(7), 569-574.

Bayard, B., Nitzke, S., & Nuhlicek, D. (1994). Using problem-based learning to integrate nutrition concepts into a preclinical medical curriculum. *Academic Medicine, 69*(5), 392.

Berkson, L. (1993). Problem-based learning: Have the expectations been met? *Academic Medicine, 68*(10), S79-S88.

Bouhuijs, P. A. J., Schmidt, H. G., Snow, R. E., & Wijnen, W. H. F. W. (1978). The Rijksuniversiteit Limburg, Maastricht, Netherlands: Development of medical education. *Public Health Papers, 70*, 133-151.

Cleave-Hogg, D., & Gare, D. (1995). Development of a problem-based obstetrics and gynecology curriculum for third-year medical students. *Teaching and Learning in Medicine: An International Journal, 7*(2), 95-101.

Colby, K. K., Almy, T. P., & Zubkoff, M. (1986). Problem-based learning of social sciences and humanities by fourth-year medical students. *Journal of Medical Education, 61*(5), 413-415.

Cooksey, J. A., Davnizer, L. H., Ervin, N. E., Groves, S. L., Tyska, C., & Kirk, G. (1995). Problem-based learning in an interdisciplinary community-based primary care course. *Teaching and Learning in Medicine: An International Journal, 7*(4), 241-245.

Des Marchais, J. E., & Dumais, B. (1990). Issues in implementing a problem-based learning curriculum at the University of Sherbrooke. *Annals of Community-Oriented Education, 3*, 9-23.

Dietrich, A. J., Moore-West, M., Palmateer, D. R., Radebaugh, J., Reed, S., & Clauson, B. (1990). Adapting problem-based learning to a traditional curriculum: Teaching about prevention. *Family Practice Research Journal, 10*(1), 65-73.

Distlehorst, L. H., & Barrows, H. S. (1982). A new tool for problem-based, self-directed learning. *Journal of Medical Education, 57*, 486-488.

Engel, C. E., & Clarke, R. M. (1978). Medical education with a difference. *Programmed Learning and Educational Technology, 16*, 70-87.

Farnsworth, W. E., Medio, F., Nelson, K., Mann, D., Norwell, D., & Van Winkle, L. J. (1988). Integrating clinical problem-solving workshops and lectures in a biochemistry course. *Biochemical Education, 16*(4), 196-200.

Heestand, D. E., Templeton, B. B., & Adams, B. D. (1989). Responding to perceived needs of the twenty-first century: A case study in curriculum design. *Medical Teacher, 11*(2), 157-167.

Kaufman, A., Klepper, D., Obenshain, S. S., Voorhees, J. D., Galey, W., Duban, S., Moore-West, M., Jackson, R., Bennett, M., & Waterman, R. (1982). Undergraduate medical education for primary care: A case study in New Mexico. *Southern Medical Journal, 75*(9), 1110-1117.

Kaufman, D. M., & Mann, K. V. (1996). Students' perceptions about their courses in problem-based learning and conventional curricula. *Academic Medicine, 71*(1), S52-S54.

Kaufman, A., Mennin, S., Waterman, R., Duban, S., Hansbarger, C., Silverblatt, H., Obenshain, S. S., Kantrowitz, M., Becker, T., Samet, J., & Wiese, W. (1989). The New Mexico experiment: Educational innovation and institutional change. *Academic Medicine, 64*(6), 285-294.

Lawrence, S. L., Grosenick, D. J., Simpson, D. E., & van Susteren, T. J. (1992). A comparison of problem-based and didactic approaches to learning on an ambulatory medicine clerkship. *Teaching and Learning in Medicine: An International Journal, 4*(4), 221-224.

Loschen, E. L., & Merideth, S. (1997). Student-centered, teacher-guided medical education. In M. Wassenberg & H. Philipsen (Eds.), *Placing the Student at the Center: Current Implementations of Student-Centered Education,* (pp. 129-133). Maastricht, Netherlands: Maastricht University.

McDermott, J. F., Jr., & Anderson, A. S. (1991). Retraining faculty for the problem-based curriculum at the University of Hawaii, 1989-1991, *Academic Medicine, 66*(12), 778-779.

McLeod, P. J., & Whittemore, N. B. (1989). A problem-based clinical course in general internal medicine. *Medical Teacher, 11*(2), 169-175.

Nash, P .P., Schwartz, R. W., Middleton, J. L., White, F. M., & Young, B. (1991). A student-centered, problem-based surgery clerkship. *Academic Medicine, 66*(7), 415-416.

Neame, R. L. B. (1982). Academic roles and satisfaction in a problem-based medical curriculum. *Studies in Higher Education, 7*(2), 141-151.

Neufeld, V. R., & Barrows, H. S. (1974). The "McMaster philosophy": An approach to medical education. *Journal of Medical Education, 49*, 1040-1050.

Puett, D., & Braunstein, J. J. (1991). The endocrine module: An integrated course for first-year medical students combining lecture-based and modified problem-based curricula. *Teaching and Learning in Medicine: An International Journal 3*(3), 159-165.

Sheline, B., Gorby, M., Small, B., Schuster, T., McCollum, S., Mennin, S., & Kaufman, A. (1990). Health of the public: New Mexico's next innovation in medical education. *Teaching and Learning in Medicine: An International Journal, 2*(3), 170-175.

Silver, A., Schechter, C., Walther, V., & Deuschle, K. (1991). Development of faculty consultants in a problem-based third-year community medicine clerkship. *Journal of Community Health, 16*(3), 133-141.

Skipper, J. K., Pratto, D. J., Philip, J. R., Camp, M. G., & Hoban, D. R. (1989). Benefits of hindsight: Design problems in evaluating innovation in medical education. *Evaluation Practice, 10*(3), 7-11.

Suwanwela, C., Li Xue-Min, McKeag, D. B., Ramos, M. B., Paul, H. A., Zeitz, H. J., & Kaufman, A. (1993). Long-term outcomes of innovative curricular tracks used in four countries. *Academic Medicine, 68*(2), 128-132.

Tosteson, D. C. (1990). New pathways in general medical education. *New England Journal of Medicine, 322*(4), 234-238.

Vernon, D. T. A., & Blake, R. L. (1993). Does problem-based learning work? A meta-analysis of evaluative research. *Academic Medicine, 68*(7), 550-563.

Vincelette, J., Lalande, R., Delorme, P., Goudreau, J., Lalonde, V., & Jean P. (1997). A pilot course as a model for implementing a PBL curriculum. *Academic Medicine, 72*(8), 698-701.

Wendelberger, K. J., Simpson, D. E., & Biernat, K. A. (1996). Problem-based learning in a third-year pediatric clerkship. *Teaching and Learning in Medicine: An International Journal, 8*(1), 28-32.

PART IV

CHALLENGES FOR MEDICAL EDUCATION

CHAPTER TWENTY-FIVE

Effects of Changing Health Care Environment on Medical Education

Michael E. Whitcomb
Association of American Medical Colleges

During the past decade, there have been remarkable changes in the organization, financing, and delivery of medical care services in the United States. These changes, by restructuring the medical market place, have altered the inpatient environment of acute care hospitals, constrained payment for medical care services, and transformed the nature of medical practice. Because the patient care experiences essential for the clinical education of doctors, including both undergraduate and graduate medical education experiences, are embedded in the country's health care delivery system, it is axiomatic that the changes occurring in the delivery system have potentially serious implications for medical education.

Medical educators must understand the changes occurring in the delivery system and the implications these changes have for the design, content, and conduct of the educational programs for which they are responsible. They must determine the impact of these changes on these programs and be prepared to alter them in response. They also must recognize that coincident with the changes occurring in the health care delivery system are changes occurring in society's expectations of physicians. Therefore, as medical educators consider how to alter their educational programs in response to the changes occurring in the delivery system, they also must consider how their programs must be changed to make certain that they will prepare doctors who can meet society's changing expectations.

IMPLICATIONS OF CHANGES IN THE HOSPITAL INPATIENT ENVIRONMENT

Throughout the years, the hospital inpatient setting has been the site for most of the clinical experiences provided for both medical students and resident physicians. For the past few decades, observers of medical education both within and outside the medical education community have argued that the amount of time devoted to clinical education in ambulatory care settings should be increased. This argument has been based on the premise that the kinds of patients and the clinical conditions encountered in ambulatory settings are more relevant to the future practice activities of most physicians. Notwithstanding this argument, most of the clinical education of medical students and resident physicians continues to be based in hospital inpatient settings.

The changes now occurring in the hospital inpatient environment provide a more compelling reason for shifting more of the clinical education of students and residents to ambulatory care settings. The average length of stay for many of the conditions for which patients still are hospitalized has declined as more and more of the care once provided in hospitals has shifted to nonhospital settings. As a result, for the average hospital, the daily census of inpatients has declined, and the case-mix intensity of the inpatient population has increased. These changes have made the inpatient environment less relevant to the educational needs of medical students and most residents. Accordingly, if medical students and residents are to be prepared adequately to care for patients in the evolving health care delivery system, it is essential that they spend more time in ambulatory care settings.

This goal presents a formidable challenge to those responsible for the design and conduct of medical education programs. Identifying a sufficient number of sites to meet the needs of the program, assisting physicians at those sites in developing the skills required to meet their responsibilities to the students and residents assigned to them, maintaining consistency of the learning experiences provided at multiple sites, and identifying funding to cover the costs of providing educational experiences at those sites are the most challenging. Furthermore, it seems likely that as the care provided in ambulatory settings becomes managed in a progressively more rigorous manner by organizations and payers, it will become increasingly difficult to embed medical education experiences in those settings.

Given that there are compelling reasons why medical students and residents should spend more time in ambulatory care settings, it is important to recognize that there still is substantial educational value in the kinds of experiences that can be provided in inpatient settings. Because the educational value of different kinds of inpatient experiences will vary depending on the purpose and focus of the educational program, the appropriate balance between inpatient and ambulatory care-based experiences will vary from program to program. The appropriate balance for the education of a family physician will almost certainly be different from the appropriate balance for the education of a general surgeon. Similarly, the balance required for the clinical education of medical students will be different from that required for the education of residents.

To ensure that each educational program has the proper balance of inpatient and ambulatory care-based clinical experiences, those responsible for the program must set forth an educational rationale for each clinical experience required of students and residents enrolled in the program. To approach this in a logical fashion, they first must establish clear learning objectives to be achieved during the course of the program. Then they must design the program so that it provides the array of clinical experiences that will allow students and residents to achieve these objectives. This approach will guarantee to the degree possible that the program will achieve a proper balance between inpatient and ambulatory care-based learning experiences.

IMPLICATIONS OF CHANGES IN PAYMENT POLICIES

Since the establishment of the Medicare and Medicaid Programs in the mid-1960s, the federal government and a number of state governments have provided funds to hospitals to cover some of the direct costs of the graduate medical education (DGME) programs sponsored by these institutions. These government funds have been, and continue to be, critical in providing an explicit source of financial support for these programs. In addition, funds provided by the Medicare Indirect Medical Education Adjustment (IMEA) and the Medicare and Medicaid Disproportionate Share Hospital Payments (DSH) have represented significant contributions to the total revenues generated by teaching hospitals (although not all teaching hospitals receive DSH payments), thus augmenting the level of institutional funds available to support medical education.

During the past decade, these government funding streams have been constrained by the adoption of new policies governing the Medicare and Medicaid Programs. The impact of the constraints imposed on the funding of the direct costs of GME (primarily Medicare DGME) has not been very significant. In contrast, there have been marked reductions in the revenues provided by IMEA and DSH payments. It is too early to determine how the most recent policy changes constraining these revenues will affect the GME activity of individual institutions, but it seems almost certain that these changes, in combination with changes in private sector payment policies, will have a significant impact on the size and scope of GME activity in some hospitals. Some institutions may choose to alter the specialty mix of the residency programs they sponsor, or to decrease the number of positions funded in individual programs.

Although constraints on government funding are important, the dramatic growth in the number of persons enrolled in some form of managed care plan presents the most significant challenge to the financial stability of major teaching hospitals. Managed care arrangements have the potential to affect teaching hospitals in two ways. First, unless a hospital is willing to accept negotiated (discounted) payments for the services provided to the plan's beneficiaries, the plan may not include the hospital among its approved providers. Under these circumstances, the hospital is at risk of losing its share of hospitalized patients in the market wherein it operates. If this occurs, there will be a decrease in the number of admissions to the institution and a decrease in its revenues. Second, if the hospital accepts discounted payments, it likely will experience a decline in its operating margin. Because approximately two thirds of the costs for the GME program activities at the average hospital are covered by funds derived from private sector payers, both of these situations threaten the ability of a hospital to generate the funds required to support its graduate medical education programs.

Changes in Medicare policies governing payment to physicians providing patient care services in teaching hospitals also have the potential to affect adversely the institutions' GME activity. Recent changes in the regulations governing payment to teaching physicians place new requirements on the role of teaching physicians in the patient care activities of resident physicians and their documentation of that role in the medical record. Once again, it is too early to determine the impact that these new regulations will have on the willingness of physicians to participate in GME programs, but this is an issue that may have serious implications in the future for graduate medical education.

Although the impact of these changes affects primarily the education of resident physicians, it is important to recognize that in some circumstances they may limit the opportunities available for clinical experiences for students, thus adversely affecting medical student education. Because the clinical education experiences provided for students do not have to exist in hospital settings where students will be in contact with residents or supervised by them, changes in the size or scope of a hospital's commitment to GME does not mean that there must necessarily be a decline in the opportunities for student education in the institution. However, because the costs of medical student education are often subsidized by hospital funds that support GME, a decrease in these funds will affect the number of opportunities available for student experiences and how the costs of those experiences will be paid. Under these circumstances, the medical school will be challenged to maintain the range of educational experiences provided for students.

IMPLICATIONS OF CHANGES IN THE PHYSICIAN PRACTICE ENVIRONMENT

The changes occurring in the physician practice environment also have significant implications for the design, content, and conduct of medical education programs. In the new practice environment, physicians increasingly are employed by or under contract to group practices, institutions, or management organizations, and thus are expected to participate in a more collaborative way with other health care professionals in the delivery of patient care. They are being held more accountable than in the past for their practice behaviors, the clinical outcomes of the care they provide, and the satisfaction of the patients and the families of the patients for whom they care.

To function effectively in the evolving system, physicians must understand how health care services are being organized, financed, and delivered. They must know how to provide high-quality care to individual patients in an efficient and cost-effective manner, how to work effectively in organizations wherein certain patient care responsibilities will be delegated to other health professionals and in which participation in health care teams is essential, and how to use systematic approaches to improve the health of individuals and populations. It is incumbent on medical school deans, residency program directors, and faculties to ensure that their educational programs provide adequate opportunities for medical students and resident physicians to gain the knowledge, skills, and attitudes required to fulfill these responsibilities.

This presents a formidable challenge because, as noted earlier, changes in the hospital inpatient environment require that more of the clinical education of students and residents be conducted in a variety of nonhospital settings. This requirement results in the development of a more distributed system of clinical education. Because it may not be possible to provide adequate learning opportunities at each site, the institution responsible for administering the educational program may need to develop a core curriculum in which all students and residents could participate, regardless of the site of their clinical experience.

IMPLICATIONS OF CHANGES IN SOCIETY'S EXPECTATIONS OF PHYSICIANS

Changes in society's expectations of physicians are occurring coincident with the changes occurring in the country's health care delivery system. For most of the 20th century, medicine has focused its attention largely on the cure of disease. This focus has had a significant impact on the way doctors have been educated and on the institutions responsible for administering medical education programs.

There is now considerable evidence that the public wants doctors who are equally attentive to all aspects of health care. They want doctors who are able and willing to explain the implications of their disease for them and their families, who understand and are sensitive to the impact of the cultural and spiritual dimensions of their lives on their care, and who will continue to care for them when the cure of disease is no longer possible. These expectations must be considered in determining the knowledge, skills, and attitudes that physicians must possess to practice medicine effectively in the 21st century.

Because medical educators are so concerned about the changes occurring in the delivery system, the implications for the education of doctors concerning society's changing expectations of physicians tend to be overlooked. In addition, the changes occurring in the country's health care delivery system create significant challenges for medical educators as they consider how to alter their programs to make certain that they prepare new doctors to meet society's changing expectations. It is difficult to envision how a system that is being transformed largely by concerns about the cost of health care will accommodate society's changing expectations of physicians, or how it will make certain that medical education programs have the resources required to provide educational experiences that will allow students and resident physicians to acquire the knowledge, skills, and attitudes required to meet society's expectations.

For example, will the new organizational arrangements governing medical practice, arrangements that limit the amount of time that doctors can spend with patients, allow doctors to communicate effectively with the patients that seek their care? Will they allow opportunities for medical students and resident physicians to learn how complex social, cultural, and spiritual factors affect patients and their response to the care they receive? Will doctors recognize the potentially adverse impact on their practice behavior of some of the perverse financial incentives operating in various organizational arrangements? If so, will they meet their professional responsibility to act always in the best interest of their patients without regard for the consequences to themselves? They are more likely to do so if the educational programs that prepared them for practice provided opportunities for them to understand the issues involved and contributed in explicit ways to their professional development. These are extremely important issues that command the attention of the medical education community.

CONCLUSION

The country's preeminent historian of medical education, Ken Ludmerer, has suggested that the current period ultimately will be viewed as the second major revolution in medical education. This view reflects his understanding, derived from an historical perspective, of the significant impact that the changes occurring in the country's health care delivery system have for medical education. At issue is not simply whether there will be adequate financial support for medical education, but whether the impact of the changes on the practice of medicine will allow students and resident physicians to gain the experience needed to prepare them for practice. These are serious concerns that will plague medical educators well into the 21st century.

These concerns should not be limited to medical educators. At a time when society's expectations of physicians are changing, the medical education community's ability to change medical education programs to ensure that new doctors will be prepared to meet those expectations is being limited by changes occurring in the country's health care delivery system. The public at large must recognize that the kind of doctors they expect may not be available to care for them unless ways are found to accommodate within the evolving health care system the particular needs of medical education. As members of the public continue to scrutinize the changes now occurring in the delivery system, they must focus some attention on how those changes are affecting the nation's medical education system, not to ensure that the education of doctors continues in its current mode, but to ensure that medical educators are able to prepare doctors to meet the public's growing expectations.

CHAPTER TWENTY-SIX

Medical Education and The Physician Workforce

Gabrielle D'Elia
Erik J. Constance
Southern Illinois University School of Medicine

In the United States, medicine as a profession has enjoyed unparalleled power and privilege (Friedson, 1973). The government has delegated to the profession itself the authority to establish training programs, to determine standards for trainee admission, to control the content and process of training, to certify the practitioner as competent, and to regulate the actual practice of medicine. Furthermore, the state has declined to exercise any centralized authority over the supply and distribution of the physician workforce. The medical profession itself, at the same time, has failed to develop any centralized authority over its constituent organizations, institutions, and members with regard to the supply and distribution of the physicians. As a result, the country today is faced with the unmet goals and unanticipated consequences of policies initiated more than 25 years ago to bring the physician supply more into line with population needs.

What was seen in the 1970s as an overall shortage will be seen in the 2000s as an oversupply. What was sought in the 1970s as an appropriate primary care-specialty care balance will remain an issue in the 2000s. What was designed in the 1970s to cause a dispersal of physicians to serve populations in need is recognized as inadequate, and brings the country to the 2000s with a safety net under severe strain. What was seen in the 1970s as a necessary goal for racial and ethnic equity in access to membership in the profession itself will be seen in the 2000s as a major challenge.

The medical education issue for the 2000s perhaps ought to be whether the profession of medicine can in fact make the physician production process more responsive to public need rather than to the interests of its constituent organizations and members. This chapter contains a description of changes in the physician supply over the past 25 years. It follows the physician production process from medical school through residency training and into professional activity.

MEDICAL EDUCATION

The 1960s were a time of many federal initiatives to address the very significant social needs facing large segments of the population. Health care, previously considered a federal responsibility for only a quite limited set of requirements, became defined as one more of the social challenges in need of intervention. Major legislation (Medicare and Medicaid) established the federal role as a powerful purchaser of care. Other legislation (Title VII of the Public Health Service Act) greatly expanded the amount and type of support the federal government could use to increase the availability of health care resources in the country. The medical education sector of the medical profession was one of the targets or beneficiaries of the federal activity. Therefore, as Table 26.1 indicates, the major change in medical education over the past 25 years was a greatly increased capacity to train physicians.

The figure of approximately 16,000 matriculants per year represents a doubling of the number of physicians produced yearly in the 1960s in medical schools in the United States. The rate of growth has now stabilized with 125 medical schools and an annual production of approximately 16,000 new physicians. The number of students seeking admission to medical school also has stabilized at approximately 46,500, although a sizable percentage (one third) of the applicants are repeating the search for admission for the second-year or more (Association of American Medical Colleges [AAMC], 1997).

If the most significant change in medical education has been the greatly increased production capacity, the second most significant change should probably be described as the diversity in the matriculant cohort. In the United States over the past 25 years, the demographic criteria of gender, racial/ethnic background, financial disadvantage, age, and disability have been the focus of initiatives that both enhance and protect the status of individuals with these characteristics.

TABLE 26.1
Medical Schools: First Year Enrollment and Graduates
During Selected Years, 1976-1996

Academic Year	No. of Schools	First-Year Enrollment	Graduates
1976-1977	116	15,667	13,607
1986-1987	127	16,779	15,836
1990-1991	126	16,803	15,481
1994-1995	125	17,048	15,911
1996-1997	125	16,904	15,904

Source: Barzansky, B., Jonas, H. S., & Etzel, S. I. (1997). Educational Programs in U.S. Medical Schools, 1996-1997. *Journal of the American Medical Association, 278*, 744-749.

In terms of medical education, gender changes have been the most visible. In 1970, women represented 11% of the matriculants in U.S. medical schools. By 1980, the comparable proportion was 28.7%, and by 1997, the proportion had risen to 43.3%. The impact of the gender shift is complex. Specialties traditionally attracting women have continued to be most popular among the new female cohort, but women are now entering fields previously filled predominantly with male physicians as well (AAMC, 1997).

Racial-ethnic disparities represent a different pattern of change. In spite of governmental and professional initiatives to increase medical school access among under represented racial and ethnic minorities, the percentage of African American and Hispanic students has remained at approximately 10%. In terms of both equal access to the profession and provision of physician choice to the growing minority population, the efforts of medical schools have fallen short. The admissions criteria in medical schools, however, have prompted a significant increase in students who identify their ethnic background as Asian American, and students from this background now constitute 19% of the first-year medical students in the United States. A variety of judicial rulings (e.g., Hopwood v. Texas and Bakke v. California) have made it more difficult for medical schools using traditional admissions criteria to recruit members of underrepresented racial and ethnic minorities.

Recruiting students from disadvantaged financial backgrounds remains a challenge, and the high cost of medical education has become a problem even for students not qualifying for disadvantaged status. The number of students securing loans (currently 59%) and the amount of indebtedness both have increased. The impact that levels of debt have on specialty choice and practice opportunity is being debated.

The third most significant change involves the medical school response to pressure stressing the need for more physicians in what are called the primary care disciplines: family medicine, general internal medicine, general pediatrics, and more recently, obstetrics/gynecology. Plans called for having half of the medical schools' graduates seeking first-year residency positions in these fields. Medical schools developed a variety of initiatives to encourage student interest in primary care over the past 25 years. The choice of specialty, however, is something the individual student seeks to negotiate, and the existing system of graduate medical education provides many opportunities in fields other than the targeted primary care disciplines.

According to the annual AAMC Medical School Graduation Questionnaire, which surveys plans of graduating medical students, only 27.6% of the 1995 graduates indicated a choice of a field initially defined as one of the primary care targets: family medicine, internal medicine, and pediatrics. If obstetrics/gynecology were included, the proportion of the graduates interested in the primary care fields rises to 31.6%. These percentages are not significantly different from those obtained for the 1985 graduating cohort, although there is a shift of students interested in primary care toward family medicine (AAMC, 1997).

Finally, from the standpoint of physician supply and distribution, medical schools have developed a variety of initiatives to influence and prepare students for practice among underserved populations. Because graduate medical education intervenes between the medical school effort and the actual practice location of the physician, assessing the effectiveness of these initiatives is difficult.

GRADUATE MEDICAL EDUCATION

The changes in medical education can be seen as a response to pressures to bring the physician workforce more into line with governmental, professional, market, and public concerns about an available, accessible, cost-effective, quality health care system. The changes were filtered, however, by the process of graduate medical education, which itself was reshaped over the past quarter century.

The major change in graduate medical education was a vast increase in the capacity to produce physicians. Residency programs grew in number, range of specialties, and number of available positions. Furthermore, control over graduate medical education shifted toward academic medical centers, as previously unaffiliated internship and residency programs either closed or aligned themselves with existing medical schools, and the newly organized medical schools created their own set of graduate programs. As a result, by the mid-1990s, the number of residency programs stood at 7,787, an increase of more than 60% from 20 years earlier.

Not only did the number of programs increase, but the range of specialties also increased. At the same time that the primary care disciplines, especially the new field of family medicine, were receiving emphasis, new fellowships and residency programs were approved in traditional specialties, in new subspecialties (e.g., cardiovascular disease and medical genetics), and in new combined specialties (e.g., medicine-pediatrics or medicine-psychiatry).

Along with the expansion of programs came the expansion of available slots for trainees. Whereas in the 1970s approximately 49,000 residents were on duty in a year, in 1996 the comparable number was 98,000. Residents were not only learning a specialty, but also providing patient care in academic health center hospitals and clinics. Residency programs and their affiliated hospitals had strong financial incentives (e.g., clinical fees and graduate medical education direct and indirect funding) for filling available training slots. The need for program applicants could not be met even by the greatly increased supply of physicians graduating from medical schools in the United States. Residency programs filled their available slots with physicians who graduated from schools in other countries. Fig. 26.1 depicts this growth.

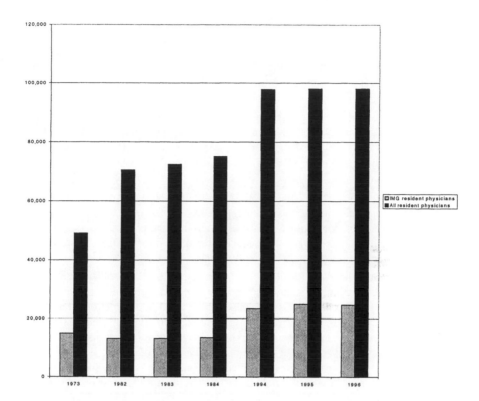

FIG. 26.1 Total number of resident physicians on duty in accredited programs and total number of resident physicians on duty who were graduates of international medical schools, selected years 1973-1997.

Sources: Fenninger, L. D., & Tracy, R. H. (1975). Section III. Graduate medical education: Annual report on graduate medical education in the U.S. *Journal of the American Medical Association*, (Suppl) *231*, 34-50.

Crowley, A. (1985). Graduate medical education in the United States, 1984-85. *Journal of the American Medical Association, 254*, 1585-1593.

Dunn, M. R., & Miller, R. S. (1997). U.S. Graduate Medical Education. *Journal of the American Medical Association, 278*, 750-754.

PROFESSIONAL ACTIVITY

At the end of the medical education and graduate medical education process, the physician is able to begin professional activity in a variety of capacities. Although providing care directly to patients is the predominant activity, some physicians choose careers in administration, research, and industry, to mention only a few of the options. In addition to graduates from the U.S. education pipeline, the physician supply has been augmented by international medical graduates hired directly into practice in a variety of settings.

As Table 26.2 indicates, the total supply of physicians in the United States has more than doubled from 1970 to the present. This rate of growth is four times the rate of growth in the U.S. population and results in a ratio of 380 persons per one physician.

The actual number of physicians in specialties defined as primary care has increased significantly, but primary care specialties as a percentage of all specialties, at 34%, have not yet regained the share they constituted in 1970. Given the figures presented in the sections on medical and graduate medical education, the goal of 50% may be elusive.

If the physician supply lacks a desired balance between primary care and nonprimary care fields, it also has a geographic distribution imbalance. The 10 states with the greatest number of physicians in 1980 also had the greatest number in 1994. Other states, although showing increases in absolute numbers, still had physician-population ratios below the 1975 national average.

Within states, the trend for physician concentration in metropolitan areas, in all specialties, has continued. Although family and general practitioners were more likely than physicians in other specialties to be located in nonmetropolitan areas, even in these two fields, the percentage of practitioners in nonmetropolitan areas has been decreasing. Even in metropolitan areas, significant variations in resource distribution and access exist. The U.S. Bureau of Health Professions (BHPr) in 1996 had 2,617 areas designated as Primary Medical Health Professional Shortage Areas, estimating the population in these areas to be more than 46 million people (BHPr, 1996).

TABLE 26.2

Federal and nonfederal physicians in the United States, by major categories, selected Years 1970-1994

Category	1970	1980	1990	1994
Total physicians	334,028	467,679	615,421	684,414
Percentage of increase	–	40%	32%	11%
Federal employment	29,501	17,787	20,475	22,454
Nonfederal employment	301,323	443,502	592,166	660,582
Patient care	278,535	376,512	503,870	562,456
Nonpatient care	32,310	38,404	43,440	43,012
Primary care*	134,354	170,705	213,514	323,651
Percentage of primary care	40%	37%	35%	34%
Ratio of male to female physicians	12.2:1	7.6:1	4.9:1	4.1:1
International medical school graduates as a percentage of all graduates	17%	21%	21%	23%

*family practice, general practice, internal medicine, pediatrics, and obstetrics/gynecology.

Source: American Medical Association. (1997). *AMA physician characteristics and distribution in the United States.* Chicago.

Finally, the characteristics of the physicians themselves reflect a number of major changes, many of which began with changes in medical school admissions. Women physicians as a percentage of all physicians increased from 7.6% in 1970 to 19.5% in 1994. Physicians from underrepresented racial and ethnic minority groups are not keeping pace with the growth of their respective minorities in the population at large. Physicians trained in countries other than the United States, however, have made a significant contribution to the physician workforce. International medical school graduates accounted for more than one fourth of the increase in the physician supply over the past 30 years.

ADEQUACY OF THE PHYSICIAN SUPPLY

In medical education, the 25-year period of growth has reached a height, has stabilized, and is beginning to feel pressure to downsize. The nation has 125 medical schools that together graduate approximately 16,000 new physicians a year. The PEW Commission Report (1995), among others, is recommending that the United States should reduce its physician training capacity by closing entire medical schools.

In graduate medical education, the 25-year period of growth, while not yet halted, is resulting in selective change. During the 1996-1997 academic year, the Accreditation Committee on Graduate Medical Education approved 213 new residency programs. Many of these programs are in emerging medical fields such as medical genetics and cardiac electrophysiology. At the same time, in response to a complex set of market conditions and projected shifts in program financing (Miller, Dunn, & Whitcomb, 1997), a number of existing programs have closed, and an even greater number have reduced their number of available positions. Table 26.3 provides some of these data for selected specialties.

Even with the current reductions, the graduate medical education capacity far outbalances the available supply of medical school graduates. Grossly calculated, 16,000 new physicians per year and 7,800 programs would still yield an average of two new physicians per program per year. Six years of medical school graduating classes would be required to equal the total number of residents currently on duty in a single year. The Council on Graduate Medical Education (1995, 1996) has recommended that the number of first-year residency positions be limited to 110% of the output of U.S. medical schools. These changes are predicated on a reduction in the supply from graduates from international medical schools.

Finally, in terms of professional activity, the overall physician supply has grown significantly and will continue to grow significantly. Concerns arise about an excess of physicians and a situation in which supply creates demand. The emphasis on managed care models, which attempt to control the number and specialty balance of physicians serving a defined population, fuels arguments that physician-induced demand has a negative effect on quality and cost of care. Furthermore, comparisons between primary care and specialty care physician distribution in the United States and other countries support arguments that specialist physicians in the United States are managing patients' primary care needs with specialty practice styles and reimbursement levels. Finally, a survey of physicians by age reveals that the number of new graduates from medical schools and residency programs will more than replace physicians expected to be lost to the supply by virtue of age. In the category of professional activity, a number of more specific considerations require attention.

Federal and Nonfederal Activity.

Physician activity can be categorized by employment status. Federal physicians are employed by the Department of Defense and by a variety of other agencies. The adequacy of the supply of federal physicians (Table 26.3) depends on federal government ability to address the overall health and safety needs of the nation (e.g., U.S. Public Health Service), and also to provide health care to specific populations for which it is directly responsible (e.g., military personnel, Indian Health Service, and Veteran's Administration). Little attention has been paid to the adequacy of the civilian health force as a supplement to the federal supply for an array of national emergencies or problems.

Primary Care and Nonprimary Care

In the category of professional specialization, the issue of which specialties grow and receive funding reflects the existing organization and power of the medical specialty groups. The emphasis on public health relative to surgical subspecialties, psychiatry relative to oncology-hematology, and family medicine relative to the medical subspecialties, for example, reflects a decision-making process not based on any systematic assessment of the health needs of the population.

TABLE 26.3
Changes in number of accredited graduate medical education programs and in number of residents in program year 1 from 1994 to 1996 by selected specialty

Specialty	Change in Number of Programs	Change in Number of Residents
Family medicine	+ 44	+ 245
Emergency medicine	+ 14	+ 86
Internal medicine	+ 2	- 804
Obstetrics/gynecology	- 6	- 129
General surgery	- 4	- 336
Orthopedics	- 3	- 78

Source: Dunn, M. R, & Miller, R. S. (1997). U.S. graduate medical education 1996-1997. *Journal of the American Medical Association, 278*, 750-754.

Distribution

Despite a vast increase in the supply of physicians, the United States has not been able to distribute resources to meet needs. The whole issue of a managed care-oriented market system for the "mainstream" and a "safety net" for an increasing number of different groups in the face of such a surplus will be one of the major health policy debates in the coming century.

FORWARD THROUGH THE PAST

Patterns of physician supply and distribution result from the complex set of influences depicted in Table 26.4. To the extent that the different sectors have had different, and frequently competing, needs and different, and frequently competing, sources of control, financing, and regulation, no coordinated plan for the workforce has been possible. A look at some of the forces in play may serve to illustrate the dynamic. Throughout the past 25 to 30 years, a number of policy recommendations about needed changes in medical education have been presented to the government, the profession, and the public. Many of these reports called for changes that emphasized primary care, a shift of the locus for training to ambulatory sites, and an addition of learning areas previously ignored in the curricula of medical schools and residency programs. In support of policy recommendations, a series of provisions were added to the U.S. Public Health Service Act. Title VII of this Act provided funding for the creation of new medical schools, increases in medical school enrollment, scholarship support for trainees, and funding to support the creation of medical school departments, residency programs, curricula, and faculty development in family medicine. A number of other medical education and service initiatives were supported by foundations such as Robert Wood Johnson and W. K. Kellogg.

At the same time, these changes had to be introduced into medical schools whose existing departmental structure, budgeting, and faculty reward process, for example, reflected a prior emphasis on tertiary care-focused, hospital-based learning. Whereas Title VII monies supported primary care residency training, particularly in family medicine, a larger share of federal money (graduate medical education direct and indirect payment from Medicare) supported tertiary care, hospital-based learning. Finally, physician reimbursement, regardless of the payment source, favored procedural specialties and hospital-based care.

Proposals to change the physician production process also were filtered through the existing mechanisms of professional control over program accreditation and learner certification. These mechanisms exist at the medical education (e.g., Liaison Committee on Medical Education [LCME]), graduate medical education (e.g., Accreditation Committee on Graduate Medical Education [ACGME]), specialty (e.g., American Board of Medical Specialties [ABMS]), and practice levels (e.g., National Board of Medical Examiners [NBME]).

Table 26.4
Influences on the supply of physicians

Medical Education	Graduate Medical Education	Professional Activity
Ownership	*Ownership*	*Ownership*
Trustees as agents of taxpayers for public schools Trustees as agents of corporation for private schools	Academic health centers Sponsoring hospitals Sponsoring corporation	Individual practice arrangement Employing organization (e.g., clinic, hospital, health maintenance organization (HMO), government, university)
Financing	*Financing*	*Financing*
State appropriations Federal grants Practice income Endowments, foundations, sponsored activity Tuition	Medicare graduate medical education funding Hospital contribution Practice income Federal grants Sponsored activity grants, contracts	Private practice payment for service (e.g.,) Medicare, Medicaid, health maintenance organization (HMO), organization, insurance, etc.) Salaried activity (financial base for employer: e.g., taxes, profits, investments)
Accreditation/Certification of Medical School	*Accreditation/Certification of Residency Program*	*Accreditation/Certification of Clinical (and Other) Site*
Liaison Committee on Medical Education (LCME)	Accreditation Committee on Graduate Medical Education (ACGME)	State licensure Joint Commission on the Accreditation of Health care organization
Certification of the MD	*Certification of the MD*	*Certification of the MD*
Medical school criteria United States Medical Licensing Examination (USMLE)	Residency program criteria	State licensure American Board of Medical Specialties
Scope of Activity	*Scope of Activity*	*Scope of Activity*
Curriculum set by school Shaped by LCME	Curriculum set by residency Shaped by specialty of ACGME	Privileges set by hospital Shaped by purchasers
Career Path	*Career Path*	*Career Path*
Individual choice of school constrained by admission criteria, financial ability individual choice of specialty constrained by performance and financial obligation	Individual choice of residency constrained by available slot, competitive performance	Individual choice of activity, location, and arrangement constrained by prior commitments, competitive performance

The practice environment exerted another set of influences on physician specialty and practice decisions. In spite of federal initiatives to increase physician reimbursement for cognitive contributions (e.g., RVRBS), physician reimbursement, regardless of the payment source favored procedural specialties and hospital-based care.

What may be different about the 2000s is the possible convergence of some of the external forces affecting the physician supply and distribution process. The physician supply is described as being in surplus rather than in need. The managed care market is looking to make the allocation of resources more rational and the delivery of services more cost efficient. The strains on the safety net will put more pressure on the public sector at the federal and state levels to address need. Graduate medical education funding will be redirected in ways that shape the production of number and type of specialists being produced. Faculty practice plans will not be competitive in the market and will need to explore new initiatives to attract patients or to be reimbursed for care. Medical schools competing for public funding, generally from state governments, will face more pressure to demonstrate their accountability and effectiveness in providing services to a more narrowly defined public than in the past. Individual students will find their choice of specialty, residency, and practice location much more constrained. The autonomy of the medical profession in controlling the production and distribution of the physician supply will be channeled if not directly challenged.

REFERENCES

American Medical Association. (1997). *AMA physician characteristics and distribution in the United States.* Chicago.

Association of American Medical Colleges (AAMC). (1997). *AAMC Data Book.* Washington, DC.

Barzansky, B., Jonas, H. S., & Etzel, S. I. (1997). Educational Programs in U.S. Medical Schools, 1996-1997. *Journal of the American Medical Association, 278,* 744-749.

Council on Graduate Medical Education. (1995, 1996).

Crowley, A. (1985). Graduate medical education in the United States, 1984-85. *Journal of the American Medical Association, 254,* 1585-1593.

Dunn, M. R., & Miller, R. S. (1997). U.S. Graduate Medical Education. *Journal of the American Medical Association, 278,* 750-754.

Fenninger, L. D., & Tracy, R. H. (1975). Section III. Graduate medical education: Annual report on graduate medical education in the U.S. *Journal of the American Medical Association,* (Suppl) *231,* 34-50.

Friedson, E. (1973). *Profession of medicine.* New York: Dodd Mead.

Miller, R .S., Dunn, M. R., & Whitcomb, M. E. (1997). Initial employment status of resident physicians completing training in 1995. *Journal of the American Medical Association,* 277:1699-1704.

PEW Commission Report. (1995).

United States Bureau of Health Professions (BHPr). (1996).

CHAPTER TWENTY-SEVEN

Supporting Medical Education

John H. Shatzer
John Hopkins University School of Medicine

M. Brownell Anderson
Association of American Medical Colleges

There is a long-recognized distinction in medical education between the clinical or scientific competence of faculty and their ability to teach. George Miller (1990), in his book *Educating Medical Teachers* chronicles the development of educational support in medicine. He reports that as early as the 1800s, European medical schools called for specific teacher training of their medical faculty. Similar early concerns were voiced in the United States as well (Holmes, 1892; American Medical Association, 1892). Abraham Flexner (1910) also recognized the need for formal educational organization in medical training in his 1910 report to the Carnegie Foundation, but left it to the individual institution to determine how the organization would structure this support.

Academics in medicine continued the call to reform well into the 1900s (Haggerty, 1929; Klapper, 1950; Meyers, 1954). Their messages were remarkably similar: Teachers in medicine should be guided by educational philosophy and theory, follow sound educational principles, and demonstrate a willingness to adopt contemporary teaching methods. This need was largely left unanswered until the Commonwealth Fund supported the Project in Medical Education at the University of Buffalo, beginning in December, 1955 (Miller, 1980, pp. 21-43). This was the first attempt by educational professionals to structure support formally for the teaching faculty. In that attempt, the medical school at Buffalo called on their school of education to help guide its thinking in training physicians to become better teachers. Other medical schools, also funded by the Commonwealth Fund, soon followed

Buffalo's lead. Internal educational support systems were created at the Medical College of Virginia, Case Western Reserve, and the University of Illinois at Chicago during the 1958-1959 academic year.

Since then, systems for the internal support of medical education have developed into a variety of forms. The organizational format has been shaped by concerns regarding budgetary administrative oversight of educational programs, educational policy implementation, and necessary logistical support for courses, as well as by the desire to provide educational expertise to faculty in fulfilling their roles as teachers, such as that offered by the Buffalo model.

External influences also have played an important role, both in creating a need for internal educational support systems, and in supporting the educational program of medical schools themselves. These influences--a veritable alphabet soup--include the Liaison Committee on Medical Education (LCME), the body that accredits U.S. and Canadian medical schools; the Association of American Medical Colleges (AAMC), particularly its professional development Group on Educational Affairs (GEA); the Generalists in Medical Education conference; the Research in Medical Education (RIME) Conference; and the National Board of Medical Examiners (NBME).

For example, the LCME (1998, p. 13) requires that "there must be integrated institutional responsibility for the design and management of a coherent and coordinated curriculum. The chief academic officer must have sufficient available resources and authority provided by the institution to fulfill this responsibility." The AAMC's 1984 Report on the General Professional Education of the Physician (GPEP) and its 1992 Assessing Change in Medical Education-The Road to Implementation (ACME-TRI) report both advocated that schools develop educational support in redesigning their curriculum and establish oversight for the educational program, vested in a department or office of medical education. Similarly, foundations such as the Robert Wood Johnson Foundation and the Macy Foundation have regularly requested proposals calling for innovative health care training programs, providing the impetus to seek educational expertise to assist in their implementation.

As a result, educational support systems, in one form or another, are now part of all LCME-accredited medical schools. During the 40 years that have followed the Buffalo experiment, two basic models have emerged. The purposes of this chapter are to review the current organizational models that have developed internally to support medical education, to describe the external systems that support medical education, and to suggest how each may fare in the 21st century.

CURRENT ORGANIZATIONAL PROTOCOLS

Administrative Model

The administrative model provides the most fundamental support for educational programs. Education-related decisions are made through either an administrative leader, usually an associate dean, or a faculty committee on curriculum, or both. Staffing typically is limited to a single individual, often an MD who has chosen to work in the administration of the educational program. Support built on this model may address such areas as educational policy, instructional budget allocations, curriculum oversight, course staffing and support, and other aspects of maintaining the delivery of instruction. Instructional services that provide test scoring, audiovisual assistance, space allocations or room scheduling, and curriculum document reproduction also may be subsumed under this model. However, there is seldom any explicit goal to help educate faculty in instructional methods, to provide faculty with resources in educational methods and theory, or to support educational research as an institutional mission.

Although the kind of educational support associated with the administrative model facilitates the delivery of its curriculum, it typically does not provide the expertise needed to solve educational problems of the faculty. Of course, skillful and experienced faculty can offer innovative ideas and design creative educational strategies, but their approaches can be based on personal experience ("That's how I was educated") rather than on substantive educational theory or principles.

The educational environment of today's academic health care institutions is vastly different from that of even 10 years ago, and personal models of teaching may no longer be effective. Furthermore, the educational theories we will draw upon, as well as the instructional and assessment tools we must use, require new and sophisticated knowledge and skills that most medical school faculty are neither trained to provide nor supported to attain. Also, designing and interpreting new research that fosters enduring student learning will require levels of educational expertise that may challenge even the most dedicated medical faculty or educational administrators (Regehr & Norman, 1996).

The challenge is not impossible, of course, because there are individuals who provide the various functions of the administrative model, who also have developed expertise in educational principles and theory. Individuals following this pathway have immersed themselves in an educational field or have sought advanced training in education programs. Their skills have enabled them to make substantive contributions to medical education, which extend beyond their normal administrative role or purpose. Important to their success is the institution that supports their professional growth and values their educational expertise.

Educational Model

Following the lead of the project in Buffalo and its offspring, the educational model suggests that there be a separate unit for educational support, which typically reports to the dean, an associate dean for academic affairs, or some equivalent. The overall mission of this structure is to provide consultative resources to faculty in their development of curricula, instructional strategies, and assessment and evaluation tools. Typically, one or more of the staff in these units hold an advanced degree in education, educational psychology, or a related field. Consultative services may range from one-on-one discussions to large-scale faculty development efforts, all making an intellectual contribution to solving educational problems and enhancing faculty educational skills. Medical education research is either an explicit function of the unit or an implied one, depending in part on whether individuals in the unit hold faculty appointments and research is regarded as a pathway to promotion.

Teaching in the medical school curriculum, in other health science curricula, or in the individual's area of expertise (e.g., school of education), also may have a part in the unit activity. The unit also may carry out routine support services such as examination scoring as part of its overall mission. Organizationally, these units usually are structured as "offices" or "centers," although a small number have achieved departmental status. The latter, more typical of large units, are situated in an institution where they have been able to develop strong academic credentials, and that role is valued there. Understandably, departments of medical education have robust research and teaching components to their mission.

A number of educational support offices have developed at academic centers that serve several health care training missions. Here, the office may provide its expertise to schools of nursing, dentistry, allied health, and the like, in addition to the medical school. The relative strengths of these offices lie in their ability to understand the diverse educational landscapes, to pool resources efficiently, and to increase collaboration among disparate faculty, especially in interdisciplinary education.

A variation on the educational model places individuals in support of education within a single department. Department-based units typically are staffed by educational professionals, who are comparable to their schoolwide counterparts, but almost exclusively composed of a single individual. Most of these offices reside within the clinical disciplines, and they appear to be most prevalent in family medicine and surgery departments. Departmental educational support may coexist with an institutional support office. It is not clear why these two entities develop in parallel, but it likely has to do with differences between the culture of the school and the educational goals and resources of the department. Individuals who hold these offices are in a position to learn the culture of the discipline and its unique educational needs. They can become substantial contributors to their respective departments' educational mission at all training levels and often are sought for their expertise by national organizations of the disciplines they serve.

Every medical school accredited by the LCME has incorporated one or the other of these two models in its organizational structure. According to the current membership roster of the Society of Directors of Research in Medical Education (SDRME), more than half of the 125 medical schools in the United States and Canada have incorporated the educational model of organization by maintaining institution-based offices or departments of medical education. However, their roster may underestimate the prevalence of the educational model in medical schools because the SDRME membership roster includes only those units that conduct educational research as one of their missions, but excludes support units that are not responsible for conducting educational research.

EXTERNAL INFLUENCES

In 1890, 66 medical college deans, united by a common desire to elevate the standards of medical education, founded the Association of American Medical Colleges for the purpose of improving the process of medical education. Arguably, the AAMC has provided the strongest external influence on the educational support systems of our medical schools. The mission of the AAMC is to improve the health of the public by enhancing the effectiveness of the nation's medical schools and teaching hospitals. The AAMC carries out a wide range of programs, studies, and services for the better support of medical schools and medical education. In addition to the LCME, the AAMC fosters the professional growth of administrators and faculty at member institutions through constituent groups such as the Group on Educational Affairs (GEA). The GEA sponsors workshops for curriculum support units and a major meeting each fall to allow the presentation of ideas and the generation of discussion among educators nationwide. In this way, it provides support to the many units of educational support in the various medical schools.

The annual meeting of the AAMC is the largest national gathering of professionals working and learning in academic medicine. In particular, the Research in Medical Education and the Innovations in Medical Education meetings have become the standard national (if not international) forum to report new and important findings in educational research and development. Similarly, the Generalists in Medical Education Conference has met conjointly with the AAMC's annual meeting over the past 20 years to provide another venue for support of educators and a forum to share innovative educational ideas. The AAMC also serves as a liaison to various foundations interested in supporting medical education and assists foundation leaders in determining how best to expend the limited resources available to their best advantage. One other important role the AAMC plays in support of the medical schools is its representation to the public and the Congress of the need for adequate support for the initiatives of medical education.

On a different scale, technology appears to becoming an increasing external influence in support of medical education. With the introduction of the Internet and list servers such as DR-ED, medical educators of all backgrounds and training have been able to create electronic forums for instantaneous answers to their educational questions and concerns. Via the Internet, faculty, literally from all over the world, have access to expert advice and opinion. Whole programs and curricula have been shared as a result of discussions via the list servers. The interchange of ideas and educational materials undoubtedly has been beneficial to the support of medical education, but the use of this technology is not without its risks. Along with access to sound educational answers comes the potential spread of long-recognized diseases of the curriculum and the perpetuation of its myths and shibboleths (Abrahamson, 1978; Abrahamson, 1989).

OUTLOOK FOR THE 21st CENTURY

Internal support for medical education, specifically offices of medical education, has ridden the vicissitudes of the academic medical center. When education is valued and resources are available, internal support for medical education has found an integral role in the institution. When the institution sets other priorities, however, the fate of educational support often hangs in the balance. The administrative model which is well entrenched in schools' core organization structure, usually fares far better than the educational model in lean times.

Great challenges lie ahead for medical education in the foreseeable future of the health care environment. To meet these challenges, units of educational support must maintain at least three essential components to their overall mission. First and foremost, service must be their primary mission. If faculty value the support received by finding solutions to the educational problems they face, then the units that provide this support will enjoy a long and prosperous life in the 21st century. But there are two other keys necessary to survival.

Business Approach

Units of educational support can no longer function strictly as cost centers. They must function also, at least in part, as revenue centers as well. The landscape of health care has evolved toward embracing a business model. As a result, the academic health center, including the office of medical education, must be prepared to use principles of business. Strategic planning, business plans, cost accounting, cost-benefit analyses, and revenue sources will quickly become, if they are not already, integral parts of the vocabulary and function of medical education offices. Medical education already has seen concepts such as "continuous quality improvement" and "total quality management" applied in the evaluation of educational programs and services, ideas that have percolated from business theory and practice.

Functioning as a business may seem incongruent with the traditional service mission of an educational support unit. Although every office is unique in its mission and structure, those discovering creative solutions to these apparently opposing missions will find themselves in a far better position to succeed in the next millennium. The business approach may demand certain creative arrangements, for example, financial understandings among the dean, the institution, and the office of medical education, permitting a portion of generated revenues to be returned to the office to help support underfunded areas of its budget or new educational initiatives for the school.

In direct support of the idea that medical schools and academic medical centers must begin to conduct themselves as businesses, the AAMC initiated the Mission-Based Management Program, a partnership of the AAMC and CSC Healthcare. The program was created to help medical schools improve their mission effectiveness. Mission-based management is a unique approach to medical school operations and decision making aimed at enhancing mission effectiveness. It is implemented through the creation of reporting tools that measure financial performance and productivity on a mission-specific basis at three levels: the school, department, and individual faculty member. Equipped with improved measuring and accounting systems, schools are on sounder footing in identifying and supporting their most mission-critical activities, including education.

Scholarship

Even within the growing businesslike environment of the academic health care institutions, rewards are routinely bestowed on faculty for their scholarly accomplishments, and because educational scholarship is increasingly recognized as a viable pathway to promotion, it has played an increasingly important part of faculty roles. Service to support the educational scholarship of faculty should be regarded as an important key to the success of an office of medical education. The most obvious form of scholarship is the conduct of research. Organized support of research may take on several forms, but units of education should at least provide leadership in demonstrating the efficacy of educational research in solving the institution's educational challenges. As faculty are rewarded for their efforts to approach and answer their educational questions through research, the value of an office of medical education is enhanced and its survival becomes more likely. If educational staff also conduct research that is valued by the institution, their peers, and the field of medical education, the role of educational research and the utility of the office are further strengthened.

However, scholarship also must be more broadly defined than the exclusive definition of research. Ernest Boyer (1990), in his book *Scholarship Reconsidered: Priorities of the Professoriate,* argued that because more and more faculty time has been expended on research and publication, other aspects of scholarship have been neglected. He contended that scholarship must be broadly defined if faculty in all higher education settings, including medical education, are to survive and the educational mission of the school is to remain undiluted. Obviously, scholarly work should include research, and this is what Boyer referred to as the creative aspect of scholarship. However, he said scholarship also must include "the serious, disciplined work that seeks to interpret, draw together, and bring new insights to bear on original research" (p. 19) which is what Boyer terms the "scholarship of integration." In the context of medical education, this expanded definition could mean a scholarship that focuses on multidisciplinary education, meta-analyses of work within a field, or other work that pulls together findings into larger intellectual wholes.

A third form of scholarship according to Boyer describes research that applies its creative and integrative findings in the service of education, which Boyer designates the "scholarship of application." This form of scholarship uses not only knowledge in useful application within the medical field, but also knowledge from other fields to apply in the service of medical education, a dynamic currently known as "thinking outside the box."

A final aspect of scholarship suggested by Boyer is teaching. Here, the medical educator should be characterized both as a teacher, through leadership in faculty development and as one involved in teaching opportunities in the university at large. Educators in medical schools should also be involved in training and mentoring faculty whose professional goals include a career in medical education, as well as providing opportunities for medical education to become a training ground for masters and doctoral students in education. This latter function has significantly decreased over the past 20 years, leaving only large units of medical education with the luxury of offering training in medical education. A potential consequence of this decrease is a paucity of junior level PhDs, experienced in medical education who can begin to assume the leadership roles required in the next 20 to 30 years. Partially meeting this need, some institutions now offer advanced degrees in medical education, health sciences education, or a related field, and professional educators play an essential role in their staffing.

Medical education is in need of such scholarship. Even the most traditional medical schools are seriously considering or developing ways in which to reward faculty for efforts in a more broadly defined scholarship. An office of medical education that plays a leadership role in supporting faculty to fulfill their scholarly roles, which is rewarded itself by work in these areas, will be a valued part of its institution.

As evidence in support of this need, the AAMC's Council of Academic Societies, in conjunction with the Group on Educational Affairs, identified Scholarship as one of its four key projects. The purpose of the project is to define scholarship for the educational community, and to identify means of introducing it and, most importantly, valuing it in the education of medical students. This project links directly to the purpose of mission-based management. Both activities should serve medical schools and educational support units well.

To further educational scholarship in the 20th century, medical education also will require increased visibility and credibility of the journals that disseminate research findings and innovations. Only half of a half dozen journals devoted to medical education are afforded the advantage of being indexed in the National Library of Medicine. If faculty are to recognize educational research as a legitimate pathway of scholarship, then the scientific community that defines scholarship must be prepared to embrace medical education as a scientific endeavor. Unfortunately, until that time, the discipline will be viewed largely as a "social science" and educational support as an activity that any faculty can easily do.

CONCLUSIONS

The demand for the educational model appears to be on the rise. A dozen new offices of medical education, staffed by PhD-level educational specialists, have been created in the past eight years alone. Advanced-degree educational training programs for medical faculty also are increasing in number. This trend may have all the appearances of another 20-year cycle, because we saw these increases before in the 1970s when, at that time, we expanded the physician pool, opened new medical schools, and sought educational expertise to develop curricula. But, as suggested earlier, the educational environment in which faculty must function is becoming increasingly complex, and the demand on their time is greater than ever before. Moreover, it is unlikely that these pressures will abate. It makes sense, then, to look to professional educators as collaborators in the education of future physicians.

ACKNOWLEDGMENT

Dr. Shatzer thanks David Irby, Robin Harvan. and Michael Ravich for their valuable suggestions and comments in the initial preparation of this manuscript.

REFERENCES

Abrahamson, S. (1978). Diseases of the curriculum. *Journal of Medical Education, 53,* 951-957.

Abrahamson, S. (1989). Myths and shibboleths of medical education. *Teaching and Learning in Medicine: An International Journal, 1,* 4-9.

American Medical Association. (1892). Methods of instruction (editorial). *Journal of the American Medical Association, 18,* 83.

Association of American Medical Colleges (AAMC). (1984). *Physicians for the twenty-first century: The report of the Panel on the General Professional Education of the Physician and College Preparation for Medicine.*

Boyer, E. L. (1990). *Scholarship reconsidered: Priorities of the professorate.* The Carnegie Foundation for the Advancement of Teaching. San Francisco: Jossey-Bass.

Flexner, A. (1910). *Medical Education in the United States and Canada,.* The Carnegie Foundation for the Advancement of Teaching: Bulletin No. 4. New York

Haggerty, M. E. (1929). The improvement of medical instruction. *Journal of the Association of American Medical Colleges, 4,* 42-58.

Holmes, E. L. (1892). Address to the annual banquet of the Practitioners Club in Chicago. *Journal of the American Medical Association, 18*, 114-115.

Klapper, P. (1950). Medical education as education. *Journal of the Association of American Medical Colleges, 25*, 314-318.

Liaison Committee on Medical Education. (1998). *Functions and structure of a medical school: Accreditation and the Liaison Committee on Medical Education.* Association of American Colleges and the American Medical Association.

Meyers, R. (1954). Educational science in medical teaching. *Journal of the Association of American Medical Colleges, 29*, 17-34.

Miller, G. (1980). *Educating Medical Teachers. Cambridge, MA: Harvard University Press.*

Regehr, G., & Norman, G. R. (1996). Issues in cognitive psychology: Implications for professional education. *Academic Medicine, 71*, 988-1001.

CHAPTER TWENTY-EIGHT

Funding and Financial Support for Research and Development in Medical Education

William A. Anderson
Michigan State University

For the past 90 years, medical educators have relied on financial support from sources other than their institutions to conduct innovative efforts to improve the preparation of medical students. In 1910, the Carnegie Foundation for the Advancement of Teaching became one of the first external supporters of medical education by funding Abraham Flexner's now famous study of medical schooling. His report, *Bulletin Number Four: Medical Education in the United States and Canada,* has forever changed the way medical students are trained (Flexner, 1910). Most components of contemporary medical education were first introduced as a result of this externally funded study.

External financial support for medical education continues today with efforts such as the Undergraduate Medical Education of the 21st Century project, supported by the Bureau of Health Professions (U.S. Public Health Service) and the Primary Care Organizations Consortium (BHPr. 1998). This national initiative supports the collaboration of medical school primary care departments with managed care organizations to develop, implement, and evaluate new managed care curricula for third- and fourth-year medical students. Several other foundations, federal government agencies, and professional organizations currently provide funding for medical education efforts to improve the preparation of medical students to meet changing societal needs.

External funding for research and development projects in medical education, however, has not been consistent. Unlike funding for basic science and clinical research, there has not been a single funding source or historical path of external financial support for medical research and development. In the early years, external dollars for medical education demonstration projects were provided mostly by philanthropic foundations (Gunzburger, 1994, p. 8). Currently, foundations provide approximately 20% of medical education research and development funding; federal agencies provide approximately 50%; and the balance is being provided by an everchanging list of local, state, and national public and private funding sources. As will be seen, medical educators have been, and continue to be, resourceful in obtaining funding for their projects from these many different sources. The results of these efforts have allowed medical schools to adopt educational innovations that would otherwise be too expensive to develop, implement, evaluate, and disseminate at a single institution.

The remainder of this chapter is divided into three major sections. First, the major historical financial supporters of medical education research and development are reviewed. Second, the current status of funding for medical education is discussed. Finally, projections for the future of externally funded medical education efforts are proposed. Three terms used in this chapter require an operational definition. "Medical education" is defined as educational efforts designed to improve the process for the preparation of physicians. These efforts generally are undertaken by educators and clinicians working in medical schools or affiliated residency training programs. "Research and development" is defined as specific educational research and demonstration projects addressing medical education curriculum, faculty development, and learner and program evaluation innovations. Excluded from this definition is clinical, health policy, and health services research and development. "External funding" is defined as monies or in-kind support provided to an institution in support of a specific medical education research or development project. These projects generally are submitted by a medical educator at that institution to a funding agency through a written contract or grant proposal.

A BRIEF HISTORY OF FINANCIAL SUPPORT
FOR MEDICAL EDUCATION

In this section, some of the major contributions to medical education provided through external financial support are examined. Space limitations preclude a complete discussion of the topic, and those interested in a more detailed examination should refer to George Miller's book, *Educating Medical Teachers*, published incidentally with support provided by the Commonwealth Fund and Rockerfeller Foundation (Miller, 1980).

As stated earlier, initial medical education research and development efforts were funded almost exclusively by foundations. Beginning in 1910 with the Carnegie Foundation funding of Abraham Flexner's seminal study of medical schooling, medical educators spent the next 30 years implementing the Report's recommendations. Although most activity focused on revising the structure, curriculum, and faculty of medical schools, there was increasing interest in examining the methods used to prepare medical students.

In 1949, the National Fund for Medical Education (NFME) was established to improve teaching practices of U.S. medical schools (National Fund for Medical Education, 1998). This philanthropic foundation was supported by funds from several foundations and corporations. Throughout the 1950s and 1960s, the NFME provided funds to improve medical school teaching practices. In addition, NFME grants supported research and development on diffusing new teaching practices, preparing clinicians for their teaching role, and incorporating new instructional technologies (videotapes and computerized instruction) into the medical curriculum.

In 1955, The Commonwealth Fund appropriated $131,400 to support the Project in Medical Education at the University of Buffalo School of Medicine. The goals of this project were to increase awareness of fundamental educational principles among medical teachers, and to assess the changes in instruction that may result from medical teacher training programs (Miller, 1980, p. 39). The impact of this grant for medical education research and development would be long-lasting. Among the many accomplishments of the Project in Medical Education were the collaboration of medical and nonmedical professionals, a systematic examination of medical school teaching and evaluation practices, medical faculty training in effective instructional practices, and assembly of a cadre of medical educators who would later establish similar offices of medical education research and development throughout the United States and Canada.

Because of the success of the Project in Medical Education, interest in medical education as an area of inquiry and development increased throughout the nation's medical schools and attracted additional external funding for research and development activities. In 1961, the Commonwealth Fund provided support for the publication of one of the first texts addressing medical teaching issues; *Teaching and Learning in Medical School* (Miller, 1980, p. 77). The Commonwealth Fund also was instrumental in funding the establishment of several offices of medical education, notably at the Medical College of Virginia, University of Illinois-Chicago, and Michigan State University.

The Carnegie Foundation also was an early supporter of medical education. Their 1961 grant to the Association of American Medical Schools (AAMC) of $300,000 established the Division of Education. Products of this award included the establishment of the Summer Institute for Medical Teaching and the formation of the annual Conference on Research in Medical Education (RIME) (Miller, 1980, p. 123).

Several other large foundations played important roles in developing opportunities for medical education research and development. The W. K. Kellogg Foundation in 1961 began a series of grants to eight universities in the United States and Canada to assist them in establishing a school of basic medical sciences through the employment of teaching personnel and the construction of facilities (Sparks,

1978). The Josiah Macy Jr. Foundation supported efforts within medical schools to strengthen their science faculties and to broaden and improve the education of physicians (Gunzburger, 1994, p. 10). The Robert Wood Johnson Foundation in the 1970s began a series of primary care faculty development fellowship programs designed to improve new faculty teaching and research skills (Cluff, 1989).

Early foundation support had been instrumental in establishing medical education research and development as an essential contributor to the educational preparation of physicians. In the late 1970s, foundations began to shift their funding priorities away from direct support for medical education issues to broader societal problems. External funding for medical education initiatives then shifted to the federal government and professional organizations and associations.

In 1954, the National Institute of Neurological Disease and Blindness (NIH) funded a two-year project for an ophthalmology-neurology academic training program, which marked one of the first attempts by the federal government to integrate educational training into a discipline (Miller, 1980, pp. 114-115). The Heart Disease, Cancer, and Stroke Amendments of 1965 (Public Law 69-239) created the Regional Medical Programs (Rosinski, 1988). Among its many provisions, this law provided funding to hire medical educators to help develop and evaluate its continuing educational programs. Other federal legislation, enacted in mid-1960s provided grants to develop and evaluate curricula for training health personnel and to conduct research on new innovations in health professions training. The Health Manpower Act of 1968 included a wide variety of medical education research and development initiatives (Rosinski, 1988, p. 8). Thus the federal government began to play a direct role in the funding of medical education research and development. By 1970, medical education had grown considerably. Several offices of medical education had been established across the United States, which were training physicians in the application of educational principles and collaborating with physicians on research documenting the effectiveness of educational innovations.

The 1970s saw continued federal support for research and development in medical education, but with a different focus. The nation was experiencing a physician shortage, and legislation was enacted, beginning with the Comprehensive Health Manpower Training Act of 1971, to increase the number medical schools and the number of trained physicians (Miller, 1980, p. 149). Special project grants were established to train new physician faculty to apply new computer technology to make learning more efficient, and to apply sound educational practices to new medical student curricula and residency training. The U.S. Public Health Service (PHS) became a leader in these training efforts. Through the primary care training grants for faculty development and grants to establish new departments of family medicine and primary care residencies, medical educators were in high demand to assist in the development and evaluation of these new educational programs. Other PHS-funded programs included the establishment of area health education centers (AHEC), and health education training centers (HETC), and geriatric training centers (Bureau of Health Profession, 1998). With many of these training programs still active today, the U.S. Public Health Service provided medical educators with continuing venues and resources for medical education research and development.

Several other federal agencies provided funding for medical education projects, beginning in the 1970s. Examples include the National Library of Medicine, the National Science Foundation, the Office of Naval Research, and the various National Institutes of Health. These external funds can be characterized primarily as education and training efforts designed to help meet the broader funding agency objectives of improving the nation's health. Medical education research was rarely defined as a specific component of these grants, and in some cases was expressly prohibited as a funding activity. Nonetheless, these federally supported efforts did provide the opportunity for medical educators to further incorporate educational innovations and conduct in-house research to assess program effectiveness.

Professional organizations and associations also provided early support for medical education research and development. In 1961, the American Heart Association allocated funding to establish a Teaching Fellowship Program to encourage basic and clinical scientists to study educational methods and research (Miller, 1980, p. 136). Also in 1961, the American Medical Association supported a study examining lifelong learning for physicians (Miller, 1980, p. 199). An outcome of this study was the AMA funding of faculty fellowships in medical education at the University of Illinois-Chicago. Medical education research received funding from the American Board of Orthopaedic Surgeons and the American College of Emergency Physicians to explore a host of board certification methodology and physician competency issues (Miller, 1980, p. 144). The National Board of Medical Examiners (NBME) played a critical role in advancing medical education research. Beginning in 1961, the NBME supported extramural studies of alternative methods to assess physician competence using audiovisuals and computers, and studies of how to assess complex cognitive and communication skills. From 1971 to 1976, a total of $1,400,000 had been allocated for these research efforts (Miller, 1980, p. 191).

Throughout its history, the Association of American Medical Colleges (AAMC) has been a supporter of medical education research and development through a commitment of its own resources and through support of educational demonstration projects and research. Highlights include the cosponsoring of the Summer Teaching Institutes with the University of Buffalo (1959), the establishment of the Division of Education in collaboration with the Carnegie Corporation (1961), the establishment of the Research in Medical Education (RIME) component of its annual meeting (1962), and the Division of Faculty Development. Although the AAMC has not provided medical educators with extensive direct funding for research and development, it has served as a catalyst for focusing the discussion and dissemination of innovative projects and research at a national level.

To summarize this first section of external funding and financial support for medical education, three general conclusions can be drawn. First, foundation support provided crucial initial funding for demonstration projects to explore the collaboration of educators and physicians, and to incorporate the contributions of educational research to improve the process of educating medical students. Second, the federal government played a later but equally crucial role in providing large-scale funding for national initiatives to train large numbers of medical faculty in effective teaching and research practices. Third, professional organizations and associations provided important, if not extensive, focused funding for medical education research and development.

THE CURRENT STATUS OF FUNDING
FOR MEDICAL EDUCATION

In this section, the current status of financial support for medical education research and development activities is examined. Specifically, what priority does each of the three historical sources of external funding (foundations, federal government, and professional organizations/associations) currently have for medical education? Also, the emergence of new funding sources of medical education research and development is examined.

Although national philanthropic foundations played a critical role in the early development of medical education, their focus has shifted steadily from the application of educational principles in medical education to broader societal issues in medicine and medical education. The Commonwealth Fund, a frequent supporter of medical education projects, now supports research and development activities addressing the quality of health care, strategies for improving Medicare and health care insurance, delivery of health care to medically underserved areas, and improvement of health care for minority populations (The Commonwealth Fund, 1998).

The W. K. Kellogg Foundation (1998), which had previously supported the educational development of clinical and medical faculty, now identifies four themes for its involvement in medicine: leadership, information systems/technology, capitalizing on diversity, and social and economic community development. The Robert Wood Johnson Foundation (1998), which had previously funded faculty development training, now has stated priorities of access to health care, substance abuse, and chronic illnesses. The Foundation, however, still supports development activities such as its Generalist Initiative and Substance Abuse Training Grants. Finally, the National Fund for Medical Education (1998), a long-time supporter of research on the process of educating medical students, now has focused its funding priorities on interdisciplinary education, specialist retraining for primary care, and medical student teaching about cost containment and the integration of psychosocial and biomedical aspects of health. Although medical educators participate in projects related to all current foundation funding priorities, they do so in a different role. Rarely are medical educators the project directors. Rather, they are part of an interdisciplinary team assisting in the overall accomplishment of larger project objectives. Medical education research and development activities are now accomplished within the constraints of larger projects.

The various agencies of the federal government also have shifted their funding priorities to projects addressing larger national issues of improving the access to quality health care, preparing generalist physicians for the future, increasing the number of minority physicians, and incorporating technology to improve the delivery of health care and health care information. Most of the National Institutes of Health allocate their resources for biomedical research and the preparation of clinical researchers. One exception is the National Cancer Institute (1999), which since 1980 has provided funding for the Cancer Education Grant Program. The goal of these grants is to develop and sustain innovative educational approaches that ultimately have an impact in reducing cancer incidence, mortality, and morbidity, as well as improving the quality of life for cancer patients. Medical educators across the country have been active in developing these new curricula and conducting research on project effectiveness.

The Bureau of Health Professions, Health Resources and Services Administration (PHS) Progress Report, (1998), since 1978 has offered a broad range of training grants and special projects authorized by Title VII of the Public Health Service Act. The agency's goals of improving the diversity of the health care workforce, ensuring access to health care services, and ensuring access to appropriate health care in all communities are being met through a broad-based program of demonstration and training grants. Current training efforts include primary care faculty development, minority faculty development fellowships, primary care residency training, partnerships for health professions education, undergraduate medical education for the 21st century, centers of excellence, area health education centers and health education training centers, geriatric education centers, and rural interdisciplinary training. Sustained funding by the Division of Medicine for these training grants has provided medical educators with one of the few sources of large-scale federal funding for educational research and development.

Other educationally related research and development funding sources exist within various federal agencies, but, like current foundation funding, these resources are allocated as part of larger scale demonstration projects addressing national health care issues. Medical educators again work collaboratively with other project personnel to achieve the goals of the funding agency. Medical education research generally is not a fundable component of these federally supported projects, but rather a venue for collecting data for in-house research projects.

The third original source of funding for medical education, professional organizations, and associations plays a larger role today than ever before in supporting projects, with medical education research as a primary focus. These nonfederal funding sources generally have smaller project funding levels, but allow medical educators to pursue a wider range of pilot and comprehensive studies. One current example is the National Board of Medical Examiners (NBME). Since 1995, the NBME (1998) has provided funding of up to $50,000 for two years for projects that show promise in contributing new knowledge and understanding of educational measurement and curricular and program evaluation methods in medical schools. The NBME Medical Education Research Fund supports innovation in the theory, knowledge, and practice of assessment in medical education. Approximately six awards are bestowed annually.

Other examples of professional organizations providing medical education funding are the Association for Surgical Education and the American Cancer Society. The Association for Surgical Education (ASE, 1999) supports two medical education research projects annually. These awards of $10,000 are for original research seed grants for new investigators in the broad area of surgical education (ASE Call for Research Grant Proposals). The American Cancer Society (1999 Grant Funding) awards up to $15,000 to provide seed money for new educationally related projects initiated by junior faculty.

Noticeably absent is the AAMC, which does not currently offer any funding for member-initiated educational research and development activities. There are, however, literally hundreds of other professional organizations and associations. Some have stated project areas, whereas others do not but will entertain unsolicited proposals from members with projects addressing the general goals of these organizations.

During the past few years, medical educators have turned to new sources of funding for their research and development projects. These sources include managed care organizations, state government agencies, university and medical school seed grants, hospital research funds, and individual community benefactors. Blue Cross and Blue Shield, state departments of public health, and the Pew Charitable Trusts (1999) are collaborating on research and development projects to improve medical residents' knowledge and skills in delivering Medicaid-managed care services to underserved populations. These projects include curriculum development, the use of new instructional technology to deliver instruction, and research and evaluation efforts to document project effectiveness and outcome. Apple Computers has been active in providing both funding and computer technology to assist medical schools in incorporating technology into medical school curricula. Other smaller and local funding sources also have provided funding for medical educator-initiated projects.

In summarizing the current status of funding for medical education, three general conclusions can be drawn. First, at the foundation and federal level, funding priorities have moved away from projects addressing the application of educational principles and practices in medical education to projects addressing national health care and medical education issues. Although opportunities exist for medical educators to conduct scholarship, they must do so within the overall parameters of a larger project. Second, because many of these federally and foundation-funded projects are large scale and require collaborative efforts among many faculty, medical educators are rarely in positions to manage resources for their research and development activities. They must either negotiate for resources to conduct their projects or use the large-scale grant project as a venue for in-house funded research. Third, new and smaller funding sources have emerged in the past few years for the funding of medical education research and development projects. The impact for medical education has been educators who are increasingly resourceful in locating these new streams of funding and in conducting projects with fewer resources. What lies ahead for the financial support of medical education? Some trends for the future are discussed next.

PROJECTIONS FOR THE FUTURE OF
MEDICAL EDUCATION FUNDING

Predictions about future funding trends for medical education research and development are always risky. Medical educators historically have demonstrated an ability to adapt and maximize opportunities and resources available to them. However, by using history and the current status of external funding for medical education as a guide, five projections for the future can be advanced with some certainty.

First, there is likely to be an overall reduction in the dollars available for medical education research and development in the future. During the past decade, the U. S. economy has shown unprecedented growth and expansion. This robust economy has provided foundations with increasing revenues from their investments, which must be passed on as funds for existing and new grant initiatives. Even the federal government has shown modest increases in the appropriations for its various agencies. A strong economy also "trickles down" to impact favorably other sources of external funding for medical education: state government, corporations, hospital foundations, professional organizations and associations, and managed care organizations. But all good things must (and eventually will) come to an end. When the current economic growth abates, the impact will be felt by all supporters of medical education research and development. With reduced revenues, funding sources likely will reduce the scope of their extramural funding and return to core missions and goals.

Another factor having an impact on future funding available for medical education research and development is a continuation of the current transformation of the medical profession in the United States. Changes in the way medicine is organized, financed, and delivered will require an influx of new resources and a reallocation of existing resources for medical schools during a transition period. Faced with core needs such as continuing biomedical research and supporting salaries of clinical faculty, medical schools will turn to external funding sources for support. Medical education demonstration projects and research may be viewed temporarily as lesser priorities.

A second prediction for the future of external funding for medical education is a continuation of a current trend: External funding agencies will devote increasing resources to addressing national medical problems and societal issues. Medical education in the United States currently faces challenges such as increasing the number of minority physicians, preparing primary care physicians to practice in ambulatory and medically underserved settings, and providing continuous high-quality medical care. Because resources to solve these problems do not reside in individual medical schools, these institutions will turn to external funding agencies for assistance in solving national problems. This trend does not in itself mean an abandonment of educational research and development projects, but it does mean that medical educators must work within the framework of these large-scale efforts to "carve out" opportunities for educational demonstration projects and research. Medical educators likely will not serve as project directors able to initiate scholarly projects, but rather as members of a collaborative team in which educational research and development is secondary to the overall project goal.

A third prediction for the future is that medical educators will have to rely increasingly on locating funding for their research and development projects from new and varied funding sources. As stated earlier in this chapter, foundations and federal agencies currently provide approximately 70% of medical education research and development funding, with the balance provided by an ever-increasing list of other sources. If foundations and federal agencies redirect their extramural funding programs to address national and societal problems, then these other funding sources become increasingly important to medical educators. Examples of these sources include state governmental agencies, corporations, professional organizations and associations, managed care organizations, community benefactors, and hospital, medical school and university seed grants. One characteristic common to all of these new funding sources is their inability to provide large-scale project funding. Future medical education research and development projects may be characterized by their smaller scale, in-house focus.

A fourth prediction for the future of medical education research and development is that technology will make the task of locating external financial support easier in the future. As little as a decade ago, the task of locating external funding sources was an onerous task. Strategies included reading the *Catalog of Federal Domestic Assistance*, the *Foundation Directory*, and professional newsletters, and cultivating contacts in various funding agencies. Currently, with the advent of the World Wide Web, access to information about grant funding sources is available to all. Almost all major funding sources post information about their grant programs on the Web. Furthermore, many university libraries have Web search engines that allow medical educators to search for funding agencies with topic or key word searches, similar to those in doing a literature search.

A fifth and final prediction for the future of medical education research and development is a positive one. As shown earlier, medical educators have been very resourceful in obtaining funding for their projects. Although some of the previous predictions may be interpreted as having a potential negative impact on the quantity and scope of research and development in medical education, there is no reason to believe that medical educators will be any less creative and successful in obtaining funding for their projects in the future. Early medical educators began with no funding for scholarly projects, but through creativity and hard work, they were able to build and sustain a discipline for the past 40 years.

This chapter addresses three major topics: a brief history of external funding for research and development in medical education, the current status of financial support, and predictions for the future of funding for research and development in medical education. The discipline began with little or no external funding, grew because of its ability to secure external funding, and will require external financial support to sustain its presence in the future. The experiences gained by medical educators during the past four decades will no doubt serve them well in the future.

REFERENCES

American Cancer Society. *Grant funding*. Available: cancer.org/rresearch/grants/intl Fellowships html Accessed: 1999

Association for Surgical Education. (1999). *ASE call for research grant proposals*. Available: siumed.edu/surgery/grant.html

Bureau of Health Professions. (1998). *Increasing access to health care: Training tomorrow's professionals, 1998 Progress report*. Rockville, MD: Bureau of Health Professions, Health Resources and Services Administration, U.S. Public Health Service, U. S. Department of Health and Human Services.

Cluff, L. E. (1989). The Robert Wood Johnson Foundation. *Academic Medicine, 64*, 246.

Commonwealth Fund. *1998 Annual report*. Available: cmwf.org/annrcprt/1998/amdx98 asp. Accessed: 1999.

Flexner, A. (1910). *Medical education in the United States and Canada. Bulletin number four*. New York: Carnegie Foundation for the Advancement of Teaching.

Gunzburger, L. K. (1994). Foundations that support medical education and health care: Their missions, accomplishments, and unique role. *Academic Medicine, 69*, 8.

Miller, G. E. (1980). *Educating medical teachers*. Cambridge, MA: Harvard University Press and The Commonwealth Fund.

National Board of Medical Examiners. (1998). *NBME Medical Education Research Fund: 1998-1999 Call for Proposals*. Philadelphia: National Board of Medical Examiners.

National Cancer Institute. *Program Guidelines for Cancer Education Grant (R 25)*. Available: dino.nci.nih.gov/public/ ctb/guidelines/r25.html. Accessed: 1999.

National Fund for Medical Education. *1998 Program description*. Available: futurehealth. ucsf.edu/nfme.html Accessed: 1999.

Pew Charitable Trusts. Partnerships for Quality Education. Available: http://www.pewtrusts.com/ search.cfm. Accessed: 1999.

Robert Wood Johnson Foundation. 1998 *Annual report*. Available: rwjf.org/main2.html Accessed: 1999.

Rosinski, E. F. (1988). *The Society of Directors of Research in Medical Education: A brief history, 8*. (Unpublished monograph). San Francisco: The Society of Directors of Research in Medical Education.

Sparks, R. D. (1978). The W. K. Kellogg Foundation and the New Medical Schools. In A. D. Hunt & L. E. Weeks (Eds.), *Medical education since 1960: Marching to a different drummer* (pp. 10-11). East Lansing, MI: The Michigan State University Foundation.

W. K. Kellogg Foundation. *1998 Annual report*. Available: wkkf.org/98AnnualReport Accessed: 1999.

Author Index

Subject Index